Advances in Skull Base Tumor Surgery: The Practical Pearls

Advances in Skull Base Tumor Surgery: The Practical Pearls

Miguel Lopez-Gonzalez

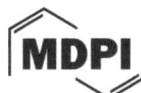

Basel • Beijing • Wuhan • Barcelona • Belgrade • Novi Sad • Cluj • Manchester

Editor
Miguel Lopez-Gonzalez
Department of Neurosurgery
Loma Linda University
Loma Linda, CA
United States

Editorial Office
MDPI AG
Grosspeteranlage 5
4052 Basel, Switzerland

This is a reprint of articles from the Special Issue published online in the open access journal *Brain Sciences* (ISSN 2076-3425) (available at: www.mdpi.com/journal/brainsci/special_issues/YUOKMX3VV1).

For citation purposes, cite each article independently as indicated on the article page online and as indicated below:

Lastname, A.A.; Lastname, B.B. Article Title. *Journal Name* **Year**, *Volume Number*, Page Range.

ISBN 978-3-7258-2612-4 (Hbk)
ISBN 978-3-7258-2611-7 (PDF)
doi.org/10.3390/books978-3-7258-2611-7

© 2024 by the authors. Articles in this book are Open Access and distributed under the Creative Commons Attribution (CC BY) license. The book as a whole is distributed by MDPI under the terms and conditions of the Creative Commons Attribution-NonCommercial-NoDerivs (CC BY-NC-ND) license.

Contents

About the Editor vii

Preface ix

Miguel Angel Lopez-Gonzalez
Editorial for Brain Sciences Special Issue: "Advances in Skull Base Tumor Surgery: The Practical Pearls"
Reprinted from: *Brain Sci.* **2024**, *14*, 352, doi:10.3390/brainsci14040352 1

Sergio Corvino, Pedro L. Villanueva-Solórzano, Martina Offi, Daniele Armocida, Motonobu Nonaka and Giorgio Iaconetta et al.
A New Perspective on the Cavernous Sinus as Seen through Multiple Surgical Corridors: Anatomical Study Comparing the Transorbital, Endonasal, and Transcranial Routes and the Relative Coterminous Spatial Regions
Reprinted from: *Brain Sci.* **2023**, *13*, 1215, doi:10.3390/brainsci13081215 3

Roberto Garcia-Navarrete, Alfonso Marhx-Bracho, Javier Terrazo-Lluch and José Luis Pérez-Gómez
The Extended-Sphenoid Ridge Approach: A New Technique for the Surgical Treatment of Skull Base Tumors in Pediatric Patients
Reprinted from: *Brain Sci.* **2023**, *13*, 888, doi:10.3390/brainsci13060888 19

Brandon Edelbach and Miguel Angel Lopez-Gonzalez
Staged Strategies to Deal with Complex, Giant, Multi-Fossa Skull Base Tumors
Reprinted from: *Brain Sci.* **2023**, *13*, 916, doi:10.3390/brainsci13060916 28

A. Karim Ahmed, Nicholas R. Rowan and Debraj Mukherjee
Operative Corridors in Endoscopic Skull Base Tumor Surgery
Reprinted from: *Brain Sci.* **2024**, *14*, 207, doi:10.3390/brainsci14030207 42

Alessandro Carretta, Matteo Zoli, Federica Guaraldi, Giacomo Sollini, Arianna Rustici and Sofia Asioli et al.
Endoscopic Endonasal Transplanum–Transtuberculum Approach for Pituitary Adenomas/PitNET: 25 Years of Experience
Reprinted from: *Brain Sci.* **2023**, *13*, 1121, doi:10.3390/brainsci13071121 59

Jorge F. Aragón-Arreola, Ricardo Marian-Magaña, Rodolfo Villalobos-Diaz, Germán López-Valencia, Tania M. Jimenez-Molina and J. Tomás Moncada-Habib et al.
Endoscopic Endonasal Approach in Craniopharyngiomas: Representative Cases and Technical Nuances for the Young Neurosurgeon
Reprinted from: *Brain Sci.* **2023**, *13*, 735, doi:10.3390/brainsci13050735 77

Lukasz Przepiorka, Katarzyna Wójtowicz, Katarzyna Camlet, Jan Jankowski, Sławomir Kujawski and Laretta Grabowska-Derlatka et al.
Postoperative Cerebral Venous Sinus Thrombosis Following a Retrosigmoid Craniotomy—A Clinical and Radiological Analysis
Reprinted from: *Brain Sci.* **2023**, *13*, 1039, doi:10.3390/brainsci13071039 89

Guilherme Finger, Kyle C. Wu, Joshua Vignolles-Jeong, Saniya S. Godil, Ben G. McGahan and Daniel Kreatsoulas et al.
A New Finding on Magnetic Resonance Imaging for Diagnosis of Hemifacial Spasm with High Accuracy and Interobserver Correlation
Reprinted from: *Brain Sci.* **2023**, *13*, 1434, doi:10.3390/brainsci13101434 101

Hossein Mahboubi, William H. Slattery, Mia E. Miller and Gregory P. Lekovic
Comparison of Surgeons' Assessment of the Extent of Vestibular Schwannoma Resection with Immediate Post Operative and Follow-Up Volumetric MRI Analysis
Reprinted from: *Brain Sci.* **2023**, *13*, 1490, doi:10.3390/brainsci13101490 110

Abdullah Keles, Burak Ozaydin, Ufuk Erginoglu and Mustafa K. Baskaya
Two-Stage Surgical Management for Acutely Presented Large Vestibular Schwannomas: Report of Two Cases
Reprinted from: *Brain Sci.* **2023**, *13*, 1548, doi:10.3390/brainsci13111548 118

Andrea L. Castillo, Ali Tayebi Meybodi and James K. Liu
Jugular Foramen Tumors: Surgical Strategies and Representative Cases
Reprinted from: *Brain Sci.* **2024**, *14*, 182, doi:10.3390/brainsci14020182 128

Steven D. Curry, Armine Kocharyan and Gregory P. Lekovic
Multi-Disciplinary Approach to Skull Base Paragangliomas
Reprinted from: *Brain Sci.* **2023**, *13*, 1533, doi:10.3390/brainsci13111533 142

Mario Sanna, Mohammed Al-Khateeb, Melcol Hailu Yilala, Mohanad Almashhadani and Giuseppe Fancello
Gruppo Otologico's Experience in Managing the So-Called Inoperable Tympanojugular Paraganglioma
Reprinted from: *Brain Sci.* **2024**, *14*, 745, doi:10.3390/brainsci14080745 153

About the Editor

Miguel Lopez-Gonzalez

Doctor Miguel Angel Lopez-Gonzalez is an Associate Professor at the Loma Linda University in Loma Linda, California, United States.

He is specialized in skull base, cerebrovascular, and complex cranial surgeries. He has contributed to the academic community through various research publications and education of the next generation of neurosurgeons.

Preface

The surgical management of skull base tumors presents one of the most formidable challenges in neurosurgery and head and neck surgery. The anatomical complexity of these regions with critical neurovascular structures demands a detailed understanding of regional anatomy, sophisticated surgical techniques and skills, and an interdisciplinary approach to minimize the potential morbidity.

This reprint has been written with the help of recognized experts in skull base surgery, and it provides a comprehensive resource for novice and experienced surgeons who seek to enhance their surgical skills in skull base surgery. The goal is to bridge the gap between foundational anatomical knowledge and advanced surgical strategies, providing readers with insights into the latest advancements and techniques.

Throughout this reprint, the reader will find detailed descriptions of various skull base tumors, the anatomical basis, and surgical planning, supported by high-quality illustrations and intraoperative images and videos in selected cases. These include open microneurosurgical procedures and nuances of minimally invasive techniques with the evolution of endoscopic approaches that have revolutionized the management of many skull base pathologies.

We hope that this reprint will inspire a deeper appreciation for the art and science of skull base surgery, motivate the young generations of surgeons for additional learning and research, and become an invaluable reference for surgeons at every stage of their careers.

Overall, the ultimate goal is to contribute to the maintenance of the meticulous delivery of microneurosurgical and endoscopic skull base surgery techniques with compassionate care for patients suffering from these complex pathologies.

Miguel Lopez-Gonzalez
Editor

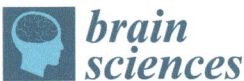

Editorial

Editorial for Brain Sciences Special Issue: "Advances in Skull Base Tumor Surgery: The Practical Pearls"

Miguel Angel Lopez-Gonzalez

School of Medicine, Loma Linda University, Loma Linda, CA 92354, USA; mlopezgonzalez@llu.edu

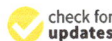

Citation: Lopez-Gonzalez, M.A. Editorial for Brain Sciences Special Issue: "Advances in Skull Base Tumor Surgery: The Practical Pearls". *Brain Sci.* **2024**, *14*, 352. https://doi.org/10.3390/brainsci14040352

Received: 21 March 2024
Accepted: 27 March 2024
Published: 1 April 2024

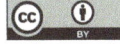

Copyright: © 2024 by the author. Licensee MDPI, Basel, Switzerland. This article is an open access article distributed under the terms and conditions of the Creative Commons Attribution (CC BY) license (https://creativecommons.org/licenses/by/4.0/).

The field of skull base surgery is unique; it involves the adequate and coordinated multidisciplinary interaction of multiple specialties, such as otorhinolaryngology, maxillofacial surgery, ophthalmology, neuro-anesthesiology, oncology, radiation oncology, neurophysiology, and neurosurgery. Young residents and fellows interested in this field need to learn and master the surgical skills required to tackle lesions located deep in the skull base with minimal morbidity.

The need to go back to the basics and learn and re-review human anatomy and classic skull base surgery approaches developed by the giants in our field cannot be overemphasized. The initial wave of skull base surgery started with approaches in sellar region developed by Schloffer in 1907 and subsequently modified by Hirsch and Cushing using the sublabial approach, and then followed by Dott, Guiot and Hardy, popularizing the transsphenoidal approach. The second wave in skull base surgery from 1980s was invigorated by the modern giants in skull base surgery, such as Yasargil, Hakuba, Al-Mefty, Dolenc, Spetzler, Kawase, Fukushima, Shekar, House, and Fisch, among others [1]. The third leap represents the endoscopic endonasal era that started in the 1990s, with the landmark paper by Jho and Carrau [2]. More knowledge has been accumulated, and now, skull base surgeons are able to access any skull base region either using a conventional lateral skull base approach, or endoscopic expanded endonasal techniques.

The trend of using minimal invasive approaches in skull base surgery is applauded, although it is critical to maintain a balanced judgement regarding when to use minimal invasive options versus the conventional skull base approaches. Current skull base surgeons need to have a good understanding of the reach of each of the approaches, profound anatomical knowledge developing via laboratory dissections, and surgical training. They also need to make an unbiased judgment on the appropriate procedure for each patient, with careful mental preparation and rehearsal to respond to all the possible intraoperative scenarios. The in-depth preoperative analysis of all the images (computed tomography, magnetic resonance, cerebral angiogram, etc.), as well as a consensus discussion with the other referred specialists when appropriate can provide an adequate and safe surgical plan. A perfectly orchestrated teamwork with surgeon leadership is mandatory. Closed and respectful communication with the entire surgical team before surgery is necessary to achieve the common goal of a successful operation. It is crucial to be versatile and provide exactly what each patient requires. There are new tools that can be utilized for preoperative planning and education, such as virtual, augmented, or mixed reality. When available, it is important to integrate these tools, although we need to keep in mind that the success of surgery comes with the adequate execution of the microneurosurgical skills, since technology, at this point, cannot perform the crucial delicate steps required for these formidable approaches.

In this Special Issue: "Advances in Skull Base Tumor Surgery: The Practical Pearls", we integrate the experience of experts in the field, describing their techniques and pearls of wisdom to improve all the areas of skull base surgery from endoscopic endonasal to lateral skull base approaches, including videos for vestibular schwannoma and craniopharyngioma resection, as well as using the sphenoid ridge approach on pediatric patients. Among others, Liu and colleagues [3] present an elegant and detailed microsurgical anatomy review and surgical examples of jugular foramen tumors, ranging from using basic retrosigmoid approaches to combined retro and infralabyrinthine transjugular transcondylar high cervical approaches. Mukherjee and colleagues [4] present the reach of endonasal endoscopic skull base surgery for pathologies in the sellar–suprasellar area, orbital apex, and anterior cranial base in detail and transpterygoid approaches, with a thorough description of their practical pearls.

Overall, all the included articles encompass all the areas of skull base surgery. I recommend adding them with the surgical approach examples to the armamentarium of different modalities of treatment for skull base surgeons to deal with complex lesions in daily practice.

Conflicts of Interest: The author declares no conflicts of interest.

References

1. Maroon, J.C. Skull base surgery: Past, present, and future trends. *Neurosurg. Focus* **2005**, *19*, E1. [CrossRef]
2. Jho, H.D.; Carrau, R.L. Endoscopic endonasal transsphenoidal surgery: Experience with 50 patients. *J. Neurosurg.* **1997**, *87*, 44–51. [CrossRef]
3. Castillo, A.L.; Meybodi, A.T.; Liu, J.K. Jugular Foramen Tumors: Surgical Strategies and Representative Cases. *Brain Sci.* **2024**, *14*, 182. [CrossRef] [PubMed]
4. Ahmed, A.K.; Rowan, N.R.; Mukherjee, D. Operative Corridors in Endoscopic Skull Base Tumor Surgery. *Brain Sci.* **2024**, *14*, 207. [CrossRef]

Disclaimer/Publisher's Note: The statements, opinions and data contained in all publications are solely those of the individual author(s) and contributor(s) and not of MDPI and/or the editor(s). MDPI and/or the editor(s) disclaim responsibility for any injury to people or property resulting from any ideas, methods, instructions or products referred to in the content.

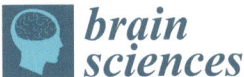

Article

A New Perspective on the Cavernous Sinus as Seen through Multiple Surgical Corridors: Anatomical Study Comparing the Transorbital, Endonasal, and Transcranial Routes and the Relative Coterminous Spatial Regions

Sergio Corvino [1,2], Pedro L. Villanueva-Solórzano [3], Martina Offi [4,5], Daniele Armocida [6], Motonobu Nonaka [7], Giorgio Iaconetta [8], Felice Esposito [1,*], Luigi Maria Cavallo [1] and Matteo de Notaris [9]

1. Division of Neurosurgery, Department of Neuroscience and Reproductive and Odontostomatological Sciences, Università di Napoli "Federico II", 80131 Naples, Italy; sercorvino@gmail.com (S.C.); lcavallo@unina.it (L.M.C.)
2. PhD Program in Neuroscience, Department of Neuroscience and Reproductive and Odontostomatological Sciences, Università di Napoli "Federico II", 80131 Naples, Italy
3. Department of Neurosurgery, National Institute of Neurology and Neurosurgery "Manuel Velasco Suarez", Mexico City 14269, Mexico; pedrovs@me.com
4. Institute of Neurosurgery, Fondazione Policlinico Universitario A. Gemelli, 00168 Rome, Italy; martinaoffi.mo@gmail.com
5. Division of Neurosurgery, Catholic University of Rome, 00153 Rome, Italy
6. Neurosurgery Division, Human Neurosciences Department, "Sapienza" University, 00185 Rome, Italy; danielearmocida@yahoo.it
7. Department of Neurosurgery, Kochi University Hospital, 185-1, Oko-cho, Kohasu, Kochi 783-8505, Japan; mtb.nonaka@gmail.com
8. Neurosurgical Clinic A.O.U. "San Giovanni di Dio e Ruggi d'Aragona", 84131 Salerno, Italy; iaconetta@libero.it
9. Neurosurgery Operative Unit, Department of Neuroscience, Coordinator Neuroanatomy Section Italian Society of Neurosurgery, G. Rummo Hospital, 82100 Benevento, Italy; matteodenotaris@gmail.com
* Correspondence: felice.esposito@unina.it

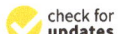

Citation: Corvino, S.; Villanueva-Solórzano, P.L.; Offi, M.; Armocida, D.; Nonaka, M.; Iaconetta, G.; Esposito, F.; Cavallo, L.M.; de Notaris, M. A New Perspective on the Cavernous Sinus as Seen through Multiple Surgical Corridors: Anatomical Study Comparing the Transorbital, Endonasal, and Transcranial Routes and the Relative Coterminous Spatial Regions. *Brain Sci.* **2023**, *13*, 1215. https://doi.org/10.3390/brainsci13081215

Academic Editors: Miguel Lopez-Gonzalez and Woon-Man Kung

Received: 5 July 2023
Revised: 27 July 2023
Accepted: 16 August 2023
Published: 17 August 2023

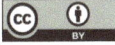

Copyright: © 2023 by the authors. Licensee MDPI, Basel, Switzerland. This article is an open access article distributed under the terms and conditions of the Creative Commons Attribution (CC BY) license (https:// creativecommons.org/licenses/by/ 4.0/).

Abstract: *Background*: The cavernous sinus (CS) is a highly vulnerable anatomical space, mainly due to the neurovascular structures that it contains; therefore, a detailed knowledge of its anatomy is mandatory for surgical unlocking. In this study, we compared the anatomy of this region from different endoscopic and microsurgical operative corridors, further focusing on the corresponding anatomic landmarks encountered along these routes. Furthermore, we tried to define the safe entry zones to this venous space from these three different operative corridors, and to provide indications regarding the optimal approach according to the lesion's location. *Methods*: Five embalmed and injected adult cadaveric specimens (10 sides) separately underwent dissection and exposure of the CS via superior eyelid endoscopic transorbital (SETOA), extended endoscopic endonasal transsphenoidal-transethmoidal (EEEA), and microsurgical transcranial fronto-temporo-orbito-zygomatic (FTOZ) approaches. The anatomical landmarks and the content of this venous space were described and compared from these surgical perspectives. *Results*: The oculomotor triangle can be clearly exposed only by the FTOZ approach. Unlike EEEA, for the exposure of the clinoid triangle content, the anterior clinoid process removal is required for FTOZ and SETOA. The supra- and infratrochlear as well as the anteromedial and anterolateral triangles can be exposed by all three corridors. The most recently introduced SETOA allowed for the exposure of the entire lateral wall of the CS without entering its neurovascular structures and part of the posterior wall; furthermore, thanks to its anteroposterior trajectory, it allowed for the disclosure of the posterior ascending segment of the cavernous ICA with the related sympathetic plexus through the Mullan's triangle, in a minimally invasive fashion. Through the anterolateral triangle, the transorbital corridor allowed us to expose the lateral 180 degrees of the Vidian nerve and artery in the homonymous canal, the anterolateral aspect of the lacerum segment of the ICA at the transition zone from the petrous horizontal to the ascending posterior cavernous segment, surrounded by the carotid sympathetic plexus, and the medial Meckel's cave. ***Conclusions***: Different regions of the cavernous sinus are better exposed by different surgical corridors. The relationship of the tumor with cranial nerves in the lateral wall guides the selection of the approach to cavernous sinus lesions. The transorbital endoscopic approach can be considered to be a safe and minimally invasive complementary surgical corridor to the well-established transcranial and endoscopic endonasal routes for the exposure of selected lesions of the cavernous sinus. Nevertheless, peer knowledge of the anatomy and a surgical learning curve are required.

Keywords: cavernous sinus triangles; endoscopic transorbital; extended endoscopic endonasal; fronto-temporo-orbito-zygomatic; middle fossa

1. Introduction

The cavernous sinus (CS) is a vulnerable venous space located deep in the center of the base of the skull, and it includes vital and highly functional neurovascular structures—e.g., the internal carotid artery (ICA) and its branches; the III, IV, and VI cranial nerves; and the ophthalmic division of the trigeminal nerve. Therefore the detailed knowledge of its anatomy is mandatory to avoid potentially life-threating iatrogenic injuries.

As already happened in the past with the advent of the endoscopic endonasal approaches (mainly addressed to the pathologies of the midline skull base through a ventral median corridor), most recently the endoscopic transorbital route has opened a new window, but mainly for the paramedian and lateral aspects of the anterior and middle cranial fossae up to the petrous apex [1,2].

Since the first pioneering work of Parkinson [3], which describes the surgical approach to a carotid-cavernous fistula, several anatomical studies [4–10] and surgical series [11–14], have provided a detailed description of this dural envelope and its safe entry zones from different routes, both transcranial [3,15–17] and endonasal [16–20], and most recently endoscopic transorbital [21–23], each of them with related pro and cons.

Nevertheless, a single approach is not sufficient to expose the entire CS and simultaneously to have the proximal and distal control of the cavernous ICA, which is necessary for a safe surgery.

Tumoral, congenital, infectious/inflammatory/granulomatous, and vascular pathologies [24], of any size and morphology, pattern of growth, and diffusion, can involve one or more compartments of the cavernous sinus and have different relationships with the structures lying within it. In this scenario, when a surgical treatment is indicated, it is mandatory for a neurosurgeon to be confident with more than one surgical route to ensure the availability of different working angles through the various triangles to maximize the tumor resection and to minimize the risk of injury to the cranial nerves and ICA, ultimately choosing the best tailored option.

The aim of the current study was to provide an anatomical description from a superior eyelid transorbital endoscopic (SETOA) perspective of the cavernous sinus and its relationship with the main neurovascular structures; furthermore, we attempted to highlight the main differences and similarities of the exposed area and its landmarks as seen from the endoscopic endonasal and transcranial routes (Figure 1). Finally, we tried to define the safe entry zones to this venous space from these three different operative corridors (Table 1) and provide indications regarding the optimal approach according to the lesion's location.

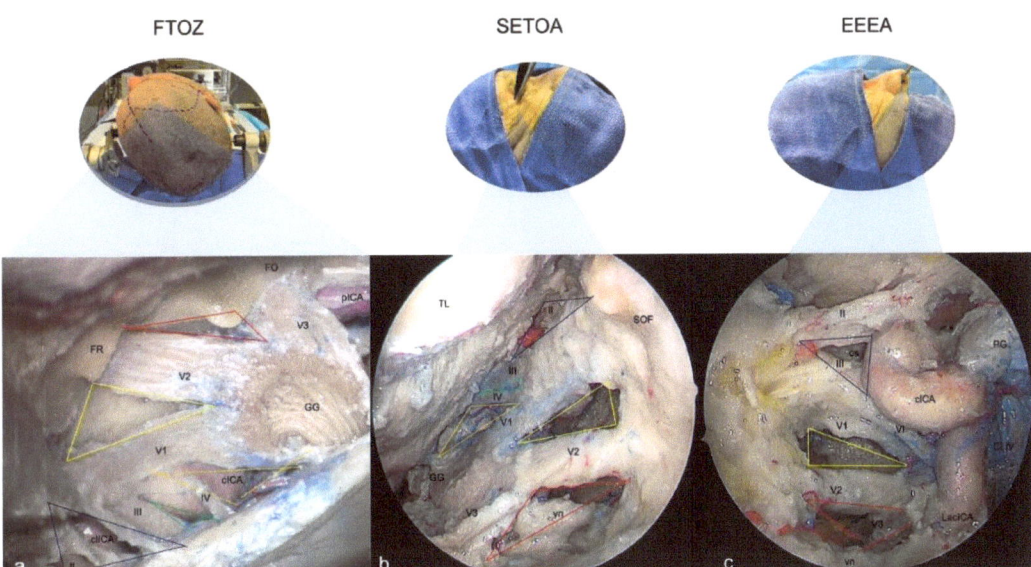

Figure 1. Exposure of the right-side cavernous sinus from different surgical perspectives: (**a**) Fronto-temporo-orbito-zygomatic (FTOZ) approach: head specimen secured in three-pin Mayfield skull clamp, 45 degrees rotated and hyperextended so that the malar eminence was the highest point at the horizon line. (**b**) Superior eyelid endoscopic transorbital approach (SETOA): head specimen in neutral supine position, 10 degrees flexed and 10 degrees rotated to the contralateral side of the operator. (**c**) Extended endoscopic endonasal transsphenoidal transethmoidal approach (EEEA): head specimen in neutral supine position, 10 degrees flexed and slightly rotated to the side of the operator. (GG: Gasserian ganglion; TL: temporal lobe; FR: foramen rotundum; FO: foramen ovale; vn: Vidian nerve; cICA: cavernous internal carotid artery; pICA: petrous internal carotid artery; LacICA: lacerum internal carotid artery; clICA: clinoidal internal carotid artery; os: optic strut; SOF: superior orbital fissure; PG: pituitary gland; CLIV: clivus; red lines: anterolateral triangle; yellow lines: anteromedial triangle; orange lines: infratrochlear triangle; green lines: supratrochlear triangle; blue lines: clinoidal triangle).

Table 1. Summary of the anatomical and surgical aspects of the cavernous sinus triangles from superior eyelid endoscopic transorbital, fronto-temporo-orbito-zygomatic, and extended endoscopic endonasal transsphenoidal-transethmoidal approaches.

Triangles	Clinoidal (Dolenc)			Supratrochlear			Infratrochlear (Parkinson)			Anteromedial (Mullan)			Anterolateral		
Boundaries	- Lower border of II c.n. superiorly; - Upper border of III c.n. inferiorly			- Lower border of III c.n. superiorly; - Upper border of IV c.n. inferiorly			- Lower border of IV c.n. superiorly; - Upper border of V1 inferiorly			- Lower border of V1 superiorly; - Upper border of V2 inferiorly			- Lower border of V2 superiorly; - Upper border of V3 inferiorly		
Approach	FTOZ	SETOA	EEEA	FTOZ	SETOA	EEEA	FTOZ	SETOA	EEEA	FTOZ	SETOA	EEEA	FTOZ	SETOA	EEEA
Surgical maneuvers for the exposition	Anterior clinoidectomy (augmented by pericavernous maneuvers)	Anterior clinoidectomy	—	Peeling of the LWCS and middle fossa	Peeling of the LWCS and middle fossa	—	Peeling of the LWCS and middle fossa	Peeling of the LWCS and middle fossa	—	Peeling of the LWCS and middle fossa	Peeling of the LWCS and middle fossa	Removal of lateral wall of the sphenoid sinus	Peeling of the LWCS and middle fossa	Peeling of the LWCS and middle fossa	Removal of lateral wall of the sphenoid sinus
Content	cl-ICA, between upper and lower dural rings	cl-ICA, between upper and lower dural rings	Optic strut or optic-carotid recess	hc-ICA and MHT, ILT	hc-ICA	—	Posterior bend of the c-ICA with MHT, VI c.n.	Superior half and posterior bend of posterior c-ICA with MHT	ILT; VI c.n.	Sphenoid sinus	Inferior half of the posterior segment of c-ICA; VI c.n.	Venous structures	Sphenoid sinus	Lacerum ICA; Sympathetic carotid plexus; FL, PLL, Vidian nerve and artery;	—
Indications	Meningioma, ACP, carotid-ophthalmic aneurysm	Meningioma, ACP	—	Schwannomas, CS tumors	Schwannomas, CS tumors	Pit-adenoma, chondrosarcomas with lateral extension up to the CS lateral wall	Aneurysm or fistula of proximal c-ICA, CS tumors	Schwannoma CS tumors	Pit-adenoma, chondrosarcomas with lateral extension up to the CS lateral wall	Middle fossa tumors with CS invasion	Small lesion involving the anteroinferior compartment of CS	Pit-adenoma, chondrosarcomas with lateral extension up to the CS lateral wall	—	Small lesion involving the anteroinferior compartment of CS	Pit-adenoma, chondrosarcomas with lateral extension up to the CS lateral wall
Safety of surgical access	Low risk	Low risk	Low risk	Mid risk	Mid risk	Mid risk	Mid risk	Mid risk	Mid risk	Low risk	Mid risk	Mid risk	Low risk	Low risk	Low risk

c.n.: cranial nerve; FTOZ: fronto-temporal-orbito-zygomatyc; SETOA: superior eyelid transorbital endoscopic approach; EEEA: extended endoscopic endonasal approach; cl: clinoid; hc: horizontal cavernous; CS: cavernous sinus; c-ICA: cavernous internal carotid artery; Pit: pituitary; LWCS: lateral wall cavernous sinus; ICA: internal carotid artery; PLL: petro-lingual ligament; MHT: meningo-hypophyseal trunk; ILT: inferolateral trunk, FL: foramen lacerum.

2. Materials and Methods

Anatomical dissections were performed at the Laboratory of Skull Base and Microneurosurgery of the Weill Cornell Neurosurgical Innovations and Training Center, New York, USA. Five adult cadaveric specimens (10 sides), embalmed and injected with red and blue latex for the arteriosus and venous blood vessels, respectively, were dissected. The fronto-temporo-orbito-zygomatic (FTOZ) approach was performed under microscopic visualization (OPMI, Zeiss, Oberkochen, Germany), whereas the extended endoscopic endonasal transsphenoidal-transethmoidal (EEEA) was performed with a rigid endoscope of 4 mm diameter, 18 cm in length, with 0° and 30° rod lenses as optical devices (Karl Storz, Tuttlingen, Germany); finally, the SETOA, after the initial step under macroscopic visualization, proceeded under endoscopic visualization. The endoscope was connected to a light source (300 W Xenon, Karl Storz) through a fiber-optic cable and to an HD camera (Endovision Telecam SL; Karl Storz).

We adopted the intracranial classification systems (C1–C7) proposed by Bouthillier et al. [25] and by Labib et al. [26] for the description of the anatomical course of the ICA during FTOZ/SETOA and EEEA, respectively, and the well-known division in triangles of the cavernous sinus [15] was used as a reference to depict the areas of exposure.

2.1. Fronto-Temporo-Orbito-Zygomatic (FTOZ) Approach

The surgical procedure started with a curvilinear skin incision extended from 1 cm anterior to the tragus and below the zygomatic arch, to the contralateral mid-pupillary line, and was followed by a subgaleal interfascial dissection [27] and a retrograde subperiosteal detachment of the temporalis muscle [28]. At this point, a two-piece orbitozygomatic craniotomy according to Zabramski's [29] technique was performed, followed by the cutting of the meningo-orbital band [30] and the extradural anterior clinoidectomy [31]. Finally, the surgical procedure was completed with the interperiosteal-dural dissection of the lateral wall of the CS and the middle cranial fossa, and with pericavernous maneuvers [32] to expand the optic–carotid and carotid–oculomotor windows.

2.2. Superior Eyelid Transorbital Endoscopic Approach (SETOA)

An SETOA to the petrous apex was performed as previously reported in the literature [33]. As previously reported in the pertinent literature [34], the orbital retraction was set at <10 mm.

A skin incision was placed in a superior eyelid wrinkle; hence, once the orbicularis oculi muscle was identified, the dissection was carried out in depth up to the superior orbital rim and extended laterally up to the frontozygomatic suture (FZS). After cutting the periosteum where it became continuous with the periorbita, the dissection continued, with endoscopic assistance, in a subperiosteum/periorbital plane within the orbit until the lateral margin of the inferior and superior orbital fissures. At this point, once the zygomatic body and the intraorbital part of the greater sphenoid wing (including the sagittal crest [35]) were drilled until the exposure of the temporal pole dura mater, an interperiosteal-dural dissection via the meningo-orbital band (MOB) [21] was performed to unlock the lateral wall of the CS up to the Gasserian ganglion (GG). After cutting the middle meningeal artery (MMA), the temporal pole was elevated in an extradural fashion and, once the mid-subtemporal ridge and the trigeminal lateral loop were identified [36], the anterolateral triangle of middle fossa was opened [37]. Finally, an extradural anterior clinoidectomy [38] completed the surgical procedure.

2.3. Extended Endoscopic Endonasal Transsphenoidal Transethmoidal Approach (EEEA)

An extended endoscopic endonasal transsphenoidal transethmoidal approach was performed as previously reported in the literature [20,39]. In contrast to the standard endoscopic endonasal transsphenoidal approach, to obtain a wider exposition of the CS, the sphenoidotomy was extended more laterally and the posterior ethmoidal cells were opened. Furthermore, to expand the operative corridor, the uncinate process was removed and the bulla ethmoidalis was opened, allowing us to reach and remove the anterior ethmoid cells. The removal of the posterior ethmoid cells and the anterior wall of the sphenoid sinus allowed us to expose the lateral wall of the sphenoid sinus with a direct trajectory, and once it was removed, the CS came into view.

3. Results

The differences and likenesses of the various regions of the CS and the related anatomical landmarks were analyzed to make a descriptive comparison from transcranial, endoscopic endonasal, and endoscopic transorbital perspectives.

3.1. Clinoid Triangle (Dolenc's Triangle)

3.1.1. FTOZ Perspective

This area is bounded by the inferior margin of the optic nerve superiorly, the superior margin of the oculomotor nerve inferiorly, and by the segment of the anterior petroclinoid dural fold between the entry point of the II and III cranial nerves. It includes the anterior clinoid process, which covers the clinoidal segment of the ICA (C5 segment [25]) between the proximal and distal dural rings. It is necessary to remove the anterior clinoidal process to expose its content (Figure 2a,b).

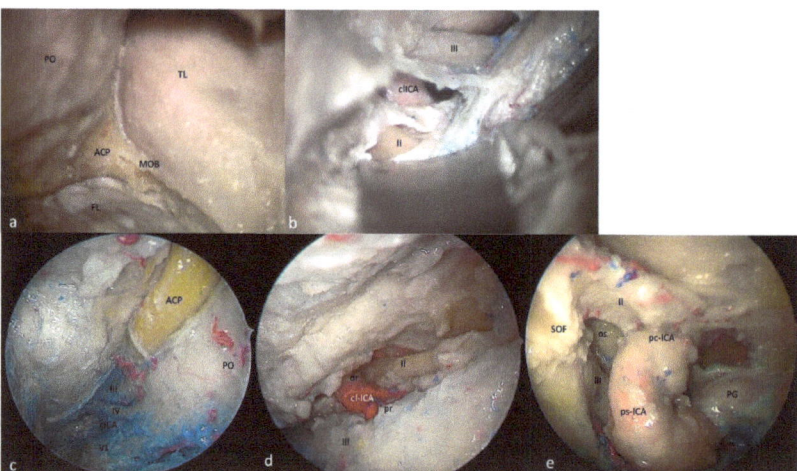

Figure 2. Right-side clinoidal (Dolenc's) triangle: FTOZ perspective (**a**) before and (**b**) after anterior clinoidal process removal. SETOA perspective (**c**) before and (**d**) after anterior clinoidal process removal. (**e**) EEEA perspective with preserved anterior clinoidal process. The boundaries of this triangles are represented by the inferior margin of the optic nerve superiorly, the superior margin of the oculomotor nerve inferiorly, and by the segment of the anterior petroclinoid dural fold between the entry point of the II and III cranial nerves (PO: periorbit; ACP: anterior clinoid process; TL: temporal lobe; MOB: meningo-orbital band; FL: frontal lobe; cl-ICA: clinoidal internal carotid artery; dr: distal ring; pr: proximal ring; SOF: superior orbital fissure; os: optic strut; ps-ICA: parasellar internal carotid artery; pc-ICA: paraclinoid internal carotid artery; PG: pituitary gland).

3.1.2. SETOA Perspective

The clinoid triangle is completely exposed through transorbital route and, after the anterior clinoidectomy, its content is also evident.

The removal of the anterior clinoid process (ACP) reveals a pyramidal dural pocket bounded by the dura on the superior surface of the lesser sphenoid wing (LSW) laterally, the dura on the superior surface of the LSW and attached to the lateral edge of the planum sphenoidale superiorly, the falciform ligament covering the proximal segment of the optic nerve (ON) after its unroofing medially, and finally, the optic nerve dural sheath and the anterior part of the distal dural ring of the ICA inferiorly.

The ON is observed along its posteromedial course toward the optic chiasm. The clinoidal segment of the ICA (C5 segment [25]) between the lower and upper dural rings is observed in the central part of the triangle, with the ophthalmic artery running inferomedially to the ON. Finally, the optic–carotid membrane and space are also evident (Figure 2c,d).

3.1.3. EEEA Perspective

This area is bounded by the optic nerve above and the oculomotor nerve below the optic strut. The base of this triangle is represented by the distal part of the parasellar and paraclinoid segments of the ICA [26]. The content of this triangle is the optic strut or optic–carotid recess (Figure 2e).

3.2. Oculomotor Triangle (Hakuba's Triangle)

3.2.1. FTOZ Perspective

This triangle forms the posterior part of the roof of the cavernous sinus. Its boundaries are the interclinoid dural fold medially and the anterior and posterior petroclinoid dural folds laterally and posteriorly, respectively.

3.2.2. SETOA Perspective

This area, even after anterior clinoidectomy, is scarcely recognizable from this surgical corridor.

3.2.3. EEEA Perspective

This triangle is also not identifiable after gentle medial displacement of the ICA.

3.3. Supratrochlear Triangle (Paramedian)

3.3.1. FTOZ Perspective

This area is bounded by the inferior border of the oculomotor nerve superiorly, the superior border of the trochlear nerve inferiorly, and the segment of the dura of the roof of the cavernous sinus between the entry points of these two nerves. Its content is represented by the horizontal cavernous ICA (Figure 3a).

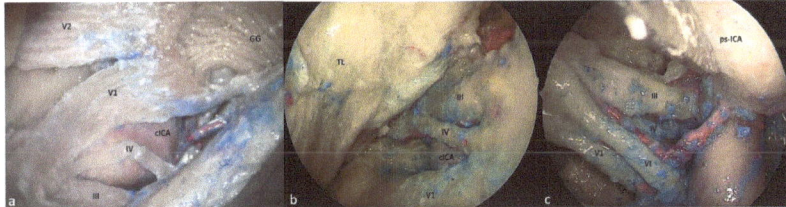

Figure 3. Right-side supra- and infratrochlear triangles: (**a**) FTOZ, (**b**) SETOA, and (**c**) EEEA perspectives. The boundaries of the supratrochlear are represented by the inferior border of the III c.n. superiorly, the superior border of the IV c.n. inferiorly, and the segment of the dura of the roof of the cavernous sinus between the entry points of these two nerves; regarding the infratrochlear triangle, it is delimited superiorly by the lower margin of the trochlear nerve, inferiorly by the upper margin of V1, and posteriorly by the line connecting the point where the trochlear nerve enters the roof of the cavernous sinus and the point where the trigeminal nerve enters the Meckel's cave (GG: Gasserian ganglion; cICA: cavernous internal carotid artery; TL: temporal lobe, ps-ICA: parasellar internal carotid artery).

3.3.2. SETOA Perspective

This triangle and its boundaries are completely exposed via the transorbital corridor just after interperiosteal-dural dissection of the lateral wall of the CS. This is a very narrow space that medially hides the horizontal segment of the cavernous ICA (C4 segment [25]) (Figure 3b).

3.3.3. EEEA Perspective

Only the apex of this triangle, where the III and IV cranial nerves converge toward the SOF, can be exposed, and the medial displacement of the ICA and/or the lateral displacement of the cranial nerves is required (Figure 3c).

3.4. Infratrochlear Triangle (Parkinson's triangle)

3.4.1. FTOZ Perspective

This triangle is delimited superiorly by the lower margin of the trochlear nerve, inferiorly by the upper margin of V1, and posteriorly by the line connecting the point where the trochlear nerve enters the roof of cavernous sinus and the point where the trigeminal nerve enters the Meckel's cave. This region hosts the posterior bend of the cavernous ICA (C4 segment [25]) with its branches (meningohypophyseal trunk) (Figure 3a).

3.4.2. SETOA Perspective

This region and its content are completely exposed via the transorbital route; just after interperiosteal-dural dissection of the lateral wall of the CS, the anterolateral aspect of the superior half of the ascending segment of the cavernous ICA is evident. Furthermore, after a gentle downward retraction of the proximal part of V1, it is possible to identify the sixth cranial neve exiting from the Dorello's canal under the Gruber's ligament and coursing anteriorly in the lateral wall of the CS medially to V1. After a gentle upward displacement of the trochlear nerve, it is possible to expose the meningohypophyseal trunk (MHT) that arises from the posterior bend of cavernous ICA (C4 segment [25]) (Figure 3b).

3.4.3. EEEA Perspective

Only the anterior narrow space of this triangle and its content, represented by the inferolateral trunk of the cavernous ICA, are evident, because of the abducens nerve that covers the ophthalmic division of the trigeminal nerve, and because of the parasellar ICA [26] that obstructs access to the posterior compartment (Figure 3c).

3.5. Anteromedial Triangle (Mullan's Triangle)

3.5.1. FTOZ Perspective

This region is delimited superiorly by the lower margin of V1, inferiorly by the upper margin of V2, and anteriorly by the line connecting the point where the ophthalmic nerve enters the superior orbital fissure and the point where the maxillary nerve enters the foramen rotundum (Figure 4a). The removal of the outer bony shell of this triangle leads into the sphenoid sinus.

3.5.2. SETOA Perspective

This region comes immediately into the endoscopic view after interperiosteal-dural dissection of the lateral wall of the CS, and it is the largest safe entry zone to the CS. Unlike the transcranial frontotemporal point of view, where no segments of the ICA are visible in this area, the SETOA allows for the in-depth disclosure, at the apex of this triangle, where V1 and V2 converge, of the inferior half of the posterior ascending segment of the cavernous ICA (C4 segment [25]), surrounded by sympathetic fibers of the carotid plexus, passing medially to the petro-lingual ligament to reach the cavernous sinus (Figure 4b). In this triangle, the VI cranial nerve courses almost horizontally, medially to V1 and laterally to the ICA, towards the SOF, and it can be visualized after gentle upward retraction of V1 (Figure 4c). One fundamental landmark that guides surgical dissection of the anteromedial triangle, avoiding entering the CS space, is the foramen rotundum, which is encountered after resection of the sagittal crest that discloses V2 inferiorly and outside the CS. Surgical dissection must be performed between the two trigeminal branches at the level of the superior edge of V2, dissecting the perineurium covering the two nerves in an anteroposterior direction to free the two branches, and mobilizing the ophthalmic nerve superiorly to expand the space between them and gain access to the posteroinferior portion of the CS.

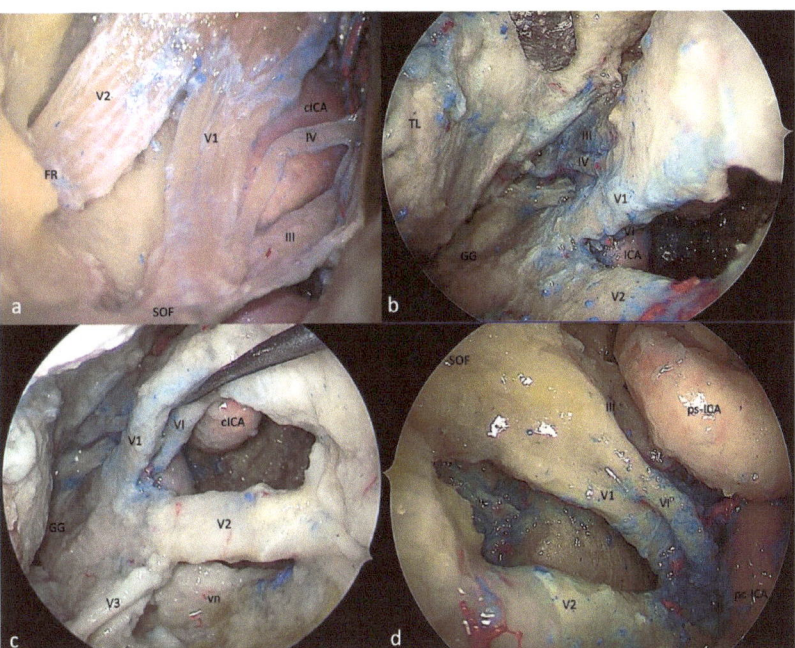

Figure 4. Right-side anteromedial (Mullan's) triangle: (**a**) FTOZ, (**b**,**c**) SETOA, and (**d**) EEEA perspectives. This region is delimited superiorly by the lower margin of V1, inferiorly by the upper margin of V2, and anteriorly by the line connecting the point where the ophthalmic nerve enters the superior orbital fissure and the point where the maxillary nerve enters the foramen rotundum (FR: foramen rotundum; SOF: superior orbital fissure; cICA: cavernous internal carotid artery; TL: temporal lobe; GG: Gasserian ganglion; vn: Vidian nerve; ps-ICA: parasellar internal carotid artery; pc-ICA: paraclival internal carotid artery).

3.5.3. EEEA Perspective

This area and its content, represented by venous structures, are completely exposed after bone removal from the lateral wall of the sphenoid sinus, with V1 partially hidden by the sixth cranial nerve. The apex of this triangle, where V1 and V2 converge, can be disclosed after medial displacement of the paraclival and parasellar segments of the ICA [26] (Figure 4d).

3.6. Anterolateral Triangle
3.6.1. FTOZ Perspective

This area is bounded by the lower border of V2 superiorly, the upper border of V3 inferiorly, and the line that connects the foramina rotundum and ovale. The drilling of its medial wall exposes the sphenoid sinus (Figure 5a).

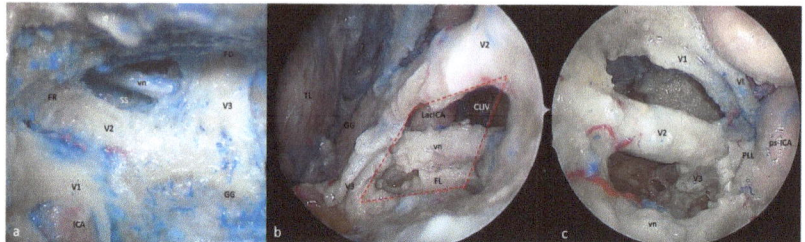

Figure 5. Right-side anterolateral triangle: (**a**) FTOZ, (**b**) SETOA, and (**c**) EEEA perspectives. This area is bounded by the lower border of V2 superiorly, the upper border of V3, inferiorly, and the line that connects the foramina rotundum and ovale (red dotted lines: quadrangular space; FO: foramen ovale; FR: foramen rotundum; GG: Gasserian ganglion; CLIV: clivus; Lac ICA: lacerum internal carotid artery; vn: Vidian nerve; FL: foramen lacerum; MC: Meckel's cave; cICA: cavernous internal carotid artery; ps-ICA: parasellar internal carotid artery).

3.6.2. SETOA Perspective

The opening of this triangle allows for the disclosure of the Vidian nerve and artery in the homonymous canal along their course up to the anterolateral edge of the foramen lacerum, where the posterior opening of the canal is filled with cartilaginous tissue that blends into the more medially positioned cartilage filling the foramen lacerum. The lacerum segment of the ICA, at its transition zone from the horizontal petrous segment to the ascending cavernous segment, located medially to the petrolingual ligament, along with the related carotid sympathetic plexus, can be also exposed (Figure 5b). As recently already described by our group [37], it is possible to appreciate a space limited by the inferior border of V2 superiorly, the superior border of V3 posteriorly, the line crossing the most anterior limit of exposure of the Vidian nerve and joining the foramen rotundum and the point where the greater wing joints the body of the sphenoid bone anteriorly, and the line between this last point and the foramen ovale posteriorly (red dotted line). This area includes two windows divided by the course of the Vidian nerve until where it blends into the cartilaginous tissue of the FL under the trigeminal nerve, and which unfold different corridors:

(a) A wider superior window ("supravidian") that discloses two corridors in relationship to the lacerum segments of the ICA: a "medial supravidian corridor" leading to the lower clivus, and a "lateral supravidian corridor" leading, after gentle lateralization of the Gasserian ganglion, to the medial aspect of the Meckel's cave and the terminal portion of the horizontal petrous ICA (pICA).
(b) A narrow inferior window ("infravidian") that includes the inferior portion of the foramen lacerum distally, and the sphenoid sinus proximally.

3.6.3. EEEA Perspective

Whereas V2 is disclosed from the origin up to the foramen rotundum, V3 is recognizable only in its course from the origin at the Gasserian ganglion up to the entrance the foramen ovale (Figure 5c).

4. Discussion

4.1. Anatomical Considerations

The oculomotor triangle can be clearly exposed and expanded by opening the optic–carotid and carotid–oculomotor windows only through the transcranial approach, whereas it is scarcely identifiable from SETOA and EEEA in normal conditions; however, Nunes et al. [40]. have described an endoscopic endonasal transoculomotor triangle approach for adenomas invading the parapeduncolar space in which the lesion created the corridor.

To expose the clinoidal triangle and its content, anterior clinoidectomy is necessary for both SETOA and FTOZ. Unlike the transcranial route, extradural clinoidectomy via the transorbital route does not have anatomical landmarks, and the limits of the ACP base drive the drilling [38]. Unlike the transcranial and transorbital approaches, during EEEA the ICA comes into the view in front of the ACP, just after exposing the posterior wall of the sphenoid sinus. We consider the access to this area to be safe from all three operative corridors ("low risk", green traffic light—Table 1).

The transorbital corridor provides the same exposure of the supra- and infratrochlear triangles' contents as the transcranial route, but with a different working angle, and provides a better control on the anterior aspect of the posterior ascending segment of the cavernous ICA. The EEEA allows for the exposure of just the apex of the supratrochlear triangle, but the medial displacement of the ICA and/or the lateral displacement of cranial nerves are required; concerning the Parkinson's triangle, the horizontal cavernous ICA and the VI nerve partially obstruct its exposure. We consider the access to both of these triangles to be relatively safe from all three corridors ("mid risk", yellow traffic light—Table 1), taking into the account the superficial course of the ICA and MHT in this region from each of the different perspectives.

The anteromedial triangle is the largest window opened on the CS from SETOA. Unlike the transcranial route, through this route, the endoscopic transorbital route allows for the exposure of the anterior aspect of the inferior half of the posterior ascending segment of the cavernous ICA, surrounded by sympathetic fibers of the carotid plexus; additionally, the VI cranial nerve, along its almost horizontal course (medially to V1 and laterally to the ICA, towards the SOF), can be visualized after gentle upward retraction of V1. We consider the access to this area from EEEA and FTOZ to be safe ("low risk", green traffic light—Table 1), whereas one should be more careful when using the transorbital corridor ("mid risk", yellow traffic light—Table 1) due to the proximity of the inferior border of the horizontal segment of the cavernous ICA, partially hidden by V2 and the inferior segment of the posterior ascending cavernous ICA deep in the triangle.

The opening of the anterolateral triangle through SETOA [37] reveals a space that can be divided into a wider superior window ("supravidian") and a narrow inferior window ("infravidian"). The supravidian window allows direct access to the lacerum segment of the ICA and the related carotid sympathetic plexus; furthermore, this space reveals two different corridors: the *medial supravidian corridor* leading to the lower clivus, and the *lateral supravidian corridor* leading to the Meckel's cave and the terminal portion of the horizontal petrous ICA, medial and lateral to the lacerum ICA, respectively. We consider the access to this area to be safe from all three (FTOZ, SETOA, and EEEA) surgical routes ("low risk", green traffic light—Table 1) (Figure 6).

4.2. Surgical Nuances

Among the more or less recent classifications of the compartments of the CS [4,41,42], in agreement with that provided by Harris et al. [4], we considered three main venous spaces in relation with the course of the cavernous ICA: posterosuperior, anteroinferior, and medial compartments.

The FTOZ route allows access to the CS through its roof and lateral wall using the clinoidal/oculomotor and the supra/infratrochlear triangles, respectively [43].

The clinoidal triangle represents the lower floor of the anterior portion of the roof of the cavernous sinus, and it is commonly used to approach paraclinoid or carotid–ophthalmic aneurysms; its exposure requires the intra- or extradural removal of the ACP, and care must be taken regarding the clinoidal ICA and the unroofing of the optic canal during this maneuver. The exposure of this area continues with the opening of the optic sheath and the distal dural ring. The oculomotor triangle represents the posterior part of the roof of the cavernous sinus, and it is usually used as corridor to access basilar tip aneurysms and tumors inside the cavernous sinus; its exposure requires the opening of the oculomotor cistern, the incision of the carotid–oculomotor membrane, and the incision of the dura of the triangle; care must be taken to identify the MHT.

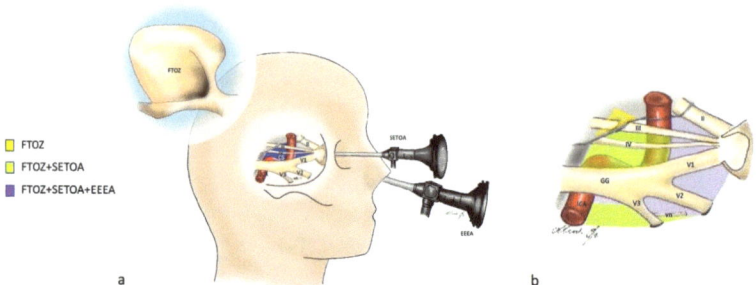

Figure 6. (**a**) Graphic showing the fronto-temporo-orbito-zygomatic (FTOZ), endoscopic transorbital (SETOA) and endoscopic endonasal (EEEA) approaches to the cavernous sinus; CS: cavernous sinus; vn: Vidian nerve; GG: Gasserian ganglion; blue = cavernous sinus; yellow: cranial nerves; red: ICA. (**b**) Graphic of the cavernous sinus and its exposure areas from the three approaches through the different triangles: yellow space: this area can be exposed only through FTOZ (oculomotor triangle); green space: these areas can be separately exposed only through FTOZ and SETOA (supra- and infratrochlear triangles, anterolateral triangle laterally to the Vidian nerve, and posteromedial and posterolateral triangles of the middle fossa, i.e., Glassock's and Kawase's triangles); purple space: these areas can be separately exposed through FTOZ, SETOA, and EEEA (clinoid, supra- and infratrochlear, and anteromedial and anterolateral triangles).

The simultaneous opening of these two triangles allows for the management of lesions involving the lateral, posterosuperior, and medial compartments of the CS.

The FTOZ allows access to the posterosuperior and anteroinferior compartments of the CS, as well as through its lateral wall by opening the supra- and/or infratrochlear triangles, just after the peeling of the middle fossa; care is recommended to identify the VI c.n. exiting the Dorello's canal in the Parkinson's triangle.

The EEEA allows access to the posterosuperior and anterior compartments of the CS through its medial (sellar) and anterior (sphenoidal) walls thanks to medial-to-lateral [44] and anterior-to-posterior trajectories [41], respectively. To access the posterior compartment, the opening of the sellar dura and the cutting of the inferior hypophyseal artery are required; access to the anteroinferior compartment is facilitated by using a transpterygoid approach.

The exposure area of the lateral wall of the CS via EEEA is greatly influenced by the ICA's position: because of its localization inside the CS, the ICA comes into the endoscopic view before the lateral wall of the CS, representing an obstacle for the visualization of the posterior content of the CS's lateral wall—mainly the supra- and infratrochlear triangles. Conversely, the anterior part of the clinoidal triangle, the entire anteromedial triangle, and the upper part of the anterolateral triangle are exposed and provide potential pathways from this route to the middle cranial fossa.

As this route is mainly indicated for midline skull-base pathologies, its main risks and drawbacks in approaching the CS are related to the lateral extension, i.e., pituitary adenomas with CS invasion, and include the injury of the ICA and the cranial nerves, CSF leakage, and limited resection rates.

The interperiosteal-dural dissection from anterior to posterior via the MOB [21] during SETOA provides a shorter and direct route, and it follows a natural sagittal plane, allowing for the exposure of the entire lateral wall of the CS without violating its neurovascular compartment, and with an optimal angle of attack [21]. The MOB represents the key landmark for identifying the CS via SETOA. If from one side the extradural endoscopic transsphenoidal and transethmoidal approaches offer direct access to the anterior portion of the cavernous sinus, from the other side the lateral and posterior walls instead represent a challenge from this route [20,45,46].

The transorbital approach respects the principles of the modern, minimally invasive skull-base techniques: flattening the skull base and using the extradural space to approach the target lesion, reducing the brain retraction [47]. Nevertheless, a mandatory consideration must be kept in mind when exposing the CS: the width of the surgical corridor. This route, while providing a wide visualization, uses a narrow (and single if compared to EEEA) surgical corridor, limited by orbital rims superiorly, laterally, and inferiorly, and by the vulnerable orbital content medially, which imposes limitations on the surgical freedom and working angles; therefore, it is mainly suitable for small lesions involving the CS at its posterosuperior and anteroinferior lateral compartments, through the supra/infratrochlear and anteromedial/anterolateral triangles, respectively [45]. Peri- and postoperative complications related to the intraoperative orbital content retraction may be avoided with careful management of the globe through the use of a corneal protector, placing the malleable ribbon retractor tangentially against the globe, while constantly monitoring the pupillary diameter during the procedure and removing the instruments from the surgical field every 20–30 min to minimize the pressure on the globe [34].

The relationship of lesion and cranial nerves in the lateral wall, the anatomical course of the ICA, and the displacement of the ICA by the pathology guide the choice of the approach [45]: lesions that displace the cranial nerves laterally are more suitable for EEEA; lesions that displace the cranial nerves medially are more suitable for FTOZ and SETOA.

The most serious and potentially life-threatening complication is represented by the iatrogenic injury of the ICA, the incidence of which ranges from 3% to 8% [48] in conventional open approaches and is less than 1% during EEEA [49]; no data are reported about the transorbital route for the recent adoption of this technique in the neurosurgical field; therefore, unnecessary exposure of the ICA must be avoided.

4.3. Limitations of This Study

Pure anatomical studies have the common limitation related to cadaveric specimens: the property of cadaveric tissue considerably differs from real anatomy, e.g., variability in size and pneumatization of the sphenoid sinus; the trajectory of the internal carotid artery and cranial nerves; bony protuberances of the skull base. However, the main anatomical relationships between the cavernous sinus and its neurovascular structures are valid and reliable, albeit there is a lack of quantitative analysis.

5. Conclusions

The three operative corridors investigated provide three different points of view of the same anatomical region; each of them has its pros and cons; some areas of the cavernous sinus are better exposed from different approaches.

In this scenario, the transorbital endoscopic approach can be considered to be a safe, complementary route to the well-established transcranial and endoscopic endonasal ones for exploring the cavernous sinus. Nevertheless, as with any new technique, it requires a learning curve, and further clinical series are expected to validate these findings.

Author Contributions: S.C.: conception, anatomical dissection, data collection, data review, drafting manuscript, reviewed and drafted manuscript, study supervision; P.L.V.-S.: anatomical dissection; M.O.: graphical drawings; M.N.: anatomical dissection; D.A.: anatomical dissection; M.d.N.: conception; G.I., F.E., and L.M.C., study supervision. All authors have read and agreed to the published version of the manuscript.

Funding: This research received no external funding.

Institutional Review Board Statement: Not applicable.

Informed Consent Statement: Not applicable.

Data Availability Statement: Data used for the current original research are available from the corresponding author upon reasonable request.

Acknowledgments: Thanks to the Laboratory of Skull Base and Micro-neurosurgery of the Weill Cornell Neurosurgical Innovations and Training Center, New York, USA.

Conflicts of Interest: All authors deny any financial and non-financial competing interest.

Abbreviations

SETOA	Superior eyelid transorbital endoscopic approach
EEEA	Extended endoscopic endonasal approach
ICA	Internal carotid artery
GG	Gasserian ganglion
MOB	Meningo-orbital band
MMA	Middle meningeal artery
CS	Cavernous sinus
FL	Foramen lacerum
PL	Petrolingual ligament
vn	Vidian nerve
pICA	Petrous internal carotid artery
FTOZ	Fronto-t'emporo-orbito-zygomatic
MC	Meckel's cave

References

1. Vural, A.; Carobbio, A.L.C.; Ferrari, M.; Rampinelli, V.; Schreiber, A.; Mattavelli, D.; Doglietto, F.; Buffoli, B.; Rodella, L.F.; Taboni, S.; et al. Transorbital endoscopic approaches to the skull base: A systematic literature review and anatomical description. *Neurosurg. Rev.* **2021**, *44*, 2857–2878. [CrossRef] [PubMed]
2. Corvino, S.; Guizzardi, G.; Sacco, M.; Corrivetti, F.; Bove, I.; Enseñat, J.; Colamaria, A.; Prats-Galino, A.; Solari, D.; Cavallo, L.M.; et al. The feasibility of three port endonasal, transorbital, and sublabial approach to the petroclival region: Neurosurgical audit and multiportal anatomic quantitative investigation. *Acta Neurochir.* **2023**, *165*, 1821–1831. [CrossRef] [PubMed]
3. Parkinson, D. A surgical approach to the cavernous portion of the carotid artery. Anatomical studies and case report. *J. Neurosurg.* **1965**, *23*, 474–483. [CrossRef] [PubMed]
4. Harris, F.S.; Rhoton, A.L. Anatomy of the cavernous sinus. A microsurgical study. *J. Neurosurg.* **1976**, *45*, 169–180. [CrossRef] [PubMed]
5. Inoue, T.; Rhoton, A.L.; Theele, D.; Barry, M.E. Surgical approaches to the cavernous sinus: A microsurgical study. *Neurosurgery* **1990**, *26*, 903–932. [CrossRef] [PubMed]
6. Xu, Z.; Wei, X.; Zhao, C. Microsurgical anatomical study of the wall of the cavernous sinus. *Zhonghua Yi Xue Za Zhi* **1996**, *76*, 855–858.
7. Jian, F.Z.; Santoro, A.; Innocenzi, G.; Wang, X.W.; Liu, S.S.; Cantore, G. Frontotemporal orbitozygomatic craniotomy to expose the cavernous sinus and its surrounding regions. Microsurgical anatomy. *J. Neurosurg. Sci.* **2001**, *45*, 19–28.
8. Yasuda, A.; Campero, A.; Martins, C.; Rhoton, A.L.; Ribas, G.C. The medial wall of the cavernous sinus: Microsurgical anatomy. *Neurosurgery* **2004**, *55*, 179–189; discussion 189–190. [CrossRef]
9. Isolan, G.R.; Krayenbühl, N.; de Oliveira, E.; Al-Mefty, O. Microsurgical Anatomy of the Cavernous Sinus: Measurements of the Triangles in and around It. *Skull Base* **2007**, *17*, 357–367. [CrossRef]
10. Sekhar, L.N.; Burgess, J.; Akin, O. Anatomical study of the cavernous sinus emphasizing operative approaches and related vascular and neural reconstruction. *Neurosurgery* **1987**, *21*, 806–816. [CrossRef]
11. Al-Mefty, O.; Smith, R.R. Surgery of tumors invading the cavernous sinus. *Surg. Neurol.* **1988**, *30*, 370–381. [CrossRef] [PubMed]
12. Cusimano, M.D.; Sekhar, L.N.; Sen, C.N.; Pomonis, S.; Wright, D.C.; Biglan, A.W.; Jannetta, P.J. The results of surgery for benign tumors of the cavernous sinus. *Neurosurgery* **1995**, *37*, 1–9; discussion 9–10. [CrossRef] [PubMed]
13. Dolenc, V. Direct microsurgical repair of intracavernous vascular lesions. *J. Neurosurg.* **1983**, *58*, 824–831. [CrossRef] [PubMed]
14. Hakuba, A.; Matsuoka, Y.; Suzuki, T.; Komiyama, M.; Jin, T.B.; Inoue, Y. Direct Approaches to Vascular Lesions in the Cavernous Sinus via the Medial Triangle. In *The Cavernous Sinus: A Multidisciplinary Approach to Vascular and Tumorous Lesions*; Dolenc, V.V., Ed.; Springer: Vienna, Austria, 1987; pp. 272–284. [CrossRef]
15. Rhoton, A.L. The cavernous sinus, the cavernous venous plexus, and the carotid collar. *Neurosurgery* **2002**, *51*, S375–S410. [CrossRef] [PubMed]
16. Doglietto, F.; Lauretti, L.; Frank, G.; Pasquini, E.; Fernandez, E.; Tschabitscher, M.; Maira, G. Microscopic and endoscopic extracranial approaches to the cavernous sinus: Anatomic study. *Neurosurgery* **2009**, *64*, 413–421; discussion 421–422. [CrossRef] [PubMed]
17. Chowdhury, F.; Haque, M.; Kawsar, K.; Ara, S.; Mohammod, Q.; Sarker, M.; Goel, A. Transcranial microsurgical and endoscopic endonasal cavernous sinus (CS) anatomy: A cadaveric study. *J. Neurol. Surg. A Cent. Eur. Neurosurg.* **2012**, *73*, 296–306. [CrossRef]

18. Alfieri, A.; Jho, H.D. Endoscopic endonasal approaches to the cavernous sinus: Surgical approaches. *Neurosurgery* **2001**, *49*, 354–360; discussion 352–360. [CrossRef]
19. Alfieri, A.; Jho, H.D. Endoscopic endonasal cavernous sinus surgery: An anatomic study. *Neurosurgery* **2001**, *48*, 827–836; discussion 827–836.
20. Cavallo, L.M.; Cappabianca, P.; Galzio, R.; Iaconetta, G.; de Divitiis, E.; Tschabitscher, M. Endoscopic transnasal approach to the cavernous sinus versus transcranial route: Anatomic study. *Neurosurgery* **2005**, *56*, 379–389; discussion 379–389. [CrossRef]
21. Dallan, I.; Di Somma, A.; Prats-Galino, A.; Solari, D.; Alobid, I.; Turri-Zanoni, M.; Fiacchini, G.; Castelnuovo, P.; Catapano, G.; de Notaris, M. Endoscopic transorbital route to the cavernous sinus through the meningo-orbital band: A descriptive anatomical study. *J. Neurosurg.* **2017**, *127*, 622–629. [CrossRef] [PubMed]
22. Santos, C.; Guizzardi, G.; Di Somma, A.; Lopez, P.; Mato, D.; Enseñat, J.; Prats-Galino, A. Comparison of Accessibility to Cavernous Sinus Areas Throughout Endonasal, Transorbital, and Transcranial Approaches: Anatomic Study With Quantitative Analysis. *Oper. Neurosurg.* **2023**, *24*, e271–e280. [CrossRef] [PubMed]
23. Jung, I.H.; Yoo, J.; Choi, S.; Lim, S.H.; Ko, J.; Roh, T.H.; Hong, J.B.; Kim, E.H. Endoscopic transorbital approach to the cavernous sinus: Cadaveric anatomy study and clinical application. *Front. Oncol.* **2022**, *12*, 962598. [CrossRef]
24. Bakan, A.A.; Alkan, A.; Kurtcan, S.; Aralaşmak, A.; Tokdemir, S.; Mehdi, E.; Özdemir, H. Cavernous Sinus: A Comprehensive Review of its Anatomy, Pathologic Conditions, and Imaging Features. *Clin. Neuroradiol.* **2015**, *25*, 109–125. [CrossRef] [PubMed]
25. Bouthillier, A.; van Loveren, H.R.; Keller, J.T. Segments of the internal carotid artery: A new classification. *Neurosurgery* **1996**, *38*, 425–432; discussion 423–432. [CrossRef]
26. Labib, M.A.; Prevedello, D.M.; Carrau, R.; Kerr, E.E.; Naudy, C.; Abou Al-Shaar, H.; Corsten, M.; Kassam, A. A road map to the internal carotid artery in expanded endoscopic endonasal approaches to the ventral cranial base. *Neurosurgery* **2014**, *10* (Suppl. S3), 448–471; discussion 471. [CrossRef]
27. Yaşargil, M.G.; Reichman, M.V.; Kubik, S. Preservation of the frontotemporal branch of the facial nerve using the interfascial temporalis flap for pterional craniotomy. Technical article. *J. Neurosurg.* **1987**, *67*, 463–466. [CrossRef]
28. Oikawa, S.; Mizuno, M.; Muraoka, S.; Kobayashi, S. Retrograde dissection of the temporalis muscle preventing muscle atrophy for pterional craniotomy. Technical note. *J. Neurosurg.* **1996**, *84*, 297–299. [CrossRef]
29. Zabramski, J.M.; Kiriş, T.; Sankhla, S.K.; Cabiol, J.; Spetzler, R.F. Orbitozygomatic craniotomy. Technical note. *J. Neurosurg.* **1998**, *89*, 336–341. [CrossRef]
30. Fukuda, H.; Evins, A.I.; Burrell, J.C.; Iwasaki, K.; Stieg, P.E.; Bernardo, A. The Meningo-Orbital Band: Microsurgical Anatomy and Surgical Detachment of the Membranous Structures through a Frontotemporal Craniotomy with Removal of the Anterior Clinoid Process. *J. Neurol. Surg. B Skull Base* **2014**, *75*, 125–132. [CrossRef]
31. Froelich, S.C.; Aziz, K.M.; Levine, N.B.; Theodosopoulos, P.V.; van Loveren, H.R.; Keller, J.T. Refinement of the extradural anterior clinoidectomy: Surgical anatomy of the orbitotemporal periosteal fold. *Neurosurgery* **2007**, *61*, 179–185; discussion 176–185. [CrossRef] [PubMed]
32. Bernardo, A.; Evins, A.I.; Barbagli, G.; Kim, M.G.; Kim, N.; Xia, J.J.; Nonaka, M.; Stieg, P.E. Tailored Surgical Access to the Cavernous Sinus and Parasellar Region: Assessment of Cavernous Sinus Entry Corridors and the Periclinoid and Pericavernous Surgical Maneuvers. *World Neurosurg.* **2023**, *171*, e253–e275. [CrossRef] [PubMed]
33. Di Somma, A.; Andaluz, N.; Cavallo, L.M.; Topczewski, T.E.; Frio, F.; Gerardi, R.M.; Pineda, J.; Solari, D.; Enseñat, J.; Prats-Galino, A.; et al. Endoscopic transorbital route to the petrous apex: A feasibility anatomic study. *Acta Neurochir.* **2018**, *160*, 707–720. [CrossRef] [PubMed]
34. Moe, K.S.; Bergeron, C.M.; Ellenbogen, R.G. Transorbital neuroendoscopic surgery. *Neurosurgery* **2010**, *67*, ons16–ons28. [CrossRef]
35. Corrivetti, F.; de Notaris, M.; Di Somma, A.; Dallan, I.; Enseñat, J.; Topczewski, T.; Solari, D.; Cavallo, L.M.; Cappabianca, P.; Prats-Galino, A. "Sagittal Crest": Definition, Stepwise Dissection, and Clinical Implications from a Transorbital Perspective. *Oper. Neurosurg.* **2022**, *22*, e206–e212. [CrossRef]
36. Wanibuchi, M.; Murakami, G.; Yamashita, T.; Minamida, Y.; Fukushima, T.; Friedman, A.H.; Fujimiya, M.; Houkin, K. Midsubtemporal ridge as a predictor of the lateral loop formed by the maxillary nerve and mandibular nerve: A cadaveric morphological study. *Neurosurgery* **2011**, *69*, ons95–ons98; discussion ons98. [CrossRef]
37. Corvino, S.; Armocida, D.; Offi, M.; Pennisi, G.; Burattini, B.; Mondragon, A.V.; Esposito, F.; Cavallo, L.M.; de Notaris, M. The anterolateral triangle as window on the foramen lacerum from transorbital corridor: Anatomical study and technical nuances. *Acta Neurochir.* **2023**. [CrossRef]
38. López, C.B.; Di Somma, A.; Cepeda, S.; Arrese, I.; Sarabia, R.; Agustín, J.H.; Topczewski, T.E.; Enseñat, J.; Prats-Galino, A. Extradural anterior clinoidectomy through endoscopic transorbital approach: Laboratory investigation for surgical perspective. *Acta Neurochir.* **2021**, *163*, 2177–2188. [CrossRef]
39. Cavallo, L.M.; de Divitiis, O.; Aydin, S.; Messina, A.; Esposito, F.; Iaconetta, G.; Talat, K.; Cappabianca, P.; Tschabitscher, M. Extended endoscopic endonasal transsphenoidal approach to the suprasellar area: Anatomic considerations—Part 1. *Neurosurgery* **2008**, *62*, 1202–1212. [CrossRef]
40. Ferrareze Nunes, C.; Lieber, S.; Truong, H.Q.; Zenonos, G.; Wang, E.W.; Snyderman, C.H.; Gardner, P.A.; Fernandez-Miranda, J.C. Endoscopic endonasal transoculomotor triangle approach for adenomas invading the parapeduncular space: Surgical anatomy, technical nuances, and case series. *J. Neurosurg.* **2018**, *130*, 1304–1314. [CrossRef]

41. Fernandez-Miranda, J.C.; Zwagerman, N.T.; Abhinav, K.; Lieber, S.; Wang, E.W.; Snyderman, C.H.; Gardner, P.A. Cavernous sinus compartments from the endoscopic endonasal approach: Anatomical considerations and surgical relevance to adenoma surgery. *J. Neurosurg.* **2018**, *129*, 430–441. [CrossRef]
42. Almeida, J.P.; de Andrade, E.; Reghin-Neto, M.; Radovanovic, I.; Recinos, P.F.; Kshettry, V.R. From Above and Below: The Microsurgical Anatomy of Endoscopic Endonasal and Transcranial Microsurgical Approaches to the Parasellar Region. *World Neurosurg.* **2022**, *159*, e139–e160. [CrossRef] [PubMed]
43. Yasuda, A.; Campero, A.; Martins, C.; Rhoton, A.L.; de Oliveira, E.; Ribas, G.C. Microsurgical anatomy and approaches to the cavernous sinus. *Neurosurgery* **2005**, *56*, 4–27; discussion 24–27. [CrossRef] [PubMed]
44. Woodworth, G.F.; Patel, K.S.; Shin, B.; Burkhardt, J.K.; Tsiouris, A.J.; McCoul, E.D.; Anand, V.K.; Schwartz, T.H. Surgical outcomes using a medial-to-lateral endonasal endoscopic approach to pituitary adenomas invading the cavernous sinus. *J. Neurosurg.* **2014**, *120*, 1086–1094. [CrossRef] [PubMed]
45. Lee, M.H.; Hong, S.D.; Woo, K.I.; Kim, Y.D.; Choi, J.W.; Seol, H.J.; Lee, J.I.; Shin, H.J.; Nam, D.H.; Kong, D.S. Endoscopic Endonasal Versus Transorbital Surgery for Middle Cranial Fossa Tumors: Comparison of Clinical Outcomes Based on Surgical Corridors. *World Neurosurg.* **2019**, *122*, e1491–e1504. [CrossRef] [PubMed]
46. Komatsu, F.; Komatsu, M.; Inoue, T.; Tschabitscher, M. Endoscopic supraorbital extradural approach to the cavernous sinus: A cadaver study. *J. Neurosurg.* **2011**, *114*, 1331–1337. [CrossRef]
47. Corvino, S.; Sacco, M.; Somma, T.; Berardinelli, J.; Ugga, L.; Colamaria, A.; Corrivetti, F.; Iaconetta, G.; Kong, D.-S.; de Notaris, M. Functional and clinical outcomes after superior eyelid transorbital endoscopic approach for spheno-orbital meningiomas: Illustrative case and literature review. *Neurosurg. Rev.* **2022**, *46*, 1–12. [CrossRef]
48. Inamasu, J.; Guiot, B.H. Iatrogenic carotid artery injury in neurosurgery. *Neurosurg. Rev.* **2005**, *28*, 239–247; discussion 248. [CrossRef]
49. AlQahtani, A.; London, N.R.; Castelnuovo, P.; Locatelli, D.; Stamm, A.; Cohen-Gadol, A.A.; Elbosraty, H.; Casiano, R.; Morcos, J.; Pasquini, E.; et al. Assessment of Factors Associated With Internal Carotid Injury in Expanded Endoscopic Endonasal Skull Base Surgery. *JAMA Otolaryngol. Head Neck Surg.* **2020**, *146*, 364–372. [CrossRef]

Disclaimer/Publisher's Note: The statements, opinions and data contained in all publications are solely those of the individual author(s) and contributor(s) and not of MDPI and/or the editor(s). MDPI and/or the editor(s) disclaim responsibility for any injury to people or property resulting from any ideas, methods, instructions or products referred to in the content.

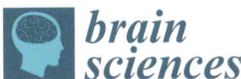

Communication

The Extended-Sphenoid Ridge Approach: A New Technique for the Surgical Treatment of Skull Base Tumors in Pediatric Patients

Roberto Garcia-Navarrete [1,2,*,†], Alfonso Marhx-Bracho [1], Javier Terrazo-Lluch [1] and José Luis Pérez-Gómez [1]

1. Neurosurgery Department, National Institute of Pediatrics of Mexico, Ciudad de Mexico 04530, Mexico; marhxalfons@yahoo.com.mx (A.M.-B.); jaterrazo@gmail.com (J.T.-L.); jlperezgomez@gmail.com (J.L.P.-G.)
2. Neurosurgery Department, Naval Medical Center, SEMAR, Ciudad de Mexico 04470, Mexico
* Correspondence: roberto.gns@gmail.com or rgarcianavarretes@pediatria.gob.mx
† Current address: Insurgentes Cuicuilco, Avenida Insurgentes Sur 3700-C, Tlalpan, Ciudad de Mexico 04530, Mexico.

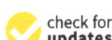

Citation: Garcia-Navarrete, R.; Marhx-Bracho, A.; Terrazo-Lluch, J.; Pérez-Gómez, J.L. The Extended-Sphenoid Ridge Approach: A New Technique for the Surgical Treatment of Skull Base Tumors in Pediatric Patients. *Brain Sci.* **2023**, *13*, 888. https://doi.org/10.3390/brainsci13060888

Academic Editor: Miguel Lopez-Gonzalez

Received: 21 April 2023
Revised: 29 May 2023
Accepted: 30 May 2023
Published: 31 May 2023

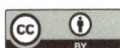

Copyright: © 2023 by the authors. Licensee MDPI, Basel, Switzerland. This article is an open access article distributed under the terms and conditions of the Creative Commons Attribution (CC BY) license (https://creativecommons.org/licenses/by/4.0/).

Abstract: The sphenoid ridge approach (SRA) was initially described as a surgical technique for treating vascular pathologies near the Sylvian fissure. However, limited studies have systematically explored the use of skull base techniques in pediatric patients. This study investigated an extended variation in the sphenoid ridge approach (E-SRA), which systematically removed the pterion, orbital walls (roof and lateral wall), greater sphenoid wing, and anterior clinoid process to access the base of the skull. Objective: This report aimed to evaluate the advantages of the extradural removal of the orbital roof, pterion, sphenoid wing, and anterior clinoid process as a complement to the sphenoid ridge approach in pediatric patients. Patients and Methods: We enrolled 36 patients with suspected neoplastic diseases in different regions. The E-SRA was performed to treat the patients. Patients were included based on the a priori objective of a biopsy or a total gross resection. The surgical time required to complete the approach, associated bleeding, and any complications were documented. Results: Our results demonstrated that the proposed a priori surgical goal, biopsy, or resection were successfully achieved in all cases. In addition, using the E-SRA technique was associated with a shorter operative time, minimal bleeding, and a lower incidence of complications. The most frequently encountered complications were related to dural closure. Conclusions: The extended sphenoid ridge approach represents a safe and effective option for managing intracranial tumors in pediatrics.

Keywords: skull base surgery; pediatric neurosurgery; craniopharyngioma; optic glioma; germinoma; Ewing's sarcoma

1. Introduction

In modern neurosurgery, minimally invasive skull base techniques are the cornerstone for treating lesions at the base of the skull [1].

The pterional approach is the gold standard technique for treating several pathologies of the skull base [2–9]. This approach offers the opportunity to treat lesions of the anterior and middle fossa and of the union of the medium and upper third of the clivus. A combination with other surgical techniques, such as the orbitozygomatic approach, allows for the treatment of neoplastic lesions that occupy large and complex skull base compartments [2,10–13].

Traditionally, minimally invasive techniques consider a careful dissection of the temporal fossa's soft tissues to avoid the inherent risk of injury from handling brain tissue and cranial nerves. However, even in the most experienced hands, these valuable techniques require a relatively longer surgical time. In addition, they will be associated with non-negligible blood loss, pain, postoperative complications, and a longer recovery, in addition to the esthetic and functional sequelae that can occur—a loss of hair on the suture line on the skin, a higher frequency of defects in the skin surface of the temporal region secondary to the atrophy of the temporalis muscle, and temporomandibular joint dysfunction.

The sphenoid ridge approach (SRA) is a minimally invasive technique commonly used to treat pathologies near the Sylvian fissure [14]. It has been demonstrated to be safe and effective in treating aneurysms of the bifurcation of the internal carotid and middle cerebral arteries. Some isolated reports have suggested that an extended variation in this approach, involving the removal of the orbital roof, pterion, sphenoid wing, and anterior clinoid process, along with an extradural anterior clinoidectomy, can further expand the surgical field and provide access to the most profound areas of the skull base [15–24].

Pediatric patients lack formal descriptions of minimally invasive techniques for treating neoplastic lesions in their supraorbital, sellar, suprasellar, and parasellar regions. Hence, this report aims to describe the benefits of the E-SRA for managing skull base tumors in pediatric patients.

Therefore, in this study, we propose a comprehensive extended approach to the sphenoid ridge (E-SRA), which includes a centered craniotomy at the pterion, in addition to the removal of the orbital walls (roof and lateral wall), greater sphenoid wing, and anterior clinoid process. This extended technique aims to reach the most profound areas of the skull base.

2. Patients and Methods

From 1 March 2015 to 30 June 2020, a total of 115 patients with presumptive diagnoses of neoplastic lesions located in their supraorbital, sellar, suprasellar, and parasellar regions were identified from the Department of Neurosurgery at the National Institute of Pediatrics of Mexico. Among these patients, 36 were selected to undergo a biopsy or gross total resection by E-SRA. The biopsy cases were considered *a priori* when a suspicion of a visual pathway glioma and germ cell tumors did not show conclusive tumor markers in the preoperative evaluation. The E-SRA procedure was followed based on a collegiate decision made by the Neurosurgery Department. In addition, informed consent from the patients' parents for the surgical procedure was obtained. The Ethics and Research Committee of the National Institute of Pediatrics evaluated and approved this study.

The criteria for selecting patients for the E-SRA procedure were as follows: (1) no history of prior surgery involving the pterion region; (2) radiological evidence of neoplastic lesions with a solid component volume of less than 50 cm^3; and (3) patients with neoplastic lesions suggestive of an optic pathway glioma. Patients who did not meet the criteria for the E-SRA were treated using conventional craniotomy and skull base surgery techniques.

E-SRA Technique: The SRA approach was performed as previously described [1]. A skin incision was made approximately 4 to 5 cm below the hairline and behind the external border of the eye, centered at the estimated location of the pterion. After the dissection of the skin and subcutaneous tissue, the superficial fascia and temporal muscle fibers were dissected along the skin incision. Next, a subperiosteal dissection was performed to expose the pterional region. A single burr hole was then made behind the pterion, followed by a small craniotomy (3×3 cm) around the visible landmarks of the sphenoid ridge. The hemostasis of the middle meningeal artery and dural vessels was achieved using a bipolar electrode after removing the bone flap. Once the pterion was removed, a triangular bone structure, defined by specific orbital points, became visible. The anterosuperior point, located at the upper and anterior angles, represented the union of the frontal bone and the internal table of the orbital roof. The posteromedial point, positioned at the medial and inferior angles, corresponded to the junction of the greater wing of the sphenoid bone and the base of the anterior clinoid process, projecting into the deep outer boundary of the superior orbital fissure. Finally, the posteroinferior point, found at the posterior and inferior angles, denoted the union of the internal table of the temporal bone and the wing of the sphenoid bone. The outer edge of the superior orbital fissure was delineated, and the meningo-orbital fold and meningo-orbital artery were dissected and coagulated to access the body and apex of the clinoid. The anterior clinoid process was drilled out and the optic strut was released at the lateral wall of the optic canal. At this stage, a dissection of the pretemporal dura allowed for an expanded surgical field of view, avoiding the use of brain retractors. Following the contour of the craniotomy edge, a dural opening was made, leaving a 5 mm free margin. After the tumor resection, the dura was sutured using a water seal technique with a 4–0 nylon suture. Sometimes, the use of a dural sealant reduces the risk of cerebrospinal fluid leakage. Next, the bone flap was repositioned and secured with non-absorbable sutures or mini plates. Finally, the temporal fascia and muscle were repaired using a 2–0 absorbable suture and the skin was closed with a 4–0 nylon suture. Subgaleal drainages were not utilized in our case (Figure 1 and Video S1).

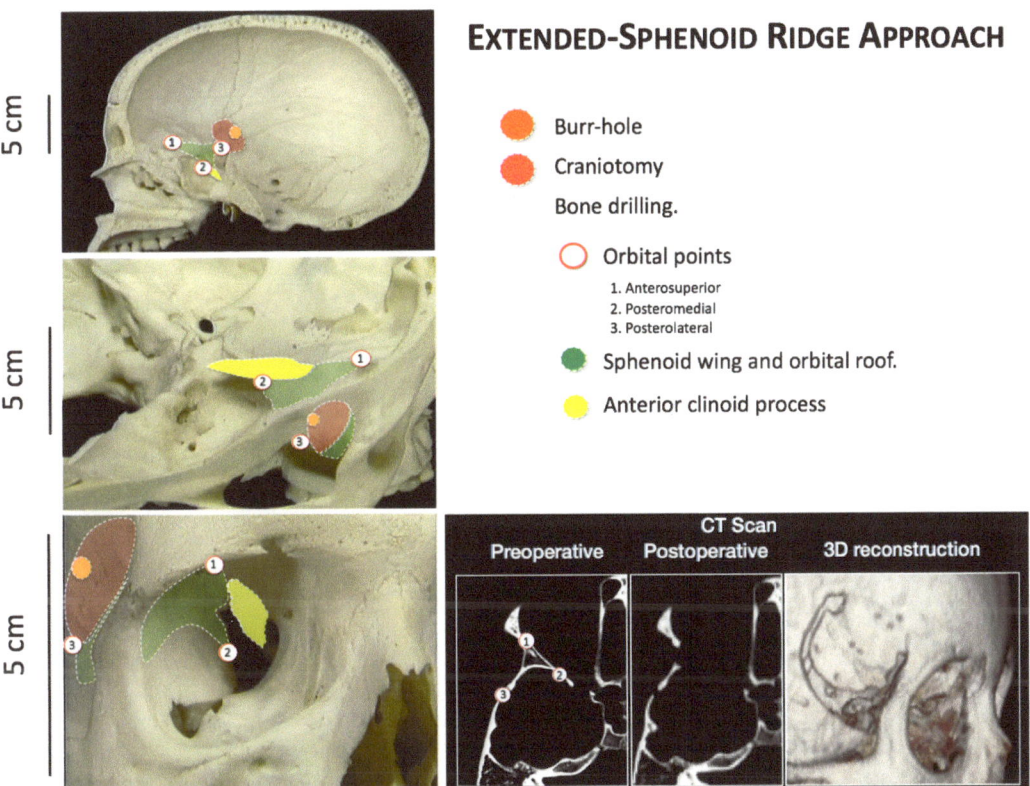

Figure 1. Surgical technique description of extended sphenoid ridge approach in pediatric patients.

The surgical objective was determined a priori based on the surgical plan established during the Department of Neurosurgery's session. The patients were categorized into two groups: those undergoing a biopsy and those undergoing an extensive resection surgery. Extensive resection surgery was considered when a neoplastic remanent accounted for less than 5% of the volume.

The evaluation of the surgical procedure included the length of the skin incision and the extension of the craniotomy, the time required to perform the E-SRA, and the associated bleeding. The complications were analyzed by reviewing all the clinical records until the patient was discharged from the institution and over a 24-month follow-up period. The statistical analysis presented the results as mean (±) standard deviation and ranges (lower and higher) for the quantitative variables and frequencies (%) for the qualitative variables.

3. Results

Patients and the Extended Sphenoid Ridge Approach Technique. We included 36 patients with a mean age of 7.8 ± 3 years; 17 male and 19 female patients were enrolled. The mean length of the skin incision was 4.2 ± 0.8 cm (3.4–5 cm) and that for the craniotomy area measured was 3.1 ± 0.5 cm^2 (2.6–3.6 cm^2). The average time taken to perform the E-SRA was 36 ± 6 min (30–42 min) and the quantified bleeding during the procedure was 20 ± 5 mL (15–25 mL). Brain retractors were not utilized in any of the cases and a dynamic retraction using cotton patties, bipolar forceps, and suction devices was preferred (Table 1).

Table 1. Demographic characteristics of patients treated with the extended-Sphenoid Ridge Approach.

Patient Characteristics.			
Age (Years)		7.8 ± 3	
Gender (Male/Female)		17/19	
Extended-Sphenoid ridge approach.			
Skin incision (cm)		4.2 ± 0.8	
Craniotomy area (cm^2)		3.1 ± 0.5	
Bleeding (mL)		20 ± 5	
Complications			
CSF Leakage		2.7%	
Subgaleal hematoma		5.5%	
Vascular injury related to the approach		0%	
Re-intervention		0%	
Histopathological diagnosis and surgical outcome.			
Diagnosis	Volume (cm^3)	Resection	
Craniopharyngioma (n = 22)	50 ± 12	Total	81% (n = 18)
		Subtotal	19% (n = 4)
Germinal tumor (n = 6)	25 ± 12	Total	33% (n = 2)
		Biopsy	66% (n = 4)
Visual pathway glioma (n = 4)	22 ± 12	Biopsy	100% (n = 4)
Pituitary adenoma (n = 3)	18 ± 12	Total	100% (n = 3)
Ewing's Sarcoma (n = 1)	12	Total	100% (n = 1)

Surgical objective. In all the patients, the objective of the surgery was accomplished: either a biopsy (22%) or a surgical excision (78%). A biopsy was performed in eight cases, when the intraoperative histopathological diagnoses were an optic pathway glioma (n = 4) or germinoma (n = 4). In 28 patients, an extensive surgical resection was performed (78%). It was considered total in 28 cases (86%) and subtotal (>90% volume) in 4 cases (14%) due to the invasion of diencephalic structures.

Histopathological diagnosis. The most common histopathological diagnosis was adamantinomatous craniopharyngioma (n = 22), followed, in order of frequency, by germinal tumors (n = 6), visual pathway gliomas (n = 4), pituitary adenoma (n = 3), and, in one case, orbital Ewing's sarcoma (n = 1).

Complications. Vascular injury. No vascular injuries related to the approach were observed—specifically, injuries to the internal carotid artery during the anterior clinoidectomy. In one case, there was a vascular injury at the origin of the contralateral posterior communicating artery during the dissection of the tumor capsule. It was controlled by applying an aneurysm clip (Video S2). One patient with Ewing's sarcoma presented a cerebrospinal fluid leak related to the infiltration of the dura mater above the orbital roof; two patients (5.5%) developed subgaleal hematomas in their temporal regions. No patient required further surgery to treat complications. Other than removing the orbital roof and lateral wall, we did not observe pulsatile exophthalmos. Despite the superior orbital fissure dissection, we did not observe clinical manifestations regarding cranial nerve paresis.

4. Discussion

The pterional approach, which was first described in the late 1970s, has become widely used for treating supratentorial neurosurgical diseases. It is considered to be the primary surgical corridor for accessing the skull base. In this study, we found that the extended sphenoid ridge approach (E-SRA) provided a safe and effective method for accessing neoplastic lesions in the skull bases of pediatric patients.

By removing the orbital roof and lateral wall, the E-SRA technique allows for transcranial access to extraconal lesions, including those with an ethmoidal extension. This expanded access enables surgeons to reach tumors in challenging locations (Figure 2).

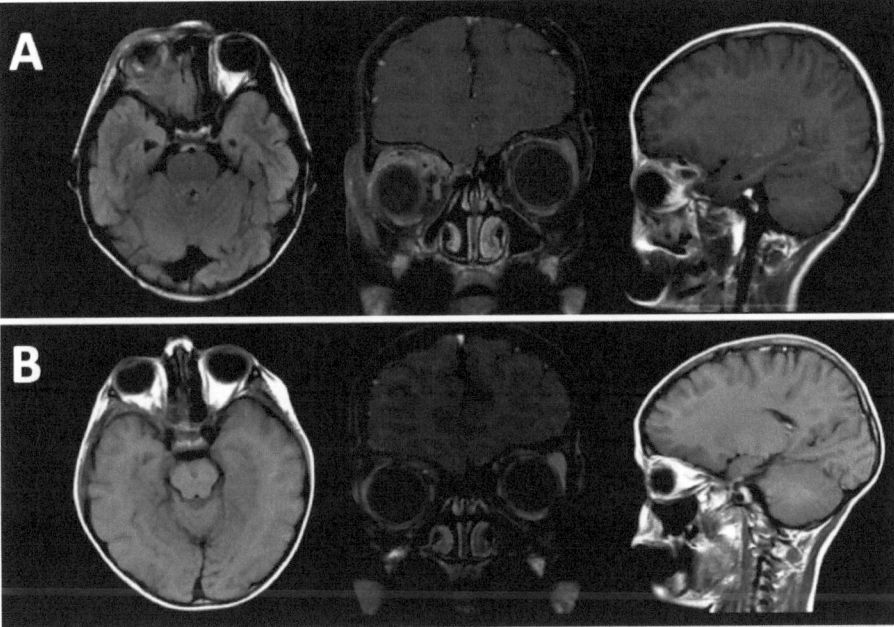

Figure 2. A 6-year-old boy was treated with orbital Ewing's sarcoma suspicion. (**A**) Pre-operative MRI shows an extraconal lesion extended medially until ethmoidal cells. (**B**) Post-operative MRI confirms the removal of tumoral tissue.

The E-SRA approach offers several advantages, including a shorter operative time, minimal bleeding, and a lower rate of complications. These benefits contribute to its improved surgical outcomes and patient recovery. However, it is essential to note that complications related to dural closure were the most frequently observed in our study.

Traditionally, various approaches, such as the supraorbital, subfrontal, pterional, and orbitozygomatic approaches, reach lesions in the sellar, suprasellar, and parasellar regions. However, these techniques pose specific risks to pediatric patients, including a longer surgical time, an increased bleeding volume, extensive soft tissue dissection, potential facial nerve injury, and a risk of temporomandibular dysfunction (Figure 3).

In this study, the extended sphenoid ridge approach (E-SRA) provided comparable exposure with other skull base approaches, while minimizing the need for extensive soft tissue dissection (Figure 4).

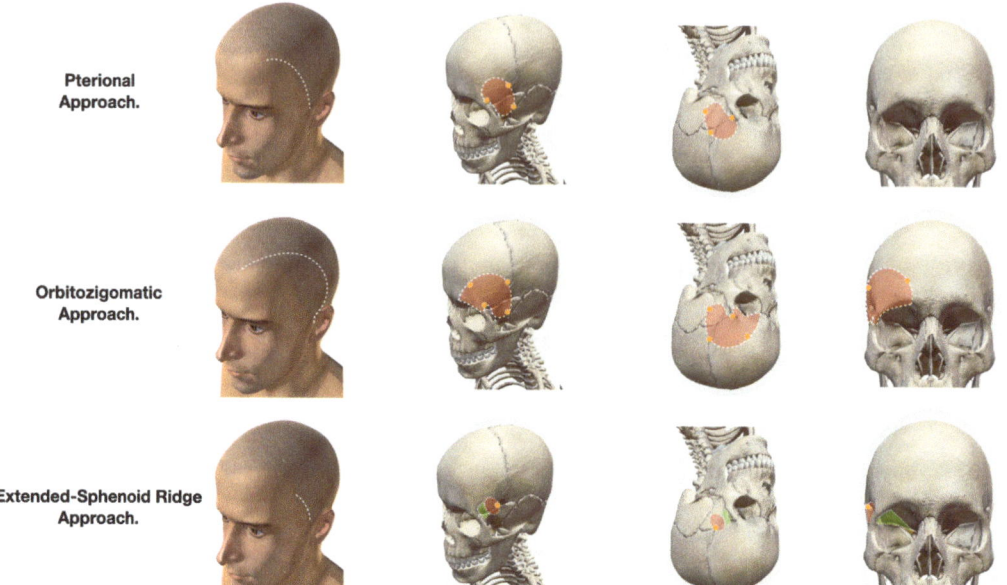

Figure 3. A graphic comparison of skin incision, craniotomy area, and orbital extension shows the benefits of the extended sphenoid ridge approach. (Modified models obtained from Atlas de Anatomía Humana Ver 2023.04.011. VISIBLE BODY® Argosy Publishing © 2007–2023).

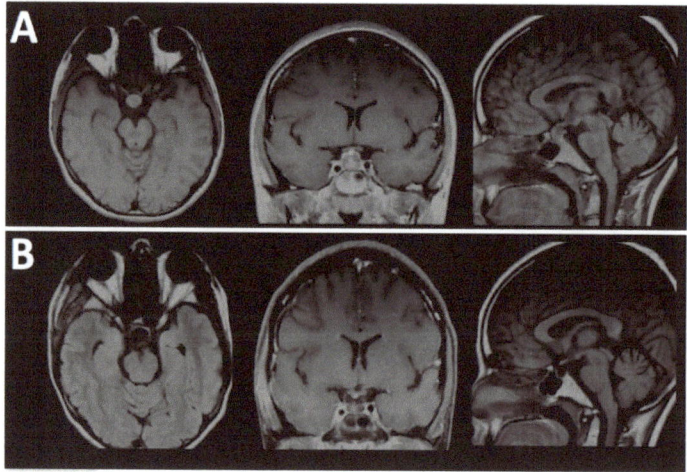

Figure 4. A 12-year-old girl admitted with diabetes insipidus and a growth delay. (**A**) Pre-operative MRI shows a sellar mass with extension to the infundibular stalk. (**B**) Postoperative MRI shows a gross-total resection.

The E-SRA technique allows for access to various structures in the skull base. The subfrontal corridor provides access to the olfactory nerves, optic nerves, inter-optic space, chiasm, lamina terminalis, A1 segment of the anterior cerebral artery, and anterior communicating artery. Dissecting Liliquist's membrane allows for access to the interpeduncular cistern, posterior cerebral arteries, superior cerebellar arteries, basilar tip, and trunk. Figures 5 and 6 and Video S2.

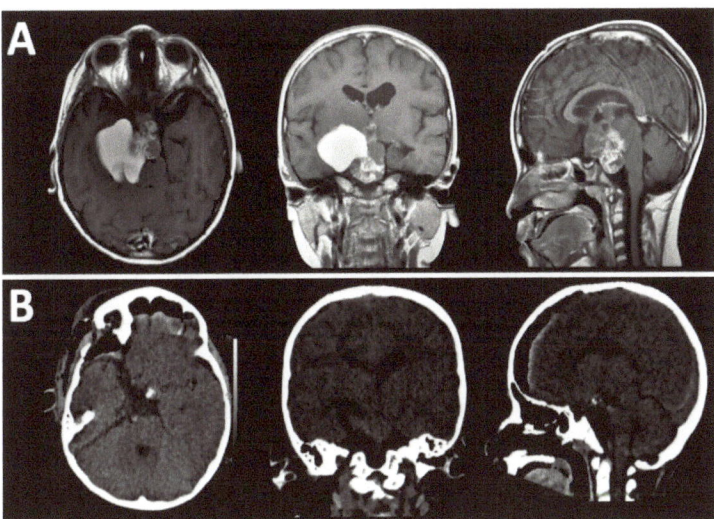

Figure 5. A 10-year-old girl with a history of headaches, visual disturbances, and panhypopituitarism. (**A**) Pre-operative MRI shows a mixed lesion with cystic and solid components. (**B**) A post-operative CT scan demonstrates the removal of tumoral tissue from sellar, parasellar, and suprasellar compartments. The histopathological analysis confirms the clinical suspicion of craniopharyngioma.

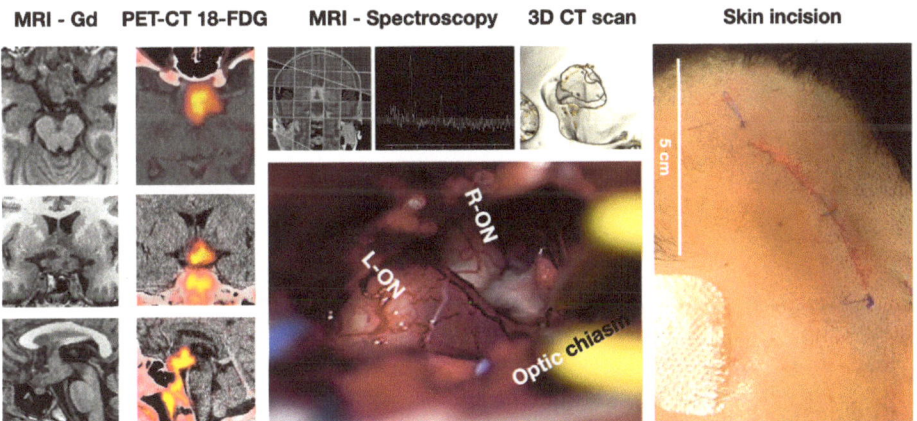

Figure 6. An 8-year-old girl with suspected optic pathway glioma was admitted. An E-SRA was performed and a sample biopsy was taken. The transoperative pathology study reported a germinal tumor. The image on the right shows the length of the skin incision behind the hair implantation.

Understanding the complex dural arrangement in the pterional region is crucial. Our observations indicate that the meningo-orbital dural fold plays a critical role as a crossroad between the superior orbital fissure, pretemporal dura, and lateral wall of the cavernous sinus. A blunt dissection initiated at the meningo-orbital fold allows for a confident dissection of the dural sheath of the superior orbital fissure and the base and lateral aspects of the anterior clinoid process. In addition, removing the anterior clinoid process tip reveals the dural transition between the pretemporal dura and the lateral wall of the cavernous sinus in an anteromedial direction. These dural folds are relevant, as their early identification and dissection create a wide corridor to the cavernous sinus and its delicate contents. Thus, an adequate dissection of the meningo-orbital fold plays a crucial role in creating a wide corridor to access the orbital fissure, pretemporal dura, and lateral wall of the cavernous sinus (Video S1).

Vascular damage, such as cavernous sinus or carotid artery injuries, was not observed during the E-SRA procedure. In one case, a vascular clip was applied at the origin of the contralateral posterior communicating artery during the craniopharyngioma's capsule dissection.

When the approach to the sphenoid ridge was described, there was significant criticism regarding fixing complications related to vascular incidents. However, the video shows that it was possible to address this complication by placing an aneurysm clip at the origin of the posterior communicating artery. Clinically, the patient did not experience any functional decline, and subsequent imaging evaluations identified circulation in the affected vessel (Video S2).

While transnasal endoscopic techniques help to treat tumors near the sphenoid sinus, their application in pediatric patients is limited and has specific challenges due to the poor pneumatization of the sphenoid sinus and an increased risk of vascular accidents. However, neuronavigation platforms can aid in directing a safe sphenoid bone removal to reach the sellar floor.

In conclusion, the extended sphenoid ridge approach is a safe and viable surgical option for treating intracranial tumors in pediatrics. This procedure should be considered among the available neurosurgical techniques, and our study provides a systematic description of skull base techniques for pediatric patients.

Supplementary Materials: The following supporting information can be downloaded at: https://www.mdpi.com/article/10.3390/brainsci13060888/s1, Video S1. E-SRA description. Video S2. Craniopharyngioma resection by E-SRA.

Author Contributions: Conceptualization, R.G.-N.; Data curation, R.G.-N., A.M.-B., J.T.-L. and J.L.P.-G.; Formal analysis, R.G.-N.; Investigation, R.G.-N.; Methodology, R.G.-N.; Visualization, R.G.-N.; Writing—original draft, R.G.-N.; Writing—review &editing, R.G.-N., A.M.-B., J.T.-L. and J.L.P.-G. All authors have read and agreed to the published version of the manuscript.

Funding: This research received no specific grant from the public, commercial, or not-for-profit funding agencies.

Institutional Review Board Statement: The study was conducted in accordance with the Declaration of Helsinki, and approved by the Ethics Committee of the National Institute of Pediatrics of Mexico (Protocol code GA143/2010, approved on 11 August 2010), for studies involving humans.

Informed Consent Statement: Informed consent was obtained from all patient´s parents involved in the study.

Data Availability Statement: No data is available due to privacy or ethical restrictions.

Conflicts of Interest: The authors declare no conflict of interest.

Abbreviations

E-SRA　Extended Sphenoid Ridge Approach
SRA　Sphenoid Ridge Approach

References

1. Yasargil, M.G.; Antic, J.; Laciga, R.; Jain, K.K.; Hodosh, R.M.; Smith, R.D. Microsurgical pterional approach to aneurysms of the basilar bifurcation. *Surg. Neurol.* **1976**, *6*, 83–91.
2. Alleyne, C.H., Jr.; Barrow, D.L.; Oyesiku, N.M. Combined transsphenoidal and pterional craniotomy approach to giant pituitary tumors. *Surg. Neurol.* **2002**, *57*, 380–390; discussion 390. [CrossRef]
3. Al-Mefty, O. Supraorbital-pterional approach to skull base lesions. *Neurosurgery* **1987**, *21*, 474–477. [CrossRef] [PubMed]
4. Anson, J.A. Treatment strategies for intracranial fusiform aneurysms. *Neurosurg. Clin. N. Am.* **1998**, *9*, 743. [PubMed]

5. Arnold, H.; Herrmann, H.D. Skull base chordoma with cavernous sinus involvement. Partial or radical tumour-removal? *Acta Neurochir.* **1986**, *83*, 31–37. [CrossRef] [PubMed]
6. Backlund, E.O. Pterional approach for orbital decompression. *Acta Ophthalmol.* **1968**, *46*, 535–540. [CrossRef] [PubMed]
7. Carmel, P.W.; Antunes, J.L.; Chang, C.H. Craniopharyngiomas in children. *Neurosurgery* **1982**, *11*, 382–389. [CrossRef]
8. Carrizo, A.; Basso, A. Current surgical treatment for sphenoorbital meningiomas. *Surg. Neurol.* **1998**, *50*, 574–578. [CrossRef]
9. Day, A.L. Aneurysms of the ophthalmic segment. A clinical and anatomical analysis. *J. Neurosurg.* **1990**, *72*, 677–691. [CrossRef]
10. Alaywan, M.; Sindou, M. Fronto-temporal approach with orbito-zygomatic removal surgical anatomy. *Acta Neurochir.* **1990**, *104*, 79–83. [CrossRef]
11. Cantore, G.; Santoro, A.; Da Pian, R. Spontaneous occlusion of supraclinoid aneurysms after the creation of extra-intracranial bypasses using long grafts: Report of two cases. *Neurosurgery* **1999**, *44*, 216–219; discussion 219–220. [CrossRef] [PubMed]
12. Day, J.D.; Giannotta, S.L.; Fukushima, T. Extradural temporopolar approach to lesions of the upper basilar artery and infrachiasmatic region. *J. Neurosurg.* **1994**, *81*, 230–235. [CrossRef]
13. Dolenc, V.V. A combined transorbital-transclinoid and transsylvian approach to carotid-ophthalmic aneurysms without retraction of the brain. *Acta Neurochir. Suppl.* **1999**, *72*, 89–97. [CrossRef] [PubMed]
14. Nathal, E.; Gomez-Amador, J.L. Anatomic and surgical basis of the sphenoid ridge keyhole approach for cerebral aneurysms. *Neurosurgery* **2005**, *56* (Suppl. S1), 178–185, discussion 178–185. [CrossRef] [PubMed]
15. Dolenc, V.V. Frontotemporal epidural approach to trigeminal neurinomas. *Acta Neurochir.* **1994**, *130*, 55–65. [CrossRef]
16. Andaluz, N.; van Loveren, H.R.; Keller, J.T.; Zuccarello, M. The One-Piece Orbitopterional Approach. *Skull Base* **2003**, *13*, 241–245. [CrossRef]
17. Chang, D.J. The "no-drill" technique of anterior clinoidectomy: A cranial base approach to the paraclinoid and parasellar region. *Neurosurgery* **2009**, *64* (Suppl. S3), ons96–105; discussion ons105–106. [CrossRef] [PubMed]
18. Takahashi, J.A.; Kawarazaki, A.; Hashimoto, N. Intradural en-bloc removal of the anterior clinoid process. *Acta Neurochir.* **2004**, *146*, 505–509. [CrossRef]
19. Bayassi, S. Fałd oponowo-oczodołowy jako kierunkowskaz zewnatrzoponowego dojścia do wyrostka pochyłego przedniego [Meningo-orbital fold (MOF) as a guiding point in extradural approach to the anterior clinoid process]. *Neurol. Neurochir. Pol.* **2005**, *39*, 49–55.
20. Lee, K.S. Extradural approach to the lateral sellar compartment. *Yonsei Med. J.* **2001**, *42*, 120–127. [CrossRef]
21. Kobayashi, M.; Yoshida, K.; Kawase, T. Inter-dural approach to parasellar tumors. *Acta Neurochir.* **2010**, *152*, 279–284; discussion 284–285. [CrossRef] [PubMed]
22. Coscarella, E.; Başkaya, M.K.; Morcos, J.J. An alternative extradural exposure to the anterior clinoid process: The superior orbital fissure as a surgical corridor. *Neurosurgery* **2003**, *53*, 162–166; discussion 166–167. [CrossRef] [PubMed]
23. Visot, A.; Boulin, A. Les voies d'abord du sphénoïde [Sphenoid bone: Surgical techniques]. *J. Neuroradiol.* **2003**, *30*, 258–267. [PubMed]
24. Acharya, R.; Shaya, M.; Kumar, R.; Caldito, G.C.; Nanda, A. Quantification of the advantages of the extended frontal approach to skull base. *Skull Base* **2004**, *14*, 133–142; discussion 141–142. [CrossRef] [PubMed]

Disclaimer/Publisher's Note: The statements, opinions and data contained in all publications are solely those of the individual author(s) and contributor(s) and not of MDPI and/or the editor(s). MDPI and/or the editor(s) disclaim responsibility for any injury to people or property resulting from any ideas, methods, instructions or products referred to in the content.

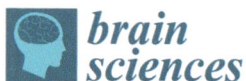

Case Report

Staged Strategies to Deal with Complex, Giant, Multi-Fossa Skull Base Tumors

Brandon Edelbach [1] and Miguel Angel Lopez-Gonzalez [2,*]

[1] School of Medicine, Loma Linda University, Loma Linda, CA 92354, USA; bedelbach@students.llu.edu
[2] Department of Neurosurgery, Loma Linda University Medical Center East Campus, Loma Linda, CA 92354, USA
* Correspondence: mlopezgonzalez@llu.edu; Tel.: +1-909-558-8723

Abstract: Given the complex and multifaceted nature of resecting giant tumors in the anterior, middle, and, to a lesser extent, the posterior fossa, we present two example strategies for navigating the intricacies of such tumors. The foundational premise of these two approaches is based on a two-stage method that aims to improve the visualization and excision of the tumor. In the first case, we utilized a combined endoscopic endonasal approach and a staged modified pterional, pretemporal, with extradural clinoidectomy, and transcavernous approach to successfully remove a giant pituitary adenoma. In the second case, we performed a modified right-sided pterional approach with pretemporal access and extradural clinoidectomy. This was followed by a transcortical, transventricular approach to excise a giant anterior clinoid meningioma. These cases demonstrate the importance of performing staged operations to address the challenges posed by these giant tumors.

Keywords: meningioma; pituitary adenoma; endonasal endoscopic transsphenoidal approach; anterior clinoidectomy; transcavernous

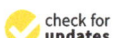

Citation: Edelbach, B.; Lopez-Gonzalez, M.A. Staged Strategies to Deal with Complex, Giant, Multi-Fossa Skull Base Tumors. *Brain Sci.* **2023**, *13*, 916. https://doi.org/10.3390/brainsci13060916

Academic Editor: N. Scott Litofsky

Received: 18 May 2023
Revised: 30 May 2023
Accepted: 4 June 2023
Published: 6 June 2023

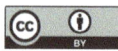

Copyright: © 2023 by the authors. Licensee MDPI, Basel, Switzerland. This article is an open access article distributed under the terms and conditions of the Creative Commons Attribution (CC BY) license (https://creativecommons.org/licenses/by/4.0/).

1. Introduction

Surgical excision of giant tumors in the anterior, middle, and partially in posterior fossa presents unique challenges due to the extension of the lesions in the sagittal, coronal, and axial planes. The extension of the lesions varies, and the surgical approach is tailored accordingly based on the size of the tumor. Several strategies have evolved for excising giant tumors in this environment. These multiple strategies include pterional craniotomy, modified pterional craniotomy, the cranio-orbitozygomatic approach, middle fossa craniotomy through anterior transpetrosal and posterior transpetrosal approaches, as well as endoscopic endonasal and expanded approaches [1–4]. Furthermore, depending on the characteristics of the tumor, a combination of these approaches may be used to ensure a thorough resection of the tumor. Giant pituitary adenomas and anterior clinoid meningiomas are two types of tumors that often require complex surgical strategies for complete resection due to their unique anatomical characteristics and potential complications [5–8].

Pituitary adenomas are intracranial tumors that account for 5–14% of surgically resected lesions [5]. Common symptoms of these tumors include bitemporal hemianopsia, headaches, and endocrine dysfunction [6]. Pituitary adenomas are graded according to the extent of invasion of local anatomical structures. Grade I represents pituitary adenomas that are limited to the sellar region. Grade II represents invasion into the cavernous sinus. Grade III is characterized by the elevation of the dura of the superior wall of the cavernous sinus. Supradiaphragmatic–subarachnoid extensions are characteristic of Grade IV pituitary adenomas [9]. Pituitary adenomas can exhibit invasive extensions that follows anatomic pathways through or around dura of the sellar region, creating diverse tumor morphology [10,11]. The structural diversity of these tumors, combined with the intricate anatomical structures present in the anterior, middle, and posterior fossa, often makes the removal of giant pituitary adenomas a complex task [12]. The removal of pituitary adenomas may be associated with postoperative complications such as cerebrospinal fluid (CSF) leak, diabetes insipidus, additional pituitary dysfunction, visual deterioration, and hydrocephalus [13], while a subtotal resection can be associated with pituitary apoplexy in up to 5.65% of cases [14]. Mitigation of these symptoms has been attempted through the use of several different surgical strategies with the intent of reducing the morbidity of this operation. The microscopic transsphenoidal approach has historically been associated with lower morbidity compared to transcranial strategies. However, with the development of endoscope-assisted microneurosurgery, surgical risks have been further reduced. As a result, the use of the endoscopic endonasal transsphenoidal (EET) approach has flourished in recent decades [15].

Contemporary methods of EET surgery involve the resection of the middle turbinate, with or without dissection of a nasoseptal flap, resection of the posterior septum, and exposure of the sphenoid ostium [16,17]. Often, the initial stage is completed by the otorhinolaryngology surgery team, and the subsequent steps are completed in collaboration with the neurosurgery team [18]. The sphenoid ostium is opened by removing the anterior wall of the sphenoid sinus, which allows access to the sella turcica [19]. Further extension may be necessary, and the choice of approach (transplanum, transclival, pterygomaxillary, or transorbital) will depend on the morphology of the pituitary adenoma to ensure proper visualization of the tumor and infundibular region.

Meningiomas originate from arachnoid cells and are classified into three WHO grades based on their histopathology [20,21]. Of significance, Grade I meningiomas have an increased likelihood of developing at the skull base [22]. The symptoms associated with meningiomas are often non-specific (headache, seizure, cognitive change, vertigo, ataxia), but may involve cranial nerve deficits dependent upon tumor morphological distribution. When it comes to skull base tumors, cranial nerve deficits are more likely to occur [7,23]. Furthermore, anterior clinoid meningiomas are known to have the propensity to present with visual impairments and exophthalmos [24]. Due to their slow growth rate and tendency to present later in life, small meningiomas (less than 3 cm) are often left untreated and followed with serial imaging. However, larger meningiomas, particularly those causing symptoms, are typically surgically resected and treated with stereotactic radiation, based on the WHO grading scale [8].

Similar to pituitary adenomas, giant anterior clinoid meningiomas present unique challenges for complete resection. A significant challenge arises from the tumor's tendency to compress the neurovascular structures associated with the anterior clinoid process [25]. The extent of tumor invasion also plays a significant role in the challenges associated with completely excising giant anterior clinoid meningiomas. The Al-Mefty classification system is based on the microanatomy of the tumor and is divided into three groups. Group I clinoid meningiomas extend over the inferior aspect of the anterior clinoid process and encircle the internal carotid artery; group II clinoid meningiomas are derived from the superior portion of the anterior clinoid process and are covered by arachnoid; group III clinoid meningiomas are derived from the optic foramen [26]. The typical method used for resecting giant anterior clinoid meningiomas consists of a pterional transsylvian approach, although alternative methods including orbitocranial or cranioorbitozygomatic approaches combining both intra- and extradural techniques have been proposed for giant anterior clinoid meningiomas [27–29]. However, the utilization of these techniques varies and is primarily dependent on the unique characteristics of the tumor and the neurosurgeon's level of expertise.

2. Results

2.1. Case 1

A 65-year-old female presented with encephalopathy secondary to a suprasellar mass with symptoms of chronic bitemporal hemianopsia, which had worsened over the course of three years. Prior to admission, she experienced a sudden deficit and could only perceive light and movement. Due to a deterioration in vision, urgent surgical intervention was recommended. A CT scan with contrast and navigation sequences revealed a heterogeneously enhancing mass measuring 6 × 2.4 × 6 cm that originated from the sella and extended inferiorly into the sphenoid sinus and anterior fossa. Additionally, there was a superior extension into the left corona radiata, clivus, and left middle fossa. The mass also encased the left internal carotid artery and extended to the bilateral cavernous sinus and also to the left crural, ambiens, and cerebellopontine cistern. A 3 mm rightward midline shift in the left lateral ventricle was noted due to mass effects, as shown in Figures 1 and 2. Given the recent visual decline, preoperative MRI was unable to be obtained and the patient was taken urgently for surgery.

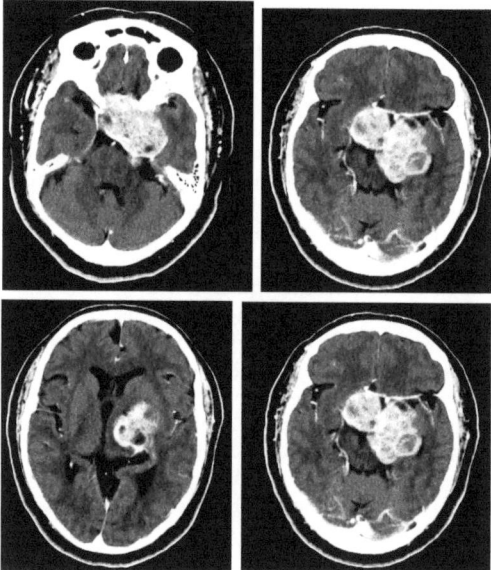

Figure 1. Case 1 giant pituitary adenoma prior to stage 1 resection. CT with contrast shows extension from anterior cranial fossa anteriorly at planum sphenoidale, evident middle fossa involvement, left cavernous sinus and cerebellopontine angle.

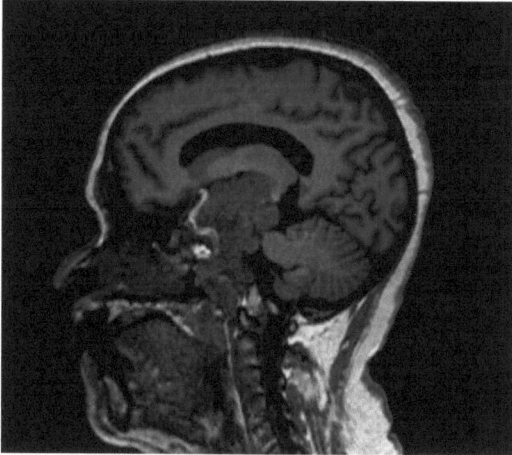

Figure 2. Case 1 giant pituitary adenoma sagittal MRI scan wo contrast.

A staged procedure was planned due to the tumor's lateral extension. Stress doses of steroids were given perioperatively and tapered to a maintenance dose. The patient continued with levothyroxine supplementation. The patient was taken to the operating room for stage 1 endoscopic endonasal tumor resection with the goal of resecting the intrasellar and suprasellar compartments of the tumor to alleviate pressure of the optic apparatus (Figure 3). The sellar component of the tumor was removed using skull base ring curettes, a side-cutting aspirator, and an ultrasonic aspirator. In the superior regions of the sellar component, patties were used to retract the arachnoid tissue, allowing for debulking of the tumor around the cavernous carotid arteries using endoscopic and microsurgical techniques. The midline segment of the tumor was removed, except the segments in the middle and posterior fossa due to the angle of approach, as shown in Figure 3.

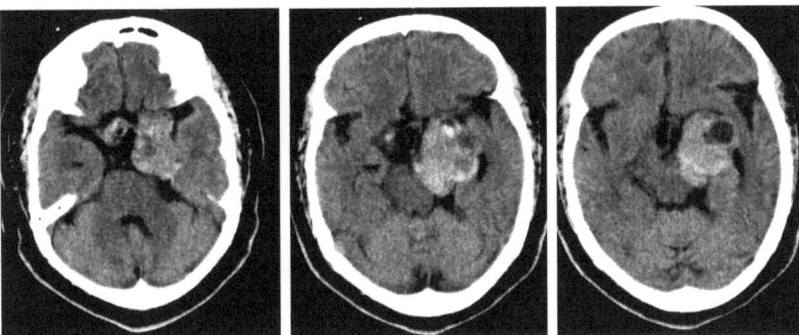

Figure 3. Poststage 1 resection CT. There are postsurgical changes related to the transsphenoidal approach debulking/partial resection of a large sellar/suprasellar mass with fat packing at the sellar floor. A large, residual, multilobulated, heterogeneously enhancing, partially cystic/partially solid mass measures 4.4 × 3.7 × 4.3 cm. The mass extends superiorly from the sella, exerting a mass effect superiorly and displacing the left basal ganglia/thalamus and laterally displacing the left temporal lobe/temporal horn. The mass is again seen within the left cavernous sinus. The residual mass extends posteriorly into the left cerebellopontine angle and perimesencephalic cistern, involves the left Meckel's cave, and exerts mass effect on the left side of midbrain. The residual mass also extends to the left orbital apex, with apparent encasement of the intracranial portion of the left optic nerve and poor delineation of the optic chiasm.

The patient was brought back into the operating room for stage 2 a week later, which involved a left-sided modified pterional transcavernous and transsylvian approach to remove the tumor from the middle and posterior fossa. The procedure required careful dissection around the left supraclinoid carotid, left middle cerebral artery, left posterior communicant artery, bilateral posterior cerebral arteries, and basilar apex. The oculomotor nerve was fully decompressed from a cavernous sinus tumor, and a small segment of fibrous tumor was left attached to the left cavernous carotid artery. The surgical site was closed using a dura substitute, surgical glue, and fat harvested from the abdomen. Postsurgical imaging of subtotal resection is shown in Figures 4 and 5, and an illustrated summary of the staged approach is presented in Figure 6. At the 6-month follow up, the patient maintained light and movement perception, and the postoperative left oculomotor palsy had improved 6 months after surgery. No further deficits were encountered.

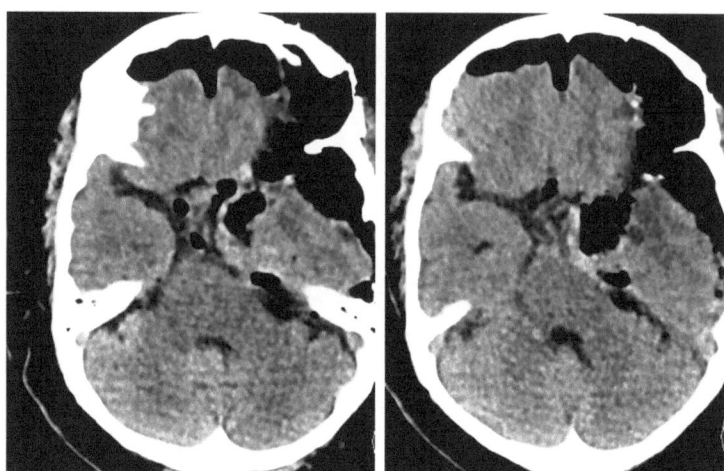

Figure 4. There is demonstration of postsurgical changes after a two-staged operation for subtotal resection of a giant pituitary macroadenoma.

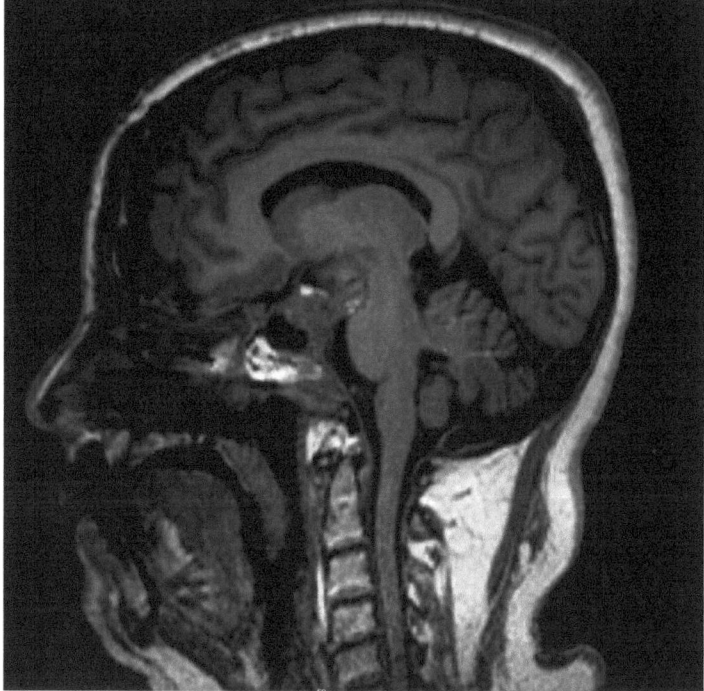

Figure 5. Poststage 2 resection. MRI. Postsurgical changes related to staged transphenoidal approach and subsequent left-sided transcranial skull base approach subtotal resection of a giant invasive pituitary macroadenoma, with fat grafting and fluid/hemorrhage within the surgical bed, with associated mass effect on the left side of the brainstem. Small residual tumor centered in the left cavernous sinus/Meckel's cave with partial encasement of the left internal carotid artery.

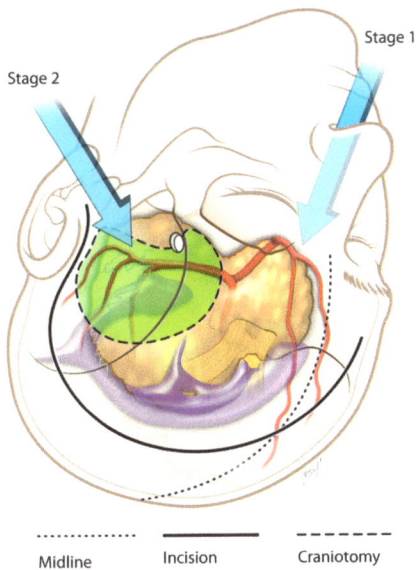

Figure 6. Giant pituitary adenoma two-staged approach illustration.

2.2. Case 2

A 74-year-old male presented with cognitive decline over several months, as well as memory and visual deficits, accompanied by a significant decline in balance. Imaging revealed a large extra-axial mass, measuring 4.3 × 6.3 cm, located at the right anterior clinoid process. The mass showed significant suprasellar and cavernous sinus extensions into the bilateral anterior fossa, middle fossa, and partially within the posterior fossa in retroclinoid space, overall resulting in significant compression of the optic chiasm apparatus and brainstem. There was significant vasogenic edema and obstructive hydrocephalus. This is illustrated in Figure 7.

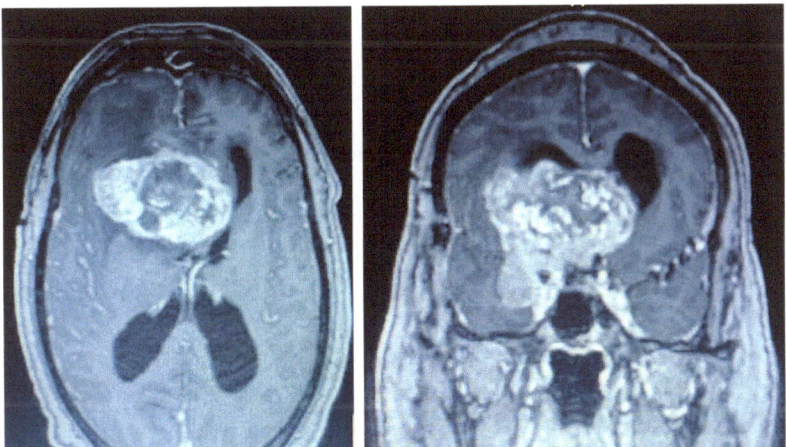

Figure 7. Preoperative axial (**left**) and coronal (**right**) MRI with contrast demonstrating a large, heterogeneously enhancing mass centered on the right anterior clinoid with cavernous sinus, suprasellar, middle fossa, anterior fossa, and intraventricular extension. It measures approximately 4.3 × 6.3 cm.

The patient was brought into the operating room, and it was planned to resect the tumor in two stages during the same operation if it showed hard consistency on the first approach. During craniotomy stage one, a modified right-sided pterional, transzygomatic, and pretemporal approach was utilized, which included extradural clinoidectomy and optic canal decompression. This was followed by transsylvian dissection. The dissection was continued to the superior aspect of the cavernous sinus, allowing visualization of the anterior cerebral arteries and optic nerves. The optic canal was decompressed, and dissection was continued toward the internal carotid arteries and middle fossa, from which a portion of the tumor was resected. The tumor was then meticulously separated from the right internal carotid artery, the right middle cerebral artery, the lateral lenticulostriate branches, the bilateral anterior cerebral arteries (A1 and A2 segments), the right anterior choroidal artery, and the right posterior communicant artery. Then, the approach continued with tumor devascularization, which was achieved by capsule electrocoagulation and by placing aneurysm clips on two main arteries that supplied the tumor. Neurophysiology monitoring was used to provide standard assistance during the procedure and confirm stable somatosensory evoked potentials and electroencephalography during temporary clipping of the vasculature.

As the entire tumor showed a hard consistency, the superior aspect of the lesion was inaccessible through this approach. Therefore, stage two was initiated with a separate right frontal craniotomy using the same incision. A transfrontal, transcortical, and transventricular microsurgical approach was performed on the right side. The giant anterior clinoid meningioma tumor was visualized through this approach and successfully debulked, exposing the anterior cerebral arteries, right internal carotid artery, and middle cerebral artery. The two large arterial tumor feeders with the temporary clips were then electrocoagulated and permanent titanium clips applied. After the tumor was sufficiently removed, fat was harvested from the abdomen and placed in the pterional area. Additionally, a right frontal external ventricular drain was left in place under direct visualization. Postoperative imaging is illustrated in Figure 8, while a summary of the staged approach is shown in Figure 9. External ventricular drain was removed on postoperative day 5. At 6 months after surgery, there was significant improvement in ambulation and cognition without additional neurological deficits.

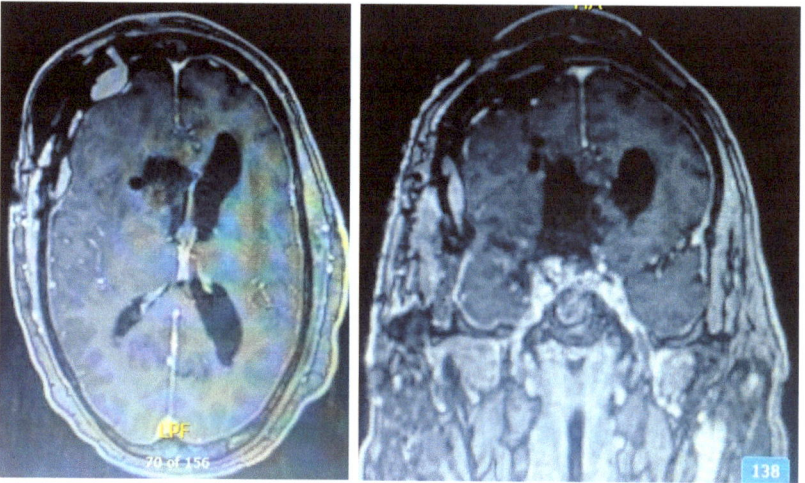

Figure 8. Postoperative axial (**left**) and coronal (**right**) MRI with contrast. Postsurgical changes related to right modified pterional, pretemporal approach and staged right frontal transcortical transventricular approach for resection of a large meningioma centered in the right anterior clinoid region.

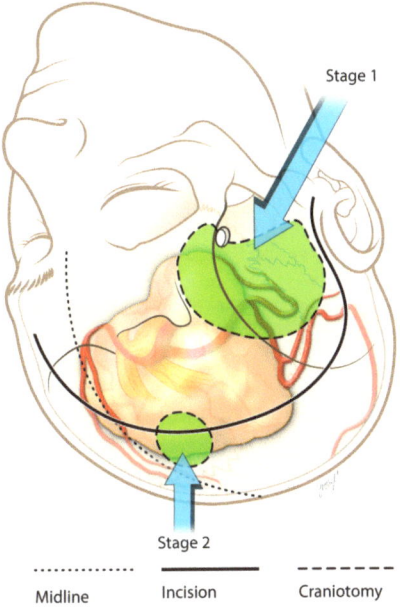

Figure 9. Giant anterior clinoid meningioma staging.

Pathologic examination of the tumor also confirmed a low-grade meningioma. The Ki67 indices were low, with mild focal elevation. E-cadherin, BAP-1, and PR stains were positive and GFAP stains indicated glial tissue along edges without any indication of brain invasion.

3. Discussion

3.1. Giant Pituitary Macroadenoma Surgery

In 1992, Jankowski et al. [30] described the first successful endonasal endoscopic resection of a pituitary adenoma in three patients. This represented a major transition from the previously popular method of microscopic transsphenoidal resection via a sublabial or endonasal approach. The endoscopic endonasal approach has been associated with significant improvements in morbidity and mortality associated with the removal of pituitary adenomas [31].

The advancements in the resection of pituitary adenoma using EET resection have been well documented [32,33]. EET surgery has been reported to achieve resection rates greater than 80% in tumors with a volume of 18 cm^3, as well as gross total resection rates up to 44% [34]. Postoperatively, there was a significant improvement in visual function (82%) and pituitary function (20–72%) in those who presented with pituitary dysfunction [33–35]. McLaughlin et al. concluded that the use of endoscopy allowed for the removal of adenomas in an additional 36% of patients, thanks to improved visualization. Furthermore, the use of endoscopy was accentuated in patients presenting with tumors larger than 2 cm, permitting the removal of 54% of pituitary adenomas [32].

However, significant complications have been reported with this procedure. As many as 37% of patients have experienced complications, which include sinusitis (13.7%), CSF leak (9.6–11.4%), and SIADH (4.1%), as well as headache, epistaxis, meningitis, and hydrocephalus in a minority of patients [33,35]. Additional clinical reports have detailed complications of diabetes insipidus at rates as high as 25–45.5%, with a minority experiencing ischemic stroke [34,35].

It is relevant to mention that the endoscopic endonasal approach, with an expanded transtubercular approach, can still be associated with a lower degree of resection when the tumor has a significant lateral extension, harder consistency, or cavernous sinus extension [36], and an open transcranial approach has a significant role in its surgical treatment [37].

3.2. Surgical Pearls

Giant pituitary macroadenomas present a significant challenge due to their extension into various anatomical compartments. In our example case, the tumor was extended into three different anatomical compartments of the skull base involving the neurovascular structures. A meticulous review of all available images is necessary to plan the different steps of the operation. After obtaining appropriate medical clearance and ensuring stability, surgery should be performed promptly. With a significant visual deficit, the initial planned step was to debulk the tumor mass inferiorly through an endoscopic endonasal approach with a transplanum sphenoidale extension to alleviate ventral compression of the optic chiasm. A combination of microsurgical and endoscopic tumor dissection techniques was required. Usually, as in this case, the capsule of a pituitary adenoma is harder in consistency, requiring careful dissection from the anterior cerebral arteries, and it is of utmost importance to maintain the anatomical landmarks respecting the trajectory of the optic apparatus. Hypervascularity is a common feature of tumors with a hard consistency. To address this, a combination of different endonasal bipolar electrocoagulators may be necessary, including long and fine-tipped regular bipolar ones. The significant lateral, superior, and posterior extension of the tumor was the deciding factor for a staged operation, where a modified pterional, extradural anterior clinoidectomy, transcavernous, and transsylvian approach allowed access to all of these compartments. After opening the intradural space, an important goal is to establish a plan for resecting a giant tumor in sectors: (a) there were multiple critical anatomical landmarks for the anterior sector of the tumor including optic nerves and chiasm, anterior cerebral arteries, and anterior communicant artery region complex; (b) the central sector with suprasellar and intercarotid space, dealing with bilateral internal carotid arteries, left posterior communicant and choroidal arteries identifying normal vasculature from feeding tumor vessels; (c) posterior sector with tumor extension to interpeduncular fossa and left cerebellopontine angle cistern, dealing with bilateral posterior cerebral arteries (P1 segments), basilar apex, and thalamo-perforating vessels. If a tumor segment exhibits tight adhesions to neurovascular structures, making it difficult to identify a clear cleavage plane, we recommend avoiding the risk of neurovascular injury, requiring leaving some tumoral tissue in place. As part of our routine, we always keep aneurysm clips, clip appliers, and cerebral bypass instruments available in the operating room in case they are needed. During the dissection of the lateral wall of the cavernous sinus, it is important to identify the normal trajectory of the nerves, especially the oculomotor and trochlear nerves, before accessing either the roof or lateral wall of the cavernous sinus. The oculomotor nerve is highly sensitive to manipulation and requires adequate release from the oculomotor cistern and lateral wall of the cavernous sinus after peeling off the dura from the middle fossa. A temporary oculomotor deficit often improves within weeks or months after surgery. This possibility should be thoroughly discussed with patients and their families prior to the operation. The consistency and vascularity of the tumor within the cavernous sinus will determine the extent of resection required. Postoperative care in the intensive care unit, along with an adequate protocol for managing diabetes insipidus and individualized hormone replacement, is essential.

3.3. Giant Anterior Clinoid Meningioma Surgery

There is significant debate regarding the most effective strategy for removing giant anterior clinoid meningiomas, mainly due to the unique challenges discussed earlier in resecting these tumors [38–42]. Two popular techniques involve either a vascular or skull base perspective. The vascular strategy of tumor debulking involves dissecting the sylvian fissure to trace the middle cerebral artery to the internal carotid artery while removing the tumor and its associated perforating arterial supply [43]. However, this school of thought is commonly criticized due to the strain placed on the sylvian fissure [26]. The alternative solution to this issue involves performing a pretemporal dissection and an anterior clinoidectomy to expand the operating field while minimizing brain retraction at the sylvian fissure [44]. This technique is associated with several advantages, such as early optic nerve decompression, early identification of the internal carotid artery, and associated devascularization of the meningioma [44]. This is associated with a decreased rate of complications. The occurrence of postoperative vascular complications has been reported in 2% of cases; cranial nerve deficits occurred in 5.5% of patients; and the overall patient mortality rate was 1.2% [45].

Further modifications to the anterior clinoidectomy have been reported. This includes extradural, intradural, and hybrid approaches to this technique. However, the merits of each of these subtechniques are still debated [45]. The use of preoperative embolization has been reported, but it is also problematic. External carotid artery branches are safer to embolize, with limited opportunities for branches arising directly from the internal carotid artery. One clinical trial found a complication rate of 12% associated with this practice, which seemed to provide little benefit to the quality of patient postsurgical recovery [46]. Additional methods are still under exploration. One such method is the Dolenc approach, which involves an extradural clinoidectomy and transdural debulking of the tumor. A study reported that 67% of patients had better vision outcome [38,39]. The gross total resection rate was 30.4%, and partial resections were achieved in 34.8% of surgeries [38,41].

When considered as a complete entity, giant anterior clinoid meningiomas had a gross total resection rate of 64.2% [45], while 25% of cases resulted in subtotal resections [41]. The reported operative mortality was 6.7%, and recurrence was observed in 11.8% of cases [40]. According to Nanda et al., four out of thirty-six patients who underwent surgery for clinoidal meningiomas experienced recurrence, with a median duration of 89 months, and one patient required repeat surgery [41]. Furthermore, it is worth noting that gross total resections of group I giant anterior clinoid meningiomas were limited to only 11.8% due to the anatomical difficulties associated with this type of tumor [45]. The minimally invasive options such as the endoscopic endonasal transtubercular approach or endoscopic-assisted supraorbital key-hole approach are ideal for midline lesions such as tuberculum sella meningiomas [46], although those options have a limited role in anterior clinoid meningioma and even less so in a giant tumor given its anatomical skull base implications [42,47].

3.4. Surgical Pearls

Meningiomas located on the anterior clinoid process may vary in size. A comprehensive surgical extension involving the anterior, middle, posterior fossa, and intraventricular areas requires a detailed analysis of preoperative imaging for effective planning. This case example involved a lesion larger than 6 cm originating from the right anterior clinoid process with a significant suprasellar and lateral cavernous sinus extension into the bilateral anterior fossa, middle fossa, and a segment of the posterior fossa, with significant compression of the optic chiasm and brainstem. A preoperative angiogram is routinely obtained for meningiomas located in this area to assess the possibility of embolizing branches from the external carotid artery. This is because branches of the internal carotid artery pose a higher risk for ischemic complications. The angiogram is obtained to define the blood supply to the tumor, regardless of whether it is possible to embolize it or not. This can provide information on the degree of displacement of the normal vasculature, collateralization, the presence of posterior communicant arteries, and cross-flow through anterior communicant arteries. All of these factors, combined with preoperative magnetic resonance imaging and computer tomography, can help define the surgical strategy. Additional tools, such as neuronavigation and neuromonitoring with techniques including somatosensory evoked potentials, brainstem auditory evoked responses, and electroencephalography, are always helpful. Given the location of the tumor, vascular proximal control measures need to be planned, either cervical carotid with prep of the cervical area, petrous carotid through the middle fossa, or clinoid carotid. Occasionally, there is the need to perform temporary clipping of some feeding tumor vessels, and neuromonitoring provides feedback on physiological stability during these episodes. The type of craniotomy, such as pterional, modified pterional, orbitocranial, or cranio-orbito-zygomatic, can be selected based on the patient's unique anatomy. Ideally, transzygomatic or cranio-orbito-zygomatic approaches can be used for tumors with significant superior extension, as in the case example presented. In addition, techniques such as pretemporal dissection and extradural clinoidectomy are recommended to partially devascularize and remove the origin of the tumor with early optic canal decompression, which can subsequently be released intradurally after opening the falciform ligament. After meticulous extradural dissection and careful attention to hemostasis, the initial intradural approach aims to explore the anatomical distortion caused by the tumor and to identify normal anatomy. This involves searching for optic nerves, oculomotor nerves, internal carotid arteries, and anterior and middle cerebral arteries. This tumor was wrapped around the right internal carotid artery and right middle cerebral artery. The goal was to divide it into sectors, starting with the lateral component in the middle fossa and around the middle cerebral artery. Central debulking was performed using high microsurgical magnification and an ultrasonic aspirator. Releasing a tumor from vascular structures such as the middle cerebral artery and towards the carotid bifurcation can be performed using constant micro-Doppler and neuronavigation to map the vascular trajectory. Once an arterial trunk is found, it can be followed proximally to remove the majority of the tumor. In cases where a tumor is calcified around the supraclinoid carotid artery or middle cerebral artery, it may be necessary to leave a cuff of the tumor to avoid causing unnecessary injury. Through the middle fossa approach, the sector adjacent to the crural and ambiens cisterns can be carefully resected while dissecting the posterior communicant artery and perforating vessels. If a tumor extends significantly in the inferior direction to the cerebellopontine angle, an anterior petrosectomy may be necessary. However, it was not required in this case. The anterior segment of the tumor is gradually dissected, following the ipsilateral and contralateral A1 segments of the anterior cerebral artery. After performing devascularization, central and superior debulking of the mass was continued, although given the hard consistency of the tumor and its capsule, it was decided to perform a staged frontal craniotomy. This procedure was conducted through a small right frontal coronal craniotomy, with a small transcortical approach used to reach the right lateral ventricle. Central debulking was then performed, followed by medial dissection of the capsule through the arachnoid plane from the anterior cerebral artery A2 and A3 segments and lateral dissection from the superior trunk of the middle cerebral artery. Finally, the dissection was carefully performed from the superior aspects of optic nerves and chiasm.

4. Conclusions

Giant tumors located in the skull base pose significant challenges due to their size, location, and proximity to critical neurovascular structures. Despite these challenges, current advances in surgical techniques and new technology have made it possible to safely remove giant skull base tumors. Neurosurgeons may employ a combination of open and minimally invasive approaches, such as endoscopic techniques, microvascular dissection, and microanastomosis, if necessary. The success of skull base surgery for giant tumors depends on several factors, including the tumor's location and size, the patient's overall health, the appropriate selection of treatment, and the expertise of the surgical team. Surgery for these patients is preferably performed at highly specialized centers with a multidisciplinary approach in order to provide a higher chance of success and long-term survival.

Author Contributions: M.A.L.-G.: completed surgical procedures, provided case notes, conceptualization, provided critical appraisal, revision and editing. B.E.: involved in drafting, revising, and critically appraising content. All authors have read and agreed to the published version of the manuscript.

Funding: This research received no external funding.

Institutional Review Board Statement: Ethical approval is not required for retrospective case report studies without identifiable information in accordance with Loma Linda University Institutional Review Board guidelines.

Informed Consent Statement: Patient's consent is not required for retrospective case report studies without identifiable information in accordance with Loma Linda University Institutional Review Board guidelines.

Data Availability Statement: Data sharing not applicable. No new data were created or analyzed in this study. Data sharing is not applicable to this article.

Acknowledgments: Jennifer Pryll for artistic illustrations.

Conflicts of Interest: The authors declare no conflict of interest.

References

1. Seçkin, H.; Avci, E.; Uluç, K.; Niemann, D.; Başkaya, M.K. The work horse of skull base surgery: Orbitozygomatic approach. Technique, modifications, and applications. *Neurosurg. Focus* **2008**, *25*, E4. [CrossRef] [PubMed]
2. Rubio, R.R.; Chae, R.; Vigo, V.; Abla, A.A.; McDermott, M. Immersive Surgical Anatomy of the Pterional Approach. *Cureus* **2019**, *11*, e5216. [CrossRef]
3. Meybodi, A.T.; Mignucci-Jiménez, G.; Lawton, M.T.; Liu, J.K.; Preul, M.C.; Sun, H. Comprehensive microsurgical anatomy of the middle cranial fossa: Part I—Osseous and meningeal anatomy. *Front. Surg.* **2023**, *10*, 1132774. [CrossRef] [PubMed]
4. Solari, D.; Villa, A.; De Angelis, M.; Esposito, F.; Cavallo, L.M.; Cappabianca, P. Anatomy and surgery of the en-doscopic endonasal approach to the skull base. *Transl. Med.@ UniSa* **2012**, *2*, 36–46.
5. Goel, A.; Nadkarni, T.; Muzumdar, D.; Desai, K.; Phalke, U.; Sharma, P. Giant pituitary tumors: A study based on surgical treatment of 118 cases. *Surg. Neurol.* **2004**, *61*, 436–445. [CrossRef] [PubMed]
6. Molitch, M.E. Diagnosis and Treatment of Pituitary Adenomas: A Review. *JAMA* **2017**, *317*, 516–524. [CrossRef]
7. Meling, T.R.; Da Broi, M.; Scheie, D.; Helseth, E. Meningiomas: Skull base versus non-skull base. *Neurosurg. Rev.* **2018**, *42*, 163–173. [CrossRef]
8. Zhao, L.; Zhao, W.; Hou, Y.; Wen, C.; Wang, J.; Wu, P.; Guo, Z. An Overview of Managements in Meningiomas. *Front. Oncol.* **2020**, *10*, 1523. [CrossRef]
9. Asa, S.L.; Mete, O.; Perry, A.; Osamura, R.Y. Overview of the 2022 WHO Classification of Pituitary Tumors. *Endocr. Pathol.* **2022**, *33*, 6–26. [CrossRef]
10. Serioli, S.; Doglietto, F.; Fiorindi, A.; Biroli, A.; Mattavelli, D.; Buffoli, B.; Ferrari, M.; Cornali, C.; Rodella, L.; Maroldi, R.; et al. Pituitary Adenomas and Invasiveness from Anatomo-Surgical, Radiological, and Histological Perspectives: A Systematic Literature Review. *Cancers* **2019**, *11*, 1936. [CrossRef]
11. Raghib, M.F.; Salim, A.; Angez, M.; Ghazi, S.M.; Hashmi, S.; Tariq, M.B.; Hashmi, F.; Bin Anis, S.; Shamim, M.S.; Tanwir, A.; et al. Prognostic implication of size on outcomes of pituitary macroadenoma: A comparative analysis of giant adenoma with non-giant macroadenoma. *J. Neuro-Oncol.* **2022**, *160*, 491–496. [CrossRef] [PubMed]
12. Agrawal, A.; Cincu, R.; Goel, A. Current concepts and controversies in the management of non-functioning giant pituitary macroadenomas. *Clin. Neurol. Neurosurg.* **2007**, *109*, 645–650. [CrossRef] [PubMed]
13. Koutourousiou, M.; Gardner, P.A.; Fernandez-Miranda, J.C.; Paluzzi, A.; Wang, E.W.; Snyderman, C.H. Endoscopic endonasal surgery for giant pituitary adenomas: Advantages and limitations. *J. Neurosurg.* **2013**, *118*, 621–631. [CrossRef]
14. Butterfield, J.T.; Araki, T.; Guillaume, D.; Tummala, R.; Caicedo-Granados, E.; Tyler, M.A.; Venteicher, A.S. Estimating Risk of Pituitary Apoplexy after Resection of Giant Pituitary Adenomas. *J. Neurol. Surg. Part B Skull Base* **2021**, *83* (Suppl. S2), e152–e159. [CrossRef] [PubMed]
15. Couldwell, W.T. Transsphenoidal and transcranial surgery for pituitary adenomas. *J. Neuro-Oncol.* **2004**, *69*, 237–256. [CrossRef]
16. Thakur, B.; Jesurasa, A.R.; Ross, R.; Carroll, T.A.; Mirza, S.; Sinha, S. Transnasal trans-sphenoidal endoscopic repair of CSF leak sec-ondary to invasive pituitary tumours using a nasoseptal flap. *Pituitary* **2011**, *14*, 163–167. [CrossRef]
17. Shah, R.N.; Surowitz, J.B.; Patel, M.R.; Huang, B.Y.; Snyderman, C.H.; Carrau, R.L.; Kassam, A.B.; Germanwala, A.V.; Zanation, A.M. Endoscopic pedicled nasoseptal flap recon-struction for pediatric skull base defects. *Laryngoscope* **2009**, *119*, 1067–1075. [CrossRef]
18. Cavallo, L.M.; Prevedello, D.M.; Solari, D.; Gardner, P.A.; Esposito, F.; Snyderman, C.H.; Carrau, R.L.; Kassam, A.B.; Cappabianca, P. Extended endoscopic endonasal transsphenoidal approach for residual or recurrent craniopharyngiomas. *J. Neurosurg.* **2009**, *111*, 578–589. [CrossRef]
19. Zhang, X.; Fei, Z.; Zhang, J.N.; Fu, L.A.; Cao, W.D.; Qu, Y. Minimally invasive neurosurgery for removal of pituitary adenomas by neuroendoscope aided with sellar floor reconstruction. *Zhonghua Yi Xue Za Zhi* **2010**, *90*, 2342–2344.

20. Torp, S.H.; Solheim, O.; Skjulsvik, A.J. The WHO 2021 Classification of Central Nervous System tumours: A practical update on what neurosurgeons need to know—A minireview. *Acta Neurochir.* **2022**, *164*, 2453–2464. [CrossRef]
21. Huntoon, K.; Toland, A.M.S.; Dahiya, S. Meningioma: A Review of Clinicopathological and Molecular Aspects. *Front. Oncol.* **2020**, *10*, 579599. [CrossRef] [PubMed]
22. Bi, W.L.; Greenwald, N.F.; Abedalthagafi, M.; Wala, J.; Gibson, W.J.; Agarwalla, P.K.; Horowitz, P.; Schumacher, S.E.; Esaulova, E.; Mei, Y.; et al. Genomic landscape of high-grade meningiomas. *NPJ Genom. Med.* **2017**, *2*, 15. [CrossRef] [PubMed]
23. Magill, S.T.; Young, J.S.; Chae, R.; Aghi, M.K.; Theodosopoulos, P.V.; McDermott, M.W. Relationship between tumor location, size, and WHO grade in meningioma. *Neurosurg. Focus* **2018**, *44*, E4. [CrossRef] [PubMed]
24. Christine, M.; Marco, H.; Karl, R.; Michele, R.; Milena, S.; Elena, M.; Charles, V. Meningioma. *Crit. Rev. Oncol. Hematol.* **2008**, *67*, 153–171. [CrossRef]
25. Attia, M.; Umansky, F.; Paldor, I.; Dotan, S.; Shoshan, Y.; Spektor, S. Giant anterior clinoidal meningiomas: Surgical technique and outcomes. *J. Neurosurg.* **2012**, *117*, 654–665. [CrossRef]
26. Al-Mefty, O. Clinoidal meningiomas. *J. Neurosurg.* **1990**, *73*, 840–849. [CrossRef]
27. De Jesús, O.; Toledo, M.M. Surgical management of meningioma en plaque of the sphenoid ridge. *Surg. Neurol.* **2001**, *55*, 265–269. [CrossRef]
28. Tomasello, F.; De Divitiis, O.; Angileri, F.; Salpietro, F.M.; D'Avella, D. Large sphenocavernous meningiomas: Is there still a role for the intradural approach via the pterional-transsylvian route? *Acta Neurochir.* **2003**, *145*, 273–282. [CrossRef]
29. van Loveren, H.R.; Keller, J.T.; El-Kalliny, M.; Scodary, D.J.; Tew, J.M., Jr. The Dolenc technique for cavernous sinus exploration (cadaveric prosection). *J. Neurosurg.* **1991**, *74*, 837–844. [CrossRef]
30. Jankowski, R.; Auque, J.; Simon, C.; Marchai, J.C.; Hepner, H.; Wayoff, M. Endoscopic Pituitary Tumor Surgery. *Laryngoscope* **1992**, *102*, 198–202. [CrossRef]
31. Liu, J.K.; Das, K.; Weiss, M.H.; Laws, E.R., Jr.; Couldwell, W.T. The history and evolution of transsphenoidal surgery. *J. Neurosurg.* **2001**, *95*, 1083–1096. [CrossRef] [PubMed]
32. McLaughlin, N.; Eisenberg, A.A.; Cohan, P.; Chaloner, C.B.; Kelly, D.F. Value of endoscopy for maximizing tumor removal in endonasal transsphenoidal pituitary adenoma surgery. *J. Neurosurg.* **2013**, *118*, 613–620. [CrossRef] [PubMed]
33. Juraschka, K.; Khan, O.H.; Godoy, B.L.; Monsalves, E.; Kilian, A.; Krischek, B.; Ghare, A.; Vescan, A.; Gentili, F.; Zadeh, G. Endoscopic endonasal transsphenoidal approach to large and giant pituitary adenomas: Institutional experience and predictors of extent of resection. *J. Neurosurg.* **2014**, *121*, 75–83. [CrossRef]
34. Elshazly, K.; Kshettry, V.R.; Farrell, C.J.; Nyquist, G.; Rosen, M.; Evans, J.J. Clinical Outcomes After Endoscopic Endonasal Resection of Giant Pituitary Adenomas. *World Neurosurg.* **2018**, *114*, e447–e456. [CrossRef]
35. Rahimli, T.; Hidayetov, T.; Yusifli, Z.; Memmedzade, H.; Rajabov, T.; Aghayev, K. Endoscopic Endonasal Approach to Giant Pituitary Adenomas: Surgical Outcomes and Review of the Literature. *World Neurosurg.* **2021**, *149*, e1043–e1055. [CrossRef] [PubMed]
36. Chibbaro, S.; Signorelli, F.; Milani, D.; Cebula, H.; Scibilia, A.; Bozzi, M.T.; Messina, R.; Zaed, I.; Todeschi, J.; Ollivier, I.; et al. Primary Endoscopic Endonasal Management of Giant Pituitary Adenomas: Outcome and Pitfalls from a Large Prospective Multicenter Experience. *Cancers* **2021**, *13*, 3603. [CrossRef] [PubMed]
37. Luzzi, S.; Lucifero, A.G.; Rabski, J.; Kadri, P.A.S.; Al-Mefty, O. The Party Wall: Redefining the Indications of Transcranial Approaches for Giant Pituitary Adenomas in Endoscopic Era. *Cancers* **2023**, *15*, 2235. [CrossRef] [PubMed]
38. Cui, H.; Wang, Y.; Yin, Y.-H.; Fei, Z.-M.; Luo, Q.-Z.; Jiang, J.-Y. Surgical management of anterior clinoidal meningiomas: A 26-case report. *Surg. Neurol.* **2007**, *68* (Suppl. S2), S6–S10. [CrossRef]
39. Sampirisi, L.; D'angelo, L.; Palmieri, M.; Pesce, A.; Santoro, A. Extradural Clinoidectomy in Clinoidal Meningiomas: Analysis of the Surgical Technique and Evaluation of the Clinical Outcome. *Tomography* **2022**, *8*, 2360–2368. [CrossRef]
40. Czernicki, T.; Kunert, P.; Nowak, A.; Marchel, A. Results of surgical treatment of anterior clinoidal meningiomas—Our experiences. *Neurol. i Neurochir. Polska* **2015**, *49*, 29–35. [CrossRef]
41. Nanda, A.; Konar, S.K.; Maiti, T.K.; Bir, S.C.; Guthikonda, B. Stratification of predictive factors to assess resectability and surgical outcome in clinoidal meningioma. *Clin. Neurol. Neurosurg.* **2016**, *142*, 31–37. [CrossRef] [PubMed]
42. Starnoni, D.; Tuleasca, C.; Giammattei, L.; Cossu, G.; Bruneau, M.; Berhouma, M.; Cornelius, J.F.; Cavallo, L.; Froelich, S.; Jouanneau, E.; et al. Surgical management of anterior clinoidal meningiomas: Consensus statement on behalf of the EANS skull base section. *Acta Neurochir.* **2021**, *163*, 3387–3400. [CrossRef]
43. Bonnal, J.; Thibaut, A.; Brotchi, J.; Born, J. Invading meningiomas of the sphenoid ridge. *J. Neurosurg.* **1980**, *53*, 587–599. [CrossRef] [PubMed]
44. Ilyas, A.; Przybylowski, C.; Chen, C.-J.; Ding, D.; Foreman, P.M.; Buell, T.J.; Taylor, D.G.; Kalani, M.Y.; Park, M.S. Preoperative embolization of skull base meningiomas: A systematic review. *J. Clin. Neurosci.* **2018**, *59*, 259–264. [CrossRef]
45. Lee, J.H.; Jeun, S.S.; Evans, J.; Kosmorsky, G. Surgical management of clinoidal meningiomas. *Neurosurgery* **2001**, *48*, 1012–1019. [PubMed]

46. Linsler, S.; Fischer, G.; Skliarenko, V.; Stadie, A.; Oertel, J. Endoscopic Assisted Supraorbital Keyhole Approach or Endoscopic Endonasal Approach in Cases of Tuberculum Sellae Meningioma: Which Surgical Route Should Be Favored? *World Neurosurg.* **2017**, *104*, 601–611. [CrossRef]
47. Giammattei, L.; Starnoni, D.; Levivier, M.; Messerer, M.; Daniel, R.T. Surgery for Clinoidal Meningiomas: Case Series and Meta-Analysis of Outcomes and Complications. *World Neurosurg.* **2019**, *129*, e700–e717. [CrossRef]

Disclaimer/Publisher's Note: The statements, opinions and data contained in all publications are solely those of the individual author(s) and contributor(s) and not of MDPI and/or the editor(s). MDPI and/or the editor(s) disclaim responsibility for any injury to people or property resulting from any ideas, methods, instructions or products referred to in the content.

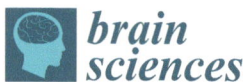 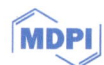

Review

Operative Corridors in Endoscopic Skull Base Tumor Surgery

A. Karim Ahmed [1], Nicholas R. Rowan [2] and Debraj Mukherjee [1,*]

[1] Department of Neurosurgery, Johns Hopkins Medical Institutions, Johns Hopkins School of Medicine, Baltimore, MD 21287, USA; aahmed33@jhmi.edu
[2] Department of Otolaryngology, Head and Neck Surgery, Johns Hopkins School of Medicine, Baltimore, MD 21287, USA
* Correspondence: dmukher1@jhmi.edu

Abstract: Advances in technology, instrumentation, and reconstruction have paved the way for extended endoscopic approaches to skull base tumors. In the sagittal plane, the endonasal approach may safely access pathologies from the frontal sinus to the craniocervical junction in the sagittal plane, the petrous apex in the coronal plane, and extend posteriorly to the clivus and posterior cranial fossa. This review article describes these modular extended endoscopic approaches, along with crucial anatomic considerations, illustrative cases, and practical operative pearls.

Keywords: endoscopic skull base surgery; transsphenoidal; transplanum; transtuberculum; transorbital; sellar; suprasellar; clivus; transpterygoid

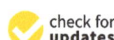

Citation: Ahmed, A.K.; Rowan, N.R.; Mukherjee, D. Operative Corridors in Endoscopic Skull Base Tumor Surgery. *Brain Sci.* **2024**, *14*, 207. https://doi.org/10.3390/brainsci14030207

Academic Editor: Miguel Lopez-Gonzalez

Received: 7 February 2024
Revised: 20 February 2024
Accepted: 22 February 2024
Published: 23 February 2024

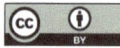

Copyright: © 2024 by the authors. Licensee MDPI, Basel, Switzerland. This article is an open access article distributed under the terms and conditions of the Creative Commons Attribution (CC BY) license (https://creativecommons.org/licenses/by/4.0/).

1. Introduction

An understanding of nasal and paranasal sinus anatomy is of paramount importance for both neurosurgeons and otolaryngologists in the endonasal approach to skull base pathologies. Endoscopic endonasal approaches were traditionally confined to paranasal sinus operations and pituitary adenomas [1]; however, with significant advances in technology, instrumentation, reconstruction, and the development of novel corridors over the past decade, the endonasal approach to the skull base is now able to safely access pathologies from the frontal sinus to the craniocervical junction in the sagittal plane, the petrous apex in the coronal plane, and posteriorly to the clivus and posterior cranial fossa [1–5]. Congenital lesions include nasal glial heterotopia, seromucinous hamartomas, encephalocele, inflammatory pseudotumor, sinonasal papilloma, polyps, and pituitary adenomas. Inflammatory lesions in this region include allergic fungal sinusitis rhinoscleroma, granulomatosis with polyangiitis, and eosinophilic granuloma and myospherulosis. Malignancy of this lesion most commonly affects the maxillary sinus, followed by the nasal cavity, nasopharynx, and ethmoid sinuses. These include epithelial-derived neoplasms such as squamous cell carcinoma, with poorly differentiated carcinoma likely arising from inverted papillomas; sinonasal undifferentiated carcinoma (SNUC), for which induction treatment is the mainstay of initial treatment; SMARCB1-deficient sinonasal carcinoma; nasopharyngeal carcinoma; HPV-related carcinoma; and salivary/non-salivary type adenocarcinomas. Mesenchymal benign tumors include glomangiopericytoma, pyogenic granuloma, myxoma, and nasopharyngeal angiofibroma—with rich blood supply commonly from the maxillary artery. Malignant mesenchymal tumors are far less frequent, including rhabdomyosarcoma, fibrosarcoma, synovial sarcoma, hemangioendothelioma, angiosarcoma, chordoma (arising from the embryological notochord), and chondrosarcoma (arising from the petroclival synchondroses). Neuroectodermal tumors comprise olfactory neuroblastoma (from the olfactory neuroepithelium), olfactory carcinoma, and Ewing family tumors. Neuroendocrine tumors, melanoma, lymphoproliferative disorders, metastatic disease, and ameloblastoma (of enamel origin) may also affect the skull base with decreasing frequency [4,5].

Endoscopic endonasal approaches may be ideally suited for ventral skull base lesions, with the ability to visualize critical anterior neurovascular structures without brain retraction and with reduced overall surgical morbidity [2]. This review article outlines the anatomic considerations and technical nuances of the endoscopic endonasal approach to the sellar, suprasellar, medial orbital apex, anterior cranial base, and transpterygoid corridors.

2. Materials and Methods

A thorough review of the literature was utilized to include all clinical and anatomic, endoscopic, and endonasal skull base approaches performed in the anterior, middle, or posterior fossa using CINAHL, PubMed, Web of Science from 1980 to 2023 in addition to the review of references in eligible articles. Studies included those describing the extended transfrontal, transplanum, transtuberculum, transcribiform, transsphenoidal, transclival, transpterygoid, and transorbital approaches for skull base tumors. Critical anatomic considerations and technical limitations are described based on a review of the literature and the authors' own experience. Illustrative cases were included for each approach as appropriate.

3. Results and Discussion

3.1. Sellar/Suprasellar

3.1.1. Anatomic Considerations

In the endonasal corridor, the Agger Nasi cells are encountered relatively early during operative dissection. Latin for 'nasal mound', these are the anterior-most ethmoidal air cells, located anterior to the frontal recess of the frontal sinus [6,7]. The turbinates are laterally situated osseous shelves which function to regulate airflow and humidification, and if removed excessively can lead to Empty nose syndrome—characterized by a paradoxical feeling of nasal obstruction [8]. The inferior turbinate originates from the maxillary and palatine bone, delineating the inferior meatus which drains the nasolacrimal duct. The middle turbinate, of the ethmoid bone, demarcates the middle meatus and attaches superiorly to the cribiform plate and laterally to the lamina paprycea at the basal lamella, separating anterior and posterior ethmoidal air cells. The superior turbinate, also of the ethmoid bone, delineates the superior meatus just anteroinferior to the sphenoethmnoidal recess [6–9]. The various lamellae attach laterally to the lamina paprycea, forming the medial orbital wall. From anterior to posterior, these include lamella of the uncinate process, lamella of the ethmoid bulla (the largest air cell of the ethmoid sinus), lamella of the middle turbinate (basal lamella), lamella of the superior turbinate, and finally the sphenoid sinus [10]. The osteomeatal complex allows for airflow and mucociliary drainage of the paranasal sinuses, providing drainage of the frontal sinus, anterior ethmoidal air cells, maxillary sinus, and middle meatus. It is composed of the maxillary ostium, infundibulum, ethmoid bulla, uncinate process, and hiatus semilunaris [9–11] As a critical component of the osteomeatal complex, the uncinate process forms the anterior–inferior border of the hiatus semilunaris, which drains the frontal recess, maxillary sinus, and anterior ethmoidal air cells. Located between the superior turbinate and sphenoid sinus, the sphenoethmoidal recess drains the posterior ethmoidal air cells and sphenoid sinus [10–13]. The sphenoid ostium may be found medial to the superior turbinate and approximately 1.5 cm superior to the choana, which demarcates the nasopharynx [14,15].

Kiesselbach's plexus supplies blood to the anterior nasal septum, receiving contributions from the superior labial anterior ethmoidal, greater palatine, and sphenopalatine arteries. The sphenopalatine artery is the main contributor to the blood supply of the nose. As a terminal branch of the internal maxillary artery, the artery originates along the lateral rostrum of the sphenoid sinus, exiting the sphenopalatine foramen. Notably, the posterior septal artery, branching from the sphenopalatine artery, is located horizontally in the sphenoethmoidal recess between the sphenoid ostium and choana to supply the septal mucosa and floor [16].

A detailed understanding of the osseous anatomy based on preoperative imaging is critical. As an important point, laterally projecting intersinus septation of the sphenoid sinus is directed toward one of the internal carotid arteries in 85% of cases [17]. Based on its ossification pattern, the sphenoid sinus may be described as conchal, presellar, sellar, or postsellar. One must also be mindful of the presence of sphenoethmoidal air cells, as Onodi Cells, located superolateral to the sphenoid sinus, may be in close proximity to the optic nerve [14,15]. The lateral opticocarotid recesses (LOCR) become important landmarks for identification of the optic nerve and anterior cavernous genu of the internal carotid artery, and these landmarks corresponds to the optic strut of the anterior clinoid. As such, a pneumatized anterior clinoid may be appreciated in the endonasal view by a deeper, more distinct LOCR [11,14]. The medial opticocarotid recess (MOCR), usually located approximately 5.6 mm medial to LOCR and just superior to the middle clinoid process, is the medial junction of the paraclinoid internal carotid artery (ICA) and optic nerve [15]. Careful preoperative planning should be undertaken to identify the presence of a carotid ring at the middle clinoid process prior to attempted removal. Anterior and superior to the tuberculum sellae, the sphenoid limbus may be visualized as an anteriorly projecting groove, serving as the anterior boundary of the chiasmatic sulcus and a landmark to identify the location of the optic chiasm [11,14,15,18].

The diaphragma sellae, a two-layer continuation of dural folds from the roof of the cavernous sinus, forms an incomplete roof over the pituitary gland with a central defect allowing for passage of the infundibulum [19]. The pituitary gland has a rich blood supply from the superior hypophyseal, inferior hypophyseal, and McConnell capsular arteries of the internal carotid arteries. Further contributors include the infundibular (from posterior communicating artery) and prechiasmatic (from the ophthalmic artery) arteries. As an important distinction, pituitary transposition frequently involves identification and careful sacrifice of the inferior hypophyseal arteries, which may be safely done; by contrast, the superior hyphophyseal arteries should be preserved whenever possible, as they supply the anterior pituitary gland, optic chiasm, and proximal optic nerves. The medial wall of the cavernous sinus is comprised of a single dural layer, separate from the pituitary capsule, with several parasellar ligaments that anchor the medial wall [20]. These include the caroticoclinoid ligament, superior parasellar ligament, inferior parasellar ligament, and posterior parasellar ligament [21].

Arising from the diaphragma sellae anteriorly, the Liliequist membrane consists of two sheets separating the suprasellar/chiasmatic cistern from the interpeduncular cistern attached to the mamillary bodies, and the interpeduncular cistern from the prepontine cistern at the junction of the midbrain and pons. The chiasmatic cistern, situated between the sella and hypothalamus, contains the proximal Sylvian veins, optic chiasm, anterior communicating artery complex, and infundibulum [18–20].

3.1.2. Illustrative Case

The present case is a 38-year-old female who presented with irregular menses and menorrhea. Lab work demonstrated a mild elevation in serum prolactin (54) consistent with mild stalk effect, along with normal adrenal, growth hormone, and thyroid axis labs. Imaging demonstrated a complex sellar lesion (Figure 1). The patient was started on cabergoline with improvement of her amenorrhea. Her visual fields examination was consistent with bitemporal, left worse than right, hemianopsia, and she agreed to proceeding with surgical resection for diagnosis and decompression of her optic apparatus.

The patient was placed supine with Mayfield cranial fixation. Both nares were decongested with two epinephrine-soaked pledgets bilaterally. Once there was adequate vasoconstriction, the inferior and middle turbinates were outfractured bilaterally. An incision was made at the caudal edge of the septum. A Cottle elevator was used to identify the submucoperichondrial plane from which mucosa was elevated from the posterior septum. A caudal strut was demarcated at the posterior aspect of the dissection with an incision and crossover cut developed with a Cottle elevator. The deviated portion of the septum was resected and removed. On the right, the superior turbinate was visualized, and its inferior one-third was resected. The sphenoid ostium was identified and cannulated. With visualization into the sphenoid sinus, a superior nasoseptal rescue flap incision was made with monopolar cautery and the mucosa was reflected inferiorly off the nasal septum, sphenoid rostrum, and arch of the choanae to protect the posterior septal artery pedicle. A posterior septectomy was then completed. Using the natural os bilaterally, the sphenoidotomies were enlarged and the entire face of the sphenoid was removed, visualizing the entire sphenoid sinus, sella, tuberculum, planum, and LOCRs.

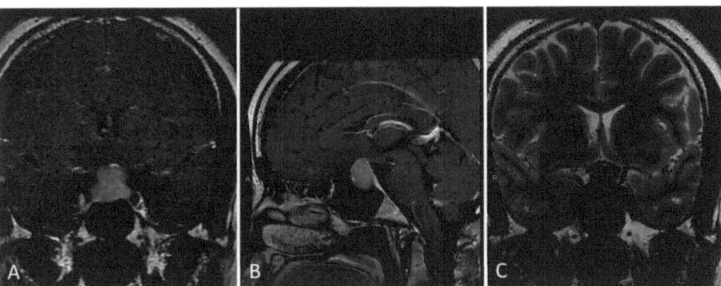

Figure 1. Preoperative imaging of a 38-year-old patient with bitemporal hemianopsia and a sellar lesion consistent with Rathke's cleft cyst. (**A**) Coronal T1 post-contrast MRI. (**B**) Sagittal T1 post-contrast MRI. (**C**) Coronal T2 MRI.

The sella was then thinned using a combination of high-speed drilling with a diamond drill bit, with the thinned shell of sellar bone subsequently peeled away from the dura using Kerrison rongeurs. The dura was opened low in the sella in an inverted horizontal and linear fashion. Fibrinous, caseous yellow debris was immediately encountered and sent for frozen and permanent pathological specimen—all consistent with Rathke's cleft cyst. Resection was performed with bimanual suctions sweeping laterally on the floor of the sella and moving upwards until the entire cyst was decompressed. The diaphragma was noted to descend following decompression, and no cerebrospinal fluid (CSF) leak was encountered. Following hemostasis, gelfoam was placed in the nasal corridor to help ensure the mucosa would remain moist during the peri-operative period, but the opening to the cyst was purposefully left unobstructed to help minimize risk of cyst recurrence. The patient was discharged home two days later without endocrine dysfunction, with a postoperative MRI demonstrating excellent decompression (Figure 2), and with recovery to full visual fields by her 2-month postoperative follow-up ophthalmology visit.

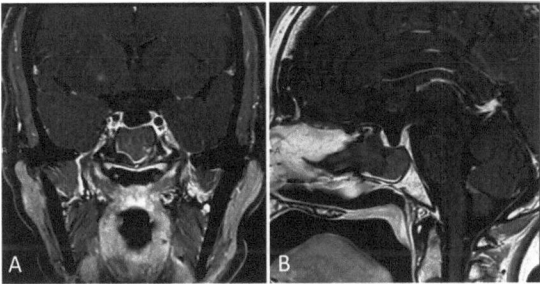

Figure 2. Postoperative imaging consistent with gross total resection of Rathke's cleft cyst. (**A**) Coronal T1 post-contrast MRI. (**B**) Sagittal T1 post-contrast MRI.

3.1.3. Practical Pearls

- An understanding of the osseous anatomy of the nasal corridor, paranasal sinuses, septum, intersinus septations, and relevant vascular structures are of paramount importance in the approach to sellar lesions.
- A pedicled nasoseptal rescue flap may be useful to obtain during the approach to the sellar lesions, particularly in cases of possible CSF leak, and should take into account the horizontal orientation of the posterior septal branch of the sphenopalatine artery.
- Dural opening of Rathke's cleft cysts, one should begin anteriorly and inferiorly to minimize the risk of inadvertent CSF leak and iatrogenic injury to the pituitary gland.
- One must be mindful of diaphragm downward migration and identification during cyst resection to avoid a CSF leak.

3.1.4. Illustrative Case

This is the case of a 57-year-old female who presented with 2 months of worsening vision loss in bitemporal fields, left worse than right, with imaging demonstrating a large cystic sellar and suprasellar lesion extending to the third ventricle (Figure 3). Admission labs were notable for mild central hypothyroidism. Given the large size of the suprasellar lesion with mass effect on the optic apparatus and vision symptom, the decision was made to proceed with surgical resection.

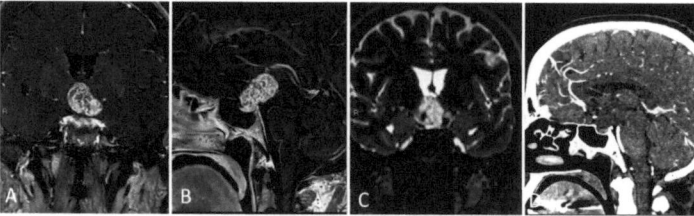

Figure 3. Preoperative imaging of a 56-year-old patient with an enhancing, partially calcified sellar and suprasellar lesion consistent with craniopharyngioma. (**A**) Coronal T1 post-contrast MRI. (**B**) Sagittal T1 post-contrast MRI. (**C**) Coronal T2-weighted MRI. (**D**) Sagittal thin cut CTA head demonstrating partial peripheral calcification.

Given the proximity of the lesion to the third ventricle, a high-flow CSF leak was anticipated, and a lumbar drain was therefore placed at the beginning of the case. Following lumbar drain placement, the patient was placed supine with Mayfield cranial fixation. The abdomen and lateral thigh were prepped for possible fat and fascia lata grafts, respectively. Both nares were decongested with two epinephrine-soaked pledgets bilaterally. Once there was adequate vasoconstriction, the inferior and middle turbinates were outfractured bilaterally. The superior turbinate was visualized on the right and its inferior third was resected. The sphenoid os was identified and a broad, right sided, pedicled nasoseptal flap was created with an anterior incision, parallel to the inferior border of the middle turbinate, transitioning superiorly along the dorsum and posteriorly to the caudal strut. Subsequently, an inferior incision was made along the vomer to the nasal floor, at the junction of the hard and soft palate, to the inferior meatus. This incision was extended to join the superior incision at the caudal strut, and the flap was raised in a circumferential fashion, with care to preserve the vascularized pedicle. Using the posteroinferior border of the uncinate process, the maxillary ostium was identified and a maxillary antrostomy was performed, alongside a total ethmoidectomy. A septoplasty was completed, a rescue flap incision was made on the left side, and a modest posterior septectomy was performed. An intersinus septation was identified coursing to the left ICA, and this septation was carefully drilled down. The bone over the sella and tuberculum sellae was carefully removed, the superior intercavernous sinus was coagulated and cut, and the dura was opened in a linear horizontal fashion at the level of the sphenoid limbus. Following sharp dissection through a soft, grey capsule located in the suprasellar cistern, gelatinous, yellow, proteinaceous material was immediately encountered and was debulked using teardrop suctures. Frozen pathological assessment of this tissue was compatible with calcified craniopharyngioma. The resection was continued superiorly into the third ventricle with removal of the posterior capsule of the tumor. The cerebral aqueduct into the fourth ventricle and bilateral foramen of Monroe were visualized. Once fenestrated into the ventricle, the remaining capsular portions of residual tumor were carefully resected eccentric to the right and left of the midline along the bilateral thalami. The eccentric portion of tumor to the left was noted to extend superiorly and inferiorly around the optic apparatus, incorporating a portion of the infundibulum, and these aspects of tumor were carefully dissected and resected, taking particular care not to manipulate the optic apparatus itself. By the end of resection, the optic nerves, superior hypophyseal arteries, and infundibulum were visualized without injury and free of tumor.

Following hemostasis, a multilayer closure, including a dural substitute inlay, dural substitute onlay, and an onlay nasoseptal flap, was created at the operative site (Figure 4). The lumbar drain was kept open to drain postoperatively at a rate of 10 cc per hour; the drain was clamped on postoperative day three, and it was removed on postoperative day. She was slowly mobilized after her drain was clamped, and she was discharged home without complication on postoperative day six. Final pathology was confirmed to be adamantinomatous craniopharyngioma, and postoperative imaging demonstrated gross total resection (Figure 5). At her 6-month postoperative ophthalmology follow-up appointment, she was noted to have significant improvement in visual fields compared to her preoperative state, with no pituitary insufficiency on endocrine follow up.

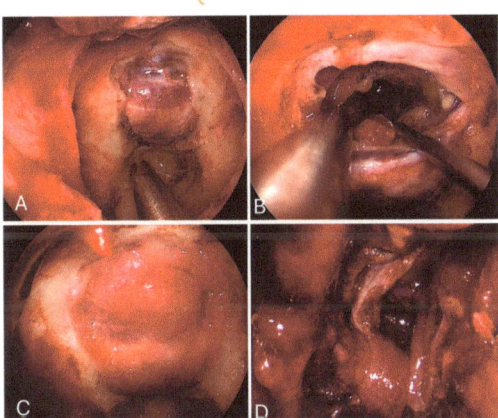

Figure 4. Intraoperative imaging of craniopharyngioma resection. (**A**) Sellar exposure. (**B**) Tumor resection. (**C**) Sellar onlay reconstruction. (**D**) Nasoseptal flap reconstruction.

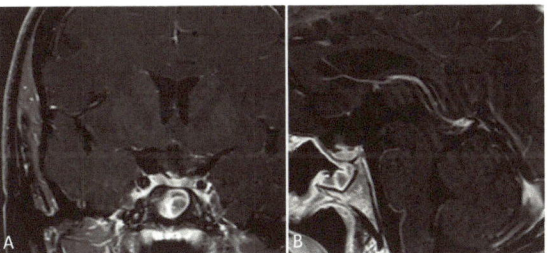

Figure 5. Postoperative imaging consistent with gross total resection of craniopharyngioma. (**A**) Coronal T1 post-contrast MRI. (**B**) Sagittal T1 post-contrast MRI.

3.1.5. Practical Pearls

- Placement of a lumbar drain is advised at the start of surgery, or preoperatively, in cases where a high-flow CSF leak is anticipated, in order to reduce immediate postoperative intracerebral pressure (ICP) and offload excessive pressure on the skull base graft.
- Upfront harvest of a nasal septal flap may be useful for skull base reconstruction in cases of anticipated high flow CSF leak.
- The sphenoid limbus serves as an important landmark for the location of the optic nerves, bridging medial to the optic canal and forming the anterior border of the prechiasmatic sulcus.
- When approaching lesions within the suprasellar region, one should be mindful of the location of the optic apparatus (i.e., pre-fixed/post-fixed chiasm) as well as relevant neurovascular structures in the chiasmatic, lamina terminalis, interpeduncular, and prepontine cisterns.
- Craniopharyngiomas may be fenestrated into a natural CSF space, such as the basal cisterns and third ventricle, to reduce long-term cystic reaccumulation/recurrence.

3.2. Orbital Apex

3.2.1. Anatomic Considerations

The optic nerve is approximately 5 cm in length and comprised of four segments: intraocular (1 mm), intraorbital (2.5–3 cm), intracanalicular, and prechiasmatic [22,23]. As an extension of the central nervous system, the optic nerve is surround by all three meningeal layers (dura, arachnoid, and pia mater) with an outer periosteal layer, the periorbita, which is continuous with the intracranial periosteal dura [22]. The average length of the bony orbit is 4 cm from base to orbital apex, separated by approximately 2.5 cm between the medial orbital wall from one side to the other. Lesions of the orbit are best characterized as intraconal/extraconal, relative to the muscular cone formed by the extraocular muscles, and intradural/extradural, relative to the periorbita, with orbital fat located in both the intraconal and extraconal spaces [24].

The bony orbit forms a pyramid comprising seven bones: frontal, ethmoid, lacrimal, sphenoid, zygomatic, palatine, and maxillary. The lamina paprycea of the ethmoid bone forms most of the medial orbital wall, articulating inferiorly with the orbital process of the palatine bone and maxilla, superiorly with the orbital plate of the frontal bone, posteriorly with the body of the sphenoid, and anteriorly with the lacrimal bone. The medial orbital rim is formed largely by the frontal process of the maxilla. The orbital roof is formed by a combination of the orbital plates of the frontal bone and the lesser wing of the sphenoid, which contain bony defects in both plates to form the anterior and posterior ethmoidal canals when joined. These canals demarcate the bulbar, retrobulbar, and apical segments of the orbit. The lateral orbital wall is formed by the greater wings of the sphenoid and the orbital surface of the zygomatic bone. The orbital floor is formed by the orbital process of the palatine bone and the orbital process of the maxillary bone. The lacrimal fossa is bordered anteriorly by the lacrimal crest of the maxillary bone and posteriorly by the lacrimal crest of the lacrimal bone, joining to form the lacrimomaxillary suture. Situated at the anteromedial and inferior portion of the orbit, the lacrimomaxillary suture serves as the site of insertion of the common canaliculus into the lacrimal sac via the valve of Rosenmuller to prevent reflux from the sac [24–28].

Blood supply to the orbit is primary through the ophthalmic artery, which passes superomedially over the intraorbital optic nerve, with several branches including the lacrimal, supraorbital, anterior ethmoidal, posterior ethmoidal, internal palpebral, supratrochlear, dorsal nasal, central retinal, anterior ciliary, posterior ciliary (long and short), central retinal, supraorbital, medial palpebral, and muscular arteries. The primary venous drainage pathway of the orbit is through the superior ophthalmic vein, draining further into the cavernous sinus, with minor tributaries to the angular and facial veins [29].

At the orbital apex, thickening of the periorbita helps to form the annulus of Zinn—a tendinous attachment for the rectus muscles, levator palpebrae superioris, and superior oblique muscles. The annulus contains the optic canal (with optic nerve and ophthalmic artery), the nasociliary nerve (V1), abducens nerve, and both superior and inferior divisions of the oculomotor nerve. The superior orbital fissure, separated from the optic canal by the optic strut, is an important landmark separating the intracranial cavernous sinus from the orbit [26–28].

The endoscopic endonasal approach allows for access to the medial orbit in the entire retrobulbar space through the annulus of Zinn and apex, limited medially the ophthalmic artery and optic nerve. In this approach, two working triangular corridors, superior and inferior, are separated by the medial rectus muscle to the superior oblique and inferior rectus muscles, respectively. The ophthalmic artery and optic nerve may be readily visualized and are the lateral limit of this approach. In the superior corridor, the retro-bulbar medial branches of the ophthalmic artery (i.e., anterior ethmoidal, posterior ethmoidal, central retinal artery) may be readily visualized; these structures are not easily accessible from the inferior corridor [30,31]. Superior and inferior oculomotor innervation is often on the ventral and medial surface of the extraocular muscles, and they are relatively well protected during gentle retraction in this approach. The superior division of the oculomotor nerve innervates the superior rectus and medial rectus muscles, with the inferior oblique and inferior rectus muscles innervated by the inferior division of the nerve. The trochlear nerve innervates the superior oblique muscle, passing extraconal from lateral to medial outside the annulus of Zinn, and then coursing superiorly above the superior rectus and levator palpebrae superioris muscles prior to reaching its point of innervation [25–29]. Medial decompression of the orbital apex in proximity to the annulus, therefore, should proceed with caution, in order to identify and preserve the trochlear nerve.

3.2.2. Illustrative Case

This is the case of a 62-year-old male with a past medical history of diffusely metastatic pancreatic neuroendocrine tumor, who presented with new onset left eye proptosis over 1 week and acute blindness in the left eye over 1 day. Imaging demonstrated a left intraconal lesion concerning for metastatic disease with optic nerve compression (Figure 6).

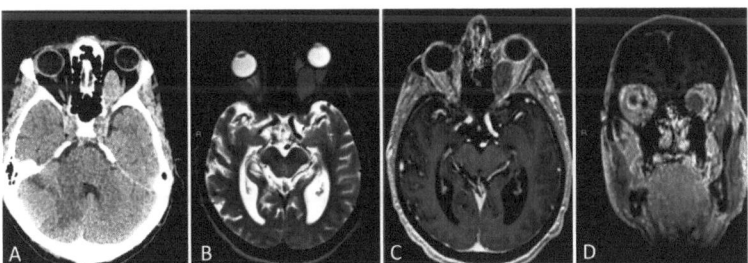

Figure 6. Preoperative imaging of a 62-year-old male with known metastatic neuroendocrine tumor presenting with left eye proptosis and a left intraconal medial orbital apex lesion with optic nerve compression. (**A**) Axial CT without contrast. (**B**) Axial T2-weighted MRI. (**C**) Axial T1 post-contrast MRI. (**D**) Coronal T1-post-contrast MRI.

Given the acuity of his vision loss and optic nerve compression, the patient was taken urgently to the operating room for endoscopic endonasal decompression of the medial orbit and pathologic diagnosis. His mean arterial pressure (MAP) was kept above 80 mm Hg and he was started on methylprednisolone for compressive optic neuropathy. The nose was decongested with epinephrine-soaked pledgets unilaterally, and the inferior and middle turbinate were fractured bilaterally. The left middle turbinate was gently medialized and the middle meatus was packed with epinephrine-soaked pledgets to ensure vasoconstriction. The uncinate process was identified and reflected anteriorly, with removal of the uncinate process revealing the maxillary ostium. A wide maxillary antrostomy was performed, followed by removal of the ethmoid bullae. The basal lamella separating anterior and posterior ethmoidal air cells was opened flush against the skull base and sphenoid, which was broadly opened to expose the orbital apex (Figure 7).

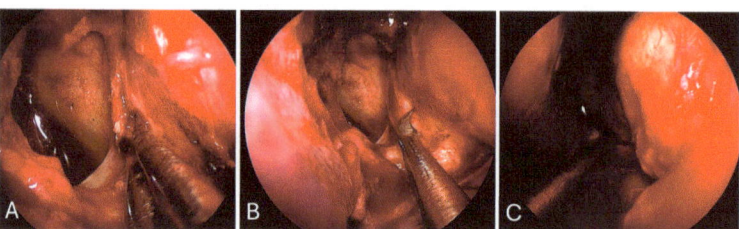

Figure 7. Intraoperative imaging demonstrating endoscopic endonasal transorbital approach. (**A**) Lamina paprycea is thinned and removed, exposing medial periorbita. (**B**) Periorbita is sharply incised with a sickle knife. (**C**) Tumor is exposed and debulked with suction and bipolar cautery.

The mucosa over the lamina paprycea was dissected and the lamina was fractured away from the orbit from anterior to posterior. The orbital strut was downfractured to reveal part of the orbital floor. The periorbita was opened parallel to the medial rectus, and the tumor was encountered between the medial rectus and inferior rectus muscles. The necrotic tumor was debulked and suctioned with decompression of the optic apparatus. Following tumor resection, there was noted mild herniation of orbital fat with an immediate decrease in left eye proptosis. No packing was used. Postoperative imaging demonstrated medial decompression of the optic nerve and orbital apex with no compression of the optic apparatus (Figure 8). He was discharged home two days after surgery with subjective improvement in left eye vision.

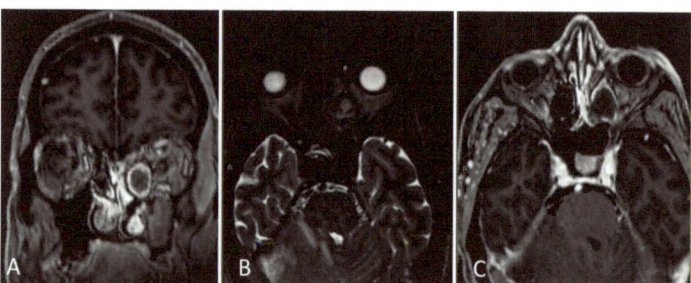

Figure 8. Postoperative imaging demonstrating complete resect of a left intraconal metastatic lesion and endoscopic endonasal optic nerve decompression. (**A**) Coronal T1 post-contrast MRI. (**B**) Axial T2-weighted MRI. (**C**) Axial T1 post-contrast MRI.

3.2.3. Practical Pearls

- The goals of surgical resection for metastatic lesions to the orbit are to obtain decompression of the optic apparatus and to obtain a diagnosis.
- The periorbita should be opened parallel to the medial rectus muscle to minimize inadvertent injury.
- In the medial endonasal approach, the two corridors include between the superior oblique and medial rectus muscles, as well as between the medial rectus and the inferior rectus muscles.

3.3. Anterior Cranial Base

3.3.1. Anatomic Considerations

The ethmoid bone comprises the anterior two-thirds of the anterior cranial fossa, with the planum sphenoidale forming the posterior third. The crista galli separates the olfactory nerves in the cribiform plate and serves as an important point of attachment for the falx cerebri. Underneath the cribiform plate, the ethmoidal labyrinth is separated from the anterior cranial fossa by fovea ethmoidalis from the orbital process of the frontal bone, which attaches to the vertical lateral lamella [32–34]. The depth of the olfactory fossa formed by the lateral lamella may be described by the Keros classification, where Type 1 is a depth of 1–3 mm, Type 2 is 4–7 mm, and Type 3 is 8–16 mm; an increased incidence of postoperative adverse events occur with higher Keros grades [35].

The anterior ethmoidal foramen, located posterior to the frontal recess, contains the anterior ethmoidal artery, anterior ethmoidal nerve, and anterior ethmoidal vein. Similarly, the posterior ethmoidal foramen contains the posterior ethmoidal artery, posterior ethmoidal nerve, and posterior ethmoidal vein. The anterior and posterior ethmoidal nerves are extraconal branches of the nasociliary nerve of V1 (ophthalmic division of the trigeminal nerve). The anterior ethmoidal artery courses between the superior oblique and medial rectus muscles, giving a nasal branch and meningeal branch to the anterior falcine artery as well as supplying the medial and inferior dura of the anterior fossa. The posterior ethmoidal artery supplies the dura of the planum, anterior clinoid process, and chiasmatic sulcus. The anterior ethmoidal artery is approximately 24 mm from the anterior lacrimal crest and 12 mm from the posterior ethmoidal artery, which is approximately 6 mm from the optic canal [32,33]. Ligation and sectioning of the anterior and posterior ethmoidal arteries should be done close to midline to avoid inadvertent artery retraction into the orbit and subsequent development of a retro-orbital hematoma [31–34].

The attachment of the uncinate process superiorly has direct implications for frontal sinus drainage. As such, when the uncinate process attaches medial to the middle turbinate, it functions as the medial wall of the frontal recess and directs drainage of the sinus to the middle meatus via the ethmoid infundibulum. When the uncinate process is attached more laterally at the lamina paprycea, it functions as the lateral wall of the frontal recess and drains directly into the middle meatus. In such cases, the ethmoid infundibulum forms a blind recess, termed the recessus terminalis [36,37].

Following completion of a Draf III frontal sinusotomy inclusive of removal of the cribiform plate and dural opening, one is able to identify the gyrus rectus located medial and adjacent to the olfactory sulcus, with the orbital frontal gyri located laterally. The blood supply to this region is via the A2 anterior cerebral artery (ACA) branches, including primarily the fronto-polar and fronto-orbital branches [32–34].

3.3.2. Illustrative Case

This is the case of a 44-year-old female with a past medical history of non-Hodgkins lymphoma, who presented with 4 months of left sided facial pain and left sided headaches with nasal congestion. On imaging, she was found to have an enhancing lesion in the left ethmoid sinus with extension to the nasal cavity, lamina paprycea, and anterior fossa floor (Figure 9). Endoscopic biopsy was consistent with squamous cell carcinoma, and PET/CT demonstrated hyperactive lymph nodes in the left neck and right inguinal region. Core biopsy of the hyperactive lymph nodes were negative for malignancy.

Given an anticipated CSF leak, a lumbar drain was placed at the beginning of the case. The nose was decongested with epinephrine-soaked pledgets bilaterally. The entire left sinonasal airway was noted to be filled with tumor on initial endoscopy, therefore the right middle turbinate was resected upfront for increased access. A maxillary antrostomy, total ethmoidectomy, and sphenoidotomy were performed on the right side. Given likely tumor involvement of the nasal septum, a nasal septal flap was designed on the right side, incorporating the pedicle of the posterior septal artery and floor of the nasal cavity. Transitioning to the left side, the tumor was debulked circumferentially with meticulous inspection of the borders for any obvious signs of invasion. The tumor was dissected from the orbit without issue and with normal appearing mucosa underlying the lesion. A Draf III frontal sinusotomy was performed, including removal of the frontal sinus floor between the orbits, anterosuperior nasal septum, frontal beak, and frontal intersinus septum. A total ethmoidectomy was performed with coagulation and sectioning of the anterior and posterior ethmoidal arteries close to midline. The cribiform plate was removed with cuts laterally on the right and left ethmoid roof, anteriorly at the frontal sinusotomy, and posteriorly at the planum sphenoidale. The dura of the anterior fossa was sharply opened at the periphery of the anterior fossa defect, and the olfactory bulbs were resected and sent for pathology alongside the dural specimen. Following circumferential removal of the tumor, a large dural substitute inlay and onlay were placed on the anterior fossa defect. The nasal septal flap was rotated from the nasopharynx and bolstered with packing material. Doyle splints were placed on the residual nasal septum (Figure 10). Postoperatively, her lumbar drain was opened to drain 5–10 cc every hour for 48 h prior to being clamped and eventually removed. Postoperative MRI demonstrated gross total resection (Figure 11). She was discharged home in good clinical condition and completed adjuvant chemoradiation consisting of 67 cGy of intensity-modulated radiation therapy (IMRT) to the resection bed atop weekly cisplatin.

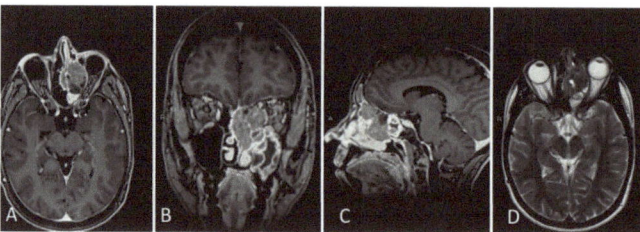

Figure 9. Preoperative imaging of a 44-year-old female with biopsy-proven squamous cell carcinoma of the left ethmoid, including invasion into the skull base and left lamina paprycea. (**A**) Axial T1 post-contrast MRI. (**B**) Coronal T1 post-contrast MRI. (**C**) Sagittal T1 post-contrast MRI. (**D**) Axial T2-weighted MRI.

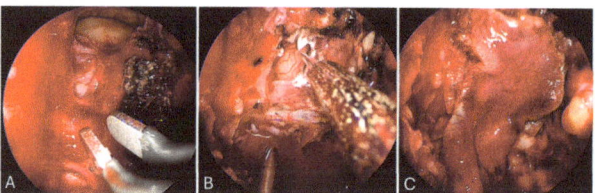

Figure 10. Intraoperative endoscopic endonasal anterior fossa approach. (**A**) Frontal sinusotomy with coagulation of the anterior and posterior ethmoidal arteries. (**B**) Draf III completed with opening of the dura over gyrus rectus and tumor removal. (**C**) Nasoseptal flap reconstruction.

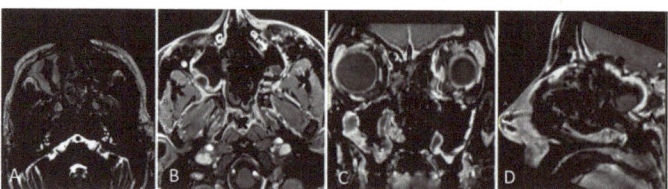

Figure 11. Postoperative imaging demonstrating gross total resection of a sinonasal squamous cell carcinoma. (**A**) Axial T2 high-resolution constructive interference steady state (CISS) T2-weighted MRI. (**B**) Axial T1 post-contrast MRI. (**C**) Coronal T1 post-contrast MRI. (**D**) Sagittal T1 post-contrast MRI.

3.3.3. Practical Pearls

- Anterior and posterior ethmoidal arteries should be ligated and cut close to midline in order to avoid retraction of these vessels into the orbit.
- The inlay dural substitute should be oversized as part of the multi-layered closure.
- Reconstruction with a nasoseptal flap should take into account sites of involved disease, which cannot be used in the flap.

3.4. Transpterygoid

3.4.1. Anatomic Considerations

The transpterygoid approach allows for more lateral access than the traditional midline endoscopic endonasal approach, which is limited laterally by the anterior genu of the ICA. This expanded approach allows for access to pathologies in the lateral recess of the sphenoid sinus, petrous apex, infratemporal fossa, middle fossa floor, and posterior fossa (Table 1). In the endoscopic endonasal approach, a maxillary antrostomy and removal of the medial posterior wall of the maxillary sinus exposes the pterygopalatine fossa [38–40]. The pterygopalatine fossa is a crucial skull base structure, particularly in cases of malignancy, with communications to the nasal cavity through the sphenopalatine foramen, infratemporal fossa through the pterygomaxillary fissure, orbit through the inferior orbital fissure, Meckel's cave through the foramen rotundum, lacerum segment of the ICA through the vidian canal, nasopharynx through the palatovaginal canal, and palate through the greater and lesser palatine canals. Formed by the palatine bone, pterygoid plates, and maxilla, this fossa additionally contains pterygopalatine fat surrounding the ganglion, the infraorbital branch of the maxillary artery, the infraorbital nerve from the maxillary nerve (V2) traveling towards the infraorbital foramen, and emissary veins with several tributaries [41–43].

The sphenopalatine artery traverses medially into the nasal cavity via the sphenopalatine foramen, formed by the orbital and sphenoid processes of the palatine bone; this artery must be cauterized and cut via the transpterygoid approach, precluding a vascularized nasoseptal flap on the ipsilateral side. The pterygopalatine ganglion is posteriorly tethered by the vidian nerve, which may be sectioned if needed (resulting in decreased lacrimation) to lateralize the ganglion and its contents. Lateral displacement of the ganglion may also put the palatine nerves on stretch, resulting in numbness of the palate. In cases where the vidian nerve is intended to be preserved, drilling of the medial pterygoid plate should remain below the border of the vidian canal and bony removal from the pterygoid wedge should be performed between foramen rotundum (superolaterally) and the vidian canal (inferomedially), which may be readily identified by following the maxillary and vidian nerves posteriorly, respectively [42–44].

Access to the masticator space requires detaching the pterygoid muscles from the pterygoid plates, with access to the post-styloid parapharyngeal space of the infratemporal fossa requiring complete resection of the plates. The lateral pterygoid muscle may be laterally detached to identify foramen ovale and V3, which descends adjacent the lateral pterygoid plate. The approach to Meckel's cave requires drilling of the pterygoid wedge and lateral pterygoid plate, following the infraorbital nerve posteriorly to the maxillary nerve to skeletonize foramen rotundum [45,46]. The 'quadrangular space', bordered by the maxillary nerve laterally and the vertical petrous ICA medially, may be opened to expose Meckel's cave [47]. The approach to the petrous apex requires identification of the clivus below the sphenoid floor, with dissection of pharyngobasilar fascia and overlying soft tissue medial to the Eustachan tube. Careful skeletonization of the vidian nerve leads to the lacerum segment of the ICA, a critical landmark in this region, and subsequent access to pathologies of the petrous apex. The petrous corridor can be laterally limited by the Eustachian tube, and the associated torus tubarus may be resected in cases of malignancy to increase lateral exposure. An alternative approach described to reach laterally along the petrous apex toward the internal acoustic canal (IAC) is the contralateral transmaxillary approach (CTM), which does not require Eustachian tube manipulation or dissection of the ICA [48].

Table 1. Landmark studies in the modular approach to endonasal skull base tumor surgery.

Authors	Approach	Study Inclusion	Outcomes
Fong et al. [49]	Sellar	Meta-analysis including eleven studies comprised of 3941 patients undergoing expanded endoscopic endonasal resection for pituitary tumors were evaluated.	Progression-free survival was significantly higher in patients who underwent gross-total resection compared to subtotal resection. Postoperative radiotherapy was associated with improved progression-free survival in patients with residual disease.
Lee et al. [50]	Suprasellar	25 articles comprising 554 pediatric patients undergoing endoscopic endonasal resection for suprasellar pathologies were included. Most common pathologies included craniopharyngiomas, adenomas, and Rathke's cleft cysts.	No significant difference in primary tumor etiology with rates of CSF leak postoperatively (8.6% overall), including craniopharyngiomas (10.6%), adenomas (6.5%), and Rathke's cleft cysts (7.2%).
Dubal et al. [51]	Orbital Apex	39 studies comprising 71 patients who underwent endoscopic endonasal resection of orbital apex pathologies were included.	Exclusively intraconal and extraconal pathologies included 51% and 30.6% of the cohort, respectively. Tumor etiology was most commonly cavernous hemangioma (45.1%), with 76.2% of complications as transient and no difference in rates of complication between intraconal or extraconal pathologies. There was only a 4.2% rate of recurrence in the pooled cohort.
Nicolai et al. [52]	Anterior Fossa	Exclusive EEA for anterior fossa sinonasal malignancies was performed in 134 patients with the remaining 50 undergoing a cranioendosopic combined approach. Malignancies included adenocarcinoma, squamous cell carcinoma, olfactory neuroblastoma, mucosal melanoma, and adenoid cystic carcinoma.	5-year disease-specific survival was 91.4% and 58.8% for EEA and CEA groups, respectively.
Hanna et al. [53]		120 patients were included with esthesioneuroblastoma, sarcoma, adenocarcinoma, melanoma, and squamous cell carcinoma. 93 select patients underwent exclusively expanded EEA and 27 underwent cranioendoscopic approach with combined open craniotomy.	No significant differences between combined nor exclusive EEA groups, with 5- and 10-year survival rates of 87% and 80%, respectively.
Battaglia et al. [46]	Transpterygoid	37 consecutive patients with who underwent transmaxillary transpterygoid approach for skull base tumor resection of the nasopharynx, middle fossa, or infratemporal fossa were included. Primary pathologies included juvenile nasopharyngeal angiofibroma, trigeminal schwannoma, cavernous hemangioma, adenoid cystic carcinoma, mucoepidermoid carcinoma, squamous cell carcinoma, adenocarcinoma, chondrosarcoma, and undifferentiated nasopharyngeal carcinoma.	One patient suffered internal carotid artery injury, and eight patients received adjuvant treatment. At most recent follow-up (30 months for malignant tumors and 60 months for benign tumors) all patients had stable disease without recurrence. Two patients of the cohort had stable intracranial disease, including one with a meningioma and one with adenoid cystic carcinoma.

3.4.2. Illustrative Case

This is the case of a 43-year-old male with a past medical history of left petrous apex cholesterol granuloma that was discovered after diagnostic workup for self-resolved diplopia, atop longstanding tinnitus and chronic sinusitis. Imaging demonstrated a 3.7 × 1.5 × 2.5 cm lesion of the left petrous apex with expansile high T1 and heterogeneous mixed T2 signal intensity in the left clival and petrous apex lesion, consistent with cholesterol granuloma (Figure 12).

The nose was decongested with epinephrine-soaked pledgets bilaterally, the inferior and middle turbinates were out-fractured bilaterally, and the left middle turbinate was resected to improve visualization. A wide sphenoidotomy was then performed, a left-sided rescue mucosal flap was created, and a right-sided vascularized nasoseptal flap was created. A modestly sized posterior septectomy was performed, and the rostrum was isolated and partially resected. A generous maxillary antrostomy was created on the left side in anticipation of possible extension of the lesion lateral to the left paraclival carotid artery.

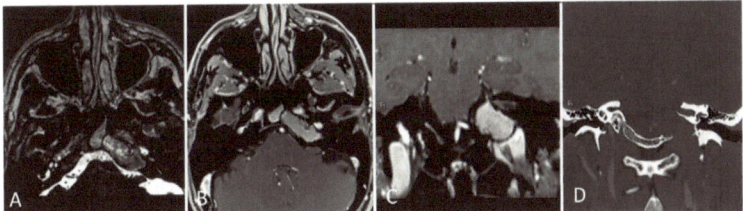

Figure 12. Preoperative imaging of a 43-year-old male with a left petroclival cholesterol granuloma. (**A**) Axial T2 high-resolution constructive interference steady state (CISS) T2-weighted MRI. (**B**) Axial T1 post-contrast MRI. (**C**) Coronal T1 post-contrast MRI. (**D**) Coronal CTA with contrast.

The mucosa was stripped from the clival recess and the intersinus septation was drilled between the well-pneumatized clival carotid protuberances. The clivus was opened medial to the left clival carotid artery to immediately encounter the cholesterol granuloma, which was sharply opened. The contents of the lesion were fully removed. The mucoperiosteum overlying the petrous internal carotid artery was similarly decompressed and visualized. The nasoseptal flap was laid into the resection cavity in an effort to allow for marsupialization of the cavity, and gelfoam was placed around this site in an attempt to minimize postoperative nasal crusting (Figure 13). Postoperative imaging demonstrated decompression of the granuloma (Figure 14) and the patient was discharged home in good condition on postoperative day two.

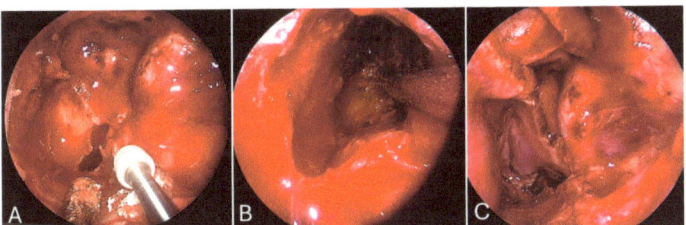

Figure 13. Intraoperative imaging of modified Denker's maxillary antrostomy and transpterygoid approach to petrous apex cholesterol granuloma, (**A**) Back wall of the maxillary sinus is opened to access the pterygopalatine fossa. (**B**) Transpterygoid approach with suction resection of the granuloma. (**C**) Nasoseptal flap reconstruction.

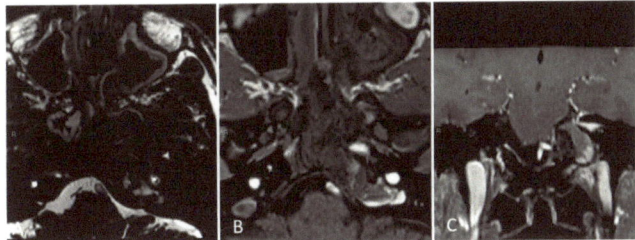

Figure 14. Postoperative imaging demonstrating decompression of a petrous apex cholesterol granuloma. (**A**) Axial T2 high-resolution constructive interference steady state (CISS) T2-weighted MRI. (**B**) Axial T1 post-contrast MRI. (**C**) Coronal T1 post-contrast MRI.

3.4.3. Practical Pearls

- Sacrifice of the sphenopalatine artery in the transpterygoid approach precludes an ipsilateral nasoseptal flap.
- Skeletonization of the maxillary nerve leads to the 'quadrangular space' and Meckel's cave.

- Skeletonization of the vidian nerve leads to the lacerum segment of the ICA.
- The contralateral transmaxillary approach may be a useful back up option for lateral petrous pathologies approaching the IAC.

Author Contributions: Conceptualization, A.K.A., N.R.R. and D.M.; data curation, A.K.A.; original draft preparation, A.K.A. and D.M.; supervision, N.R.R. and D.M.; writing—review and editing, A.K.A., N.R.R. and D.M. All authors have read and agreed to the published version of the manuscript.

Funding: This research received no external funding.

Institutional Review Board Statement: Not applicable.

Informed Consent Statement: Not applicable.

Data Availability Statement: No data were created as part of this project.

Conflicts of Interest: The authors declare no conflicts of interest.

References

1. Doglietto, F.; Prevedello, D.M.; Jane, J.A., Jr.; Han, J.; Laws, E.R., Jr. Brief history of endoscopic transsphenoidal surgery–From Philipp Bozzini to the First World Congress of Endoscopic Skull Base Surgery. *Neurosurg. Focus* **2005**, *19*, 1–6. [CrossRef]
2. Porras, J.L.; Rowan, N.R.; Mukherjee, D. Endoscopic Endonasal Skull Base Surgery Complication Avoidance: A Contemporary Review. *Brain Sci.* **2022**, *12*, 1685. [CrossRef]
3. Chakravarthi, S.; Gonen, L.; Monroy-Sosa, A.; Khalili, S.; Kassam, A. Endoscopic Endonasal Reconstructive Methods to the Anterior Skull Base. *Semin. Plast. Surg.* **2017**, *31*, 203–213. [CrossRef] [PubMed]
4. Roxbury, C.R.; Ishii, M.; Richmon, J.D.; Blitz, A.M.; Reh, D.D.; Gallia, G.L. Endonasal Endoscopic Surgery in the Management of Sinonasal and Anterior Skull Base Malignancies. *Head Neck Pathol.* **2016**, *10*, 13–22, Erratum in *Head Neck Pathol.* **2017**, *11*, 268. [CrossRef] [PubMed]
5. Castelnuovo, P.; Dallan, I.; Battaglia, P.; Bignami, M. Endoscopic endonasal skull base surgery: Past, present and future. *Eur. Arch. Otorhinolaryngol.* **2010**, *267*, 649–663. [CrossRef] [PubMed]
6. Verillaud, B.; Bresson, D.; Sauvaget, E.; Mandonnet, E.; Georges, B.; Kania, R.; Herman, P. Endoscopic endonasal skull base surgery. *Eur. Ann. Otorhinolaryngol. Head Neck Dis.* **2012**, *129*, 190–196. [CrossRef] [PubMed]
7. Patel, C.R.; Fernandez-Miranda, J.C.; Wang, W.H.; Wang, E.W. Skull Base Anatomy. *Otolaryngol. Clin. N. Am.* **2016**, *49*, 9–20. [CrossRef] [PubMed]
8. Kanjanawasee, D.; Campbell, R.G.; Rimmer, J.; Alvarado, R.; Kanjanaumporn, J.; Snidvongs, K.; Kalish, L.; Harvey, R.J.; Sacks, R. Empty Nose Syndrome Pathophysiology: A Systematic Review. *Otolaryngol. Head Neck Surg.* **2022**, *167*, 434–451. [CrossRef] [PubMed]
9. Rohr, A.S.; Spector, S.L. Paranasal sinus anatomy and pathophysiology. *Clin. Rev. Allergy* **1984**, *2*, 387–395. [PubMed]
10. Baroody, F.M. Nasal and paranasal sinus anatomy and physiology. *Clin. Allergy Immunol.* **2007**, *19*, 1–21.
11. Ferrari, M.; Mattavelli, D.; Schreiber, A.; Nicolai, P. Macroscopic and Endoscopic Anatomy of the Anterior Skull Base and Adjacent Structures. In *Anterior Skull Base Tumors*; Advances in Oto-Rhino-Laryngology; Karger Publishers: Basel, Switzerland, 2020; Volume 84, pp. 1–12. [CrossRef]
12. Jankowski, R.; Nguyen, D.T.; Poussel, M.; Chenuel, B.; Gallet, P.; Rumeau, C. Sinusology. *Eur. Ann. Otorhinolaryngol. Head Neck Dis.* **2016**, *133*, 263–268. [CrossRef]
13. Kubal, W.S. Sinonasal anatomy. *Neuroimaging Clin. N. Am.* **1998**, *8*, 143–156.
14. Campero, A.; Emmerich, J.; Socolovsky, M.; Martins, C.; Yasuda, A.; Agustín Campero, A.; Rhoton, A., Jr. Microsurgical anatomy of the sphenoid ostia. *J. Clin. Neurosci.* **2010**, *17*, 1298–1300. [CrossRef]
15. Rhoton, A.L., Jr. The sellar region. *Neurosurgery* **2002**, *51* (Suppl. 4), S335–S374. [CrossRef]
16. Patel, R.G. Nasal Anatomy and Function. *Facial Plast. Surg.* **2017**, *33*, 3–8. [CrossRef]
17. Fernandez-Miranda, J.C.; Prevedello, D.M.; Madhok, R.; Morera, V.; Barges-Coll, J.; Reineman, K.; Snyderman, C.H.; Gardner, P.; Carrau, R.; Kassam, A.B. Sphenoid septations and their relationship with internal carotid arteries: Anatomical and radiological study. *Laryngoscope* **2009**, *119*, 1893–1896. [CrossRef]
18. Ceylan, S.; Koc, K.; Anik, I. Extended endoscopic approaches for midline skull-base lesions. *Neurosurg. Rev.* **2009**, *32*, 309–319, discussion 318–319. [CrossRef] [PubMed]
19. Rejane-Heim, T.C.; Silveira-Bertazzo, G.; Carrau, R.L.; Prevedello, D.M. Surgical anatomy and nuances of the expanded endonasal transdorsum sellae and posterior clinoidectomy approach to the interpeduncular and prepontine cisterns: A stepwise cadaveric dissection of various pituitary gland transpositions. *Acta Neurochir.* **2021**, *163*, 407–413. [CrossRef] [PubMed]
20. Cironi, K.A.; Decater, T.; Iwanaga, J.; Dumont, A.S.; Tubbs, R.S. Arterial Supply to the Pituitary Gland: A Comprehensive Review. *World Neurosurg.* **2020**, *142*, 206–211. [CrossRef] [PubMed]

21. Truong, H.Q.; Lieber, S.; Najera, E.; Alves-Belo, J.T.; Gardner, P.A.; Fernandez-Miranda, J.C. The medial wall of the cavernous sinus. Part 1: Surgical anatomy, ligaments, and surgical technique for its mobilization and/or resection. *J. Neurosurg.* **2018**, *131*, 122–130. [CrossRef] [PubMed]
22. Romano, N.; Federici, M.; Castaldi, A. Imaging of cranial nerves: A pictorial overview. *Insights Imaging* **2019**, *10*, 33. [CrossRef]
23. Gentry, L.R. Anatomy of the orbit. *Neuroimaging Clin. N. Am.* **1998**, *8*, 171–194.
24. Banks, C.; Husain, Q.; Bleier, B.S. Endoscopic endonasal intraconal orbit surgery. *World J. Otorhinolaryngol. Head Neck Surg.* **2019**, *6*, 100–105. [CrossRef] [PubMed]
25. Castelnuovo, P.; Turri-Zanoni, M.; Battaglia, P.; Locatelli, D.; Dallan, I. Endoscopic Endonasal Management of Orbital Pathologies. *Neurosurg. Clin. N. Am.* **2015**, *26*, 463–472. [CrossRef] [PubMed]
26. Hayek, G.; Mercier, P.; Fournier, H.D. Anatomy of the orbit and its surgical approach. *Adv. Tech. Stand. Neurosurg.* **2006**, *31*, 35–71. [CrossRef] [PubMed]
27. Chastain, J.B.; Sindwani, R. Anatomy of the orbit, lacrimal apparatus, and lateral nasal wall. *Otolaryngol. Clin. N. Am.* **2006**, *39*, 855–864. [CrossRef]
28. Weisman, R.A. Surgical anatomy of the orbit. *Otolaryngol. Clin. N. Am.* **1988**, *21*, 1–12. [CrossRef]
29. Hayreh, S.S. Orbital vascular anatomy. *Eye* **2006**, *20*, 1130–1144. [CrossRef] [PubMed]
30. Omura, K.; Nomura, K.; Mori, R.; Ishii, Y.; Tanaka, Y.; Otori, N.; Kojima, H. Advanced Endoscopic Endonasal Approach to the Pterygopalatine Fossa and Orbit: The Endoscopic Tri-port Approach. *J. Neurol. Surg. B Skull Base* **2020**, *82*, 437–442. [CrossRef] [PubMed]
31. Chiou, C.A.; Vickery, T.W.; Reshef, E.R.; Bleier, B.S.; Freitag, S.K. Endonasal Endoscopic Approach to Orbital Tumors. *Int. Ophthalmol. Clin.* **2023**, *63*, 249–262. [CrossRef]
32. Almeida, J.P.; DE Andrade, E.J.; Vescan, A.; Zadeh, G.; Recinos, P.F.; Kshettry, V.R.; Gentili, F. Surgical anatomy and technical nuances of the endoscopic endonasal approach to the anterior cranial fossa. *J. Neurosurg. Sci.* **2021**, *65*, 103–117. [CrossRef] [PubMed]
33. Plou, P.; Serioli, S.; Leonel, L.C.P.C.; Alexander, A.Y.; Agosti, E.; Vilany, L.; Graepel, S.; Choby, G.; Pinheiro-Neto, C.D.; Peris-Celda, M. Surgical Anatomy and Approaches of the Anterior Cranial Fossa from a Transcranial and Endonasal Perspective. *Cancers* **2023**, *15*, 2587. [CrossRef]
34. Silveira-Bertazzo, G.; Li, R.; Rejane-Heim, T.C.; Martinez-Perez, R.; Albonette-Felicio, T.; Sholkamy Diab, A.G.; Mahmoud Mady, M.S.; Hardesty, D.A.; Carrau, R.L.; Prevedello, D.M. Endoscopic approaches to skull base malignancies affecting the anterior fossa. *J. Neurosurg. Sci.* **2021**, *65*, 169–180. [CrossRef] [PubMed]
35. Santosh, B. A Study of Clinical Significance of the Depth of Olfactory Fossa in Patients Undergoing Endoscopic Sinus Surgery. *Indian J. Otolaryngol. Head Neck Surg.* **2017**, *69*, 514–522. [CrossRef]
36. Srivastava, M.; Tyagi, S. Role of Anatomic variations of Uncinate Process in Frontal Sinusitis. *Indian. J. Otolaryngol. Head Neck Surg.* **2016**, *68*, 441–444. [CrossRef]
37. Zhang, L.; Han, D.; Ge, W.; Xian, J.; Zhou, B.; Fan, E.; Liu, Z.; He, F. Anatomical and computed tomographic analysis of the interaction between the uncinate process and the agger nasi cell. *Acta Otolaryngol.* **2006**, *126*, 845–852. [CrossRef]
38. Finger, G.; Gun, R.; Wu, K.C.; Carrau, R.L.; Prevedello, D.M. Endoscopic Endonasal Transpterygoid Approach: Technical Lessons. *Oper. Neurosurg.* **2023**, *25*, e272. [CrossRef]
39. Mehta, G.U.; Raza, S.M. Endoscopic endonasal transpterygoid approach to petrous pathologies: Technique, limitations and alternative approaches. *J. Neurosurg. Sci.* **2018**, *62*, 339–346. [CrossRef]
40. Hardesty, D.A.; Montaser, A.S.; Carrau, R.L.; Prevedello, D.M. Limits of endoscopic endonasal transpterygoid approach to cavernous sinus and Meckel's cave. *J. Neurosurg. Sci.* **2018**, *62*, 332–338. [CrossRef]
41. Oakley, G.M.; Harvey, R.J. Endoscopic Resection of Pterygopalatine Fossa and Infratemporal Fossa Malignancies. *Otolaryngol. Clin. N. Am.* **2017**, *50*, 301–313. [CrossRef]
42. Tashi, S.; Purohit, B.S.; Becker, M.; Mundada, P. The pterygopalatine fossa: Imaging anatomy, communications, and pathology revisited. *Insights Imaging* **2016**, *7*, 589–599. [CrossRef]
43. Ozawa, H.; Sekimizu, M.; Saito, S.; Nakamura, S.; Mikoshiba, T.; Toda, M.; Ogawa, K. Endoscopic Endonasal Management of Pterygopalatine Fossa Tumors. *J. Craniofac Surg.* **2021**, *32*, e454–e457. [CrossRef]
44. Vuksanovic-Bozaric, A.; Vukcevic, B.; Abramovic, M.; Vukcevic, N.; Popovic, N.; Radunovic, M. The pterygopalatine fossa: Morphometric, C.T. study with clinical implications. *Surg. Radiol. Anat.* **2019**, *41*, 161–168. [CrossRef]
45. Hosseini, S.M.; Razfar, A.; Carrau, R.L.; Prevedello, D.M.; Fernandez-Miranda, J.; Zanation, A.; Kassam, A.B. Endonasal transpterygoid approach to the infratemporal fossa: Correlation of endoscopic and multiplanar, C.T. anatomy. *Head Neck* **2012**, *34*, 313–320. [CrossRef]
46. Battaglia, P.; Turri-Zanoni, M.; Dallan, I.; Gallo, S.; Sica, E.; Padoan, G.; Castelnuovo, P. Endoscopic endonasal transpterygoid transmaxillary approach to the infratemporal and upper parapharyngeal tumors. *Otolaryngol. Head Neck Surg.* **2014**, *150*, 696–702. [CrossRef] [PubMed]
47. Cárdenas Ruiz-Valdepeñas, E.; Simal Julián, J.A.; Pérez Prat, G.; Arraez, M.A.; Ambrosiani, J.; Martin Schrader, I.; Soto Moreno, A.; Kaen, A. The Quadrangular Space, Endonasal Access to the Meckel Cave: Technical Considerations and Clinical Series. *World Neurosurg.* **2022**, *163*, e124–e136. [CrossRef] [PubMed]

48. Mangussi-Gomes, J.; Alves-Belo, J.T.; Truong, H.Q.; Nogueira, G.F.; Wang, E.W.; Fernandez-Miranda, J.C.; Gardner, P.A.; Snyderman, C.H. Anatomical Limits of the Endoscopic Contralateral Transmaxillary Approach to the Petrous Apex and Petroclival Region. *J. Neurol. Surg. B Skull Base* **2020**, *83*, 44–52. [CrossRef] [PubMed]
49. Fong, K.Y.; Lim, M.J.R.; Fu, S.; Low, C.E.; Chan, Y.H.; Deepak, D.S.; Xu, X.; Thong, M.; Jain, S.; Teo, K.; et al. Postsurgical outcomes of nonfunctioning pituitary adenomas: A patient-level meta-analysis. *Pituitary* **2023**, *26*, 461–473. [CrossRef] [PubMed]
50. Lee, J.A.; Cooper, R.L.; Nguyen, S.A.; Schlosser, R.J.; Gudis, D.A. Endonasal Endoscopic Surgery for Pediatric Sellar and Suprasellar Lesions: A Systematic Review and Meta-analysis. *Otolaryngol. Head Neck Surg.* **2020**, *163*, 284–292. [CrossRef]
51. Dubal, P.M.; Svider, P.F.; Denis, D.; Folbe, A.J.; Eloy, J.A. Short-term outcomes of purely endoscopic endonasal resection of orbital tumors: A systematic review. *Int. Forum Allergy Rhinol.* **2014**, *4*, 1008–1015. [CrossRef] [PubMed]
52. Nicolai, P.; Battaglia, P.; Bignami, M.; Villaret, A.B.; Delù, G.; Khrais, T.; Lombardi, D.; Castelnuovo, P. Endoscopic surgery for tumors of the sinonasal tract and adjacent skull base: A 10 year experience. *Am. J. Rhinol.* **2008**, *22*, 308–316. [CrossRef] [PubMed]
53. Hanna, E.; DeMonte, F.; Ibrahim, S.; Roberts, D.; Levine, N.; Kupferman, M. Endoscopic resection of sinonasal cancers with and without craniotomy: Oncologic results. *Arch. Otolaryngol. Head Neck Surg.* **2009**, *135*, 1219–1234. [CrossRef] [PubMed]

Disclaimer/Publisher's Note: The statements, opinions and data contained in all publications are solely those of the individual author(s) and contributor(s) and not of MDPI and/or the editor(s). MDPI and/or the editor(s) disclaim responsibility for any injury to people or property resulting from any ideas, methods, instructions or products referred to in the content.

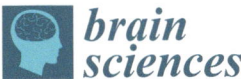

Article

Endoscopic Endonasal Transplanum–Transtuberculum Approach for Pituitary Adenomas/PitNET: 25 Years of Experience

Alessandro Carretta [1], Matteo Zoli [1,2,*], Federica Guaraldi [2], Giacomo Sollini [3], Arianna Rustici [1,4], Sofia Asioli [1,5], Marco Faustini-Fustini [2], Ernesto Pasquini [3] and Diego Mazzatenta [1,2]

1. Department of Bio-Medical and Neuromotor Sciences (DIBINEM), University of Bologna, 40138 Bologna, Italy; arianna.r87@gmail.com (A.R.); sofia.asioli3@unibo.it (S.A.); diego.mazzatenta@unibo.it (D.M.)
2. IRCCS Istituto delle Scienze Neurologiche di Bologna, Programma Neurochirurgia Ipofisi–Pituitary Unit, 40139 Bologna, Italy; federica.guaraldi@ausl.bologna.it (F.G.); marco.faustini@isnb.it (M.F.-F.)
3. ENT Unit, Bellaria Hospital, Azienda USL Bologna, 40139 Bologna, Italy; giacomo.sollini@ausl.bologna.it (G.S.); ernesto.pasquini@ausl.bologna.it (E.P.)
4. IRCCS Istituto delle Scienze Neurologiche di Bologna, Neuroradiology Unit, Ospedale Maggiore, 40139 Bologna, Italy
5. IRCCS Istituto delle Scienze Neurologiche di Bologna, 40139 Bologna, Italy
* Correspondence: matteo.zoli4@unibo.it; Tel.: +39-0516225111

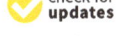

Citation: Carretta, A.; Zoli, M.; Guaraldi, F.; Sollini, G.; Rustici, A.; Asioli, S.; Faustini-Fustini, M.; Pasquini, E.; Mazzatenta, D. Endoscopic Endonasal Transplanum–Transtuberculum Approach for Pituitary Adenomas/PitNET: 25 Years of Experience. *Brain Sci.* **2023**, *13*, 1121. https://doi.org/10.3390/brainsci13071121

Academic Editor: Miguel Angel Lopez-Gonzalez

Received: 19 June 2023
Revised: 16 July 2023
Accepted: 20 July 2023
Published: 24 July 2023

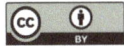

Copyright: © 2023 by the authors. Licensee MDPI, Basel, Switzerland. This article is an open access article distributed under the terms and conditions of the Creative Commons Attribution (CC BY) license (https://creativecommons.org/licenses/by/4.0/).

Abstract: The role of the endoscopic transplanum–transtuberculum approach (ETTA) in the treatment of pituitary adenomas/PitNETs (PAs) is sparsely analyzed in the literature, and its use is still debated in the current practice. The aim of this study was to report our experience with this approach. Our institutional registry was retrospectively reviewed, and patients who underwent ETTA for a PA from 1998 to 2022 were included. Fifty-seven cases were enrolled over a time span of 25 years, corresponding to 2.4% of our entire PA caseload. Radical resection was achieved in 57.9% of cases, with re-do surgery ($p = 0.033$) and vessel encasement/engulfment ($p < 0.001$) as predictors of partial resection. CSF leak incidence stood at 8.8%, with higher BMI ($p = 0.038$) as its only significant predictor. Partial or full improvement of the visual field deficits was achieved in 73.5% of cases. No surgical mortality was observed. According to our results, ETTA for the treatment of PAs is characterized by a satisfactory surgical outcome but with greater morbidity than the conventional endoscopic approach. Therefore, it should be reserved for the few selected cases otherwise unsuitable for the endoscopic trans-sphenoidal route, representing a valid alternative and an effective complementary route for the transcranial approach for these challenging PAs.

Keywords: pituitary adenoma; PitNET; extended; transplanum; transtuberculum; endoscopic endonasal; outcome; complications

1. Introduction

The introduction of the extended trans-sphenoidal transplanum/transtuberculum approach dates back to 1987, when Weiss demonstrated that this anterior expansion of the microsurgical trans-sphenoidal route would allow the surgeon to also approach suprasellar tumors, such as craniopharyngiomas, meningiomas or large pituitary adenomas/PitNET (PA) [1]. However, the lack of a panoramic vision and the restricted field granted by microscopical magnification prevented a widespread diffusion and impaired the popularity of this specific approach for decades [2–8].

Nevertheless, the introduction of the endoscope in trans-sphenoidal surgery has largely improved the intra-operative visualization of this approach, giving a panoramic and, at the same time, very detailed exposure of the nasal and skull base structures, overcoming the drawbacks associated with microscopic vision [9]. The endoscopic endonasal extended transplanum/transtuberculum approach (ETTA) has proved to be a valuable workhorse for the resection of suprasellar neoplasms (for instance, tuberculum sellae or planum meningiomas, suprasellar craniopharyngiomas—even with third ventricle involvement—suprasellar epidermoid/dermoid cysts or hypothalamic gliomas with a debulking or bioptic aim), which would otherwise require a transcranial approach, since they are not approachable through the standard endoscopic endonasal route [10–15].

A further rare and under-considered indication for an ETTA is represented by those cases of PA with an uncommon complex morphology, such as a major suprasellar or sub-frontal expansion, not manageable through a standard trans-sphenoidal approach and therefore requiring a transcranial or a combined transcranial–trans-sphenoidal approach [16–21]. Although the effectiveness of ETTA for these rare PAs has already been proposed in a few clinical series, most of them were not selectively focused on a PA population or were mainly aimed to describe the reconstruction technique [22–28].

The goal of this study was to analyze our surgical series of PAs operated through an ETTA in our center. The primary objective was the assessment of the extent of tumor resection (EOR) and the normalization rate of bio-chemical hypersecretion in functioning adenomas, identifying the factors predicting the EOR. The secondary aims were the determination of the complication rate of this approach, with particular attention to the risk of post-operative CSF leak, whose predictive factors were analyzed, and the visual and endocrinological outcomes of these patients.

2. Materials and Methods

2.1. Study Design, Settings and Inclusion Criteria

Our prospectively collected database of all consecutive patients treated surgically in our institution (Programma Neurochirurgia Ipofisi—Pituitary Unit of IRCCS Istituto delle Scienze Neurologiche di Bologna, Italy) between 1998 and September 2022 was retrospectively reviewed to consider all the PAs treated through the ETTA. The inclusion criteria consisted of (1) histologically confirmed diagnosis of functioning or non-functioning PA; (2) adoption of an ETTA; (3) minimum follow-up of 6 months; (4) availability of all clinical and radiological pre- and post-operative features. Tumors primarily involving the cavernous sinus or the clival region, therefore treated with different extended endoscopic approaches, or those lacking complete data were excluded from the study.

Ethics committee approval and informed consent were waived for this study because of its retrospective observational design.

2.2. Patient Management and Surgical Nuances

The management of every single patient referred to our institution is discussed at a multi-disciplinary skull base board comprising neurosurgeons, rhinologists, neuroendocrinologists, neuroradiologists and neuropathologists, with specific expertise in skull base diseases.

Following our management protocol, each patient underwent an endocrinological evaluation to determine the pre-operative pituitary functional status. In case of clinical suspicion of hormonal hypersecretion, specific stimulation/inhibition tests were performed. All patients also underwent ophthalmological assessment with visual acuity and visual field function determination. Clinical history was collected pre-operatively with specific attention given to previous medical, surgical or radiation treatments for the PA. Each patient performed a pre-operative contrast-enhanced MRI and a CT scan for the evaluation of nasal and paranasal sinuses' anatomy. Based on the pre-operative MRI, each case was classified according to Barazi et al. to assess the morphological indication for an ETTA instead of conventional EEA (Table 1).

Our surgical technique for ETTA has been extensively reported in previous reports, both for PAs and for other neoplasms [10,19,21,29]. In brief, the patient lies in a semi-sitted position under general anesthesia and orotracheal intubation. A lumbar drain is not routinely positioned. For normally pneumatized sphenoidal sinuses, we avoid the opening of the ethmoid, limiting the approach to a large anterior sphenoidectomy with extensive drilling of the floor of the sphenoidal sinus in order to completely expose its posterior wall up the planum sphenoidalis. Conversely, in case of presence of Onodi cells or other paranasal sinuses' variants, a posterior ethmoidectomy is also performed to achieve the satisfactory exposure of the sellar bulge and tuberculum/planum notch. After bone removal and dura incision, tumor resection is performed with the standard bimanual microsurgical technique, starting with central debulking, possibly with ultrasonic aspiration (Sonopet®, Stryker Corporation, Kalamazoo, MI, USA; CUSA® NXT or CUSA® Clarity, Integra LifeSciences, Princeton, NJ, USA) for tumors with increased consistency, followed by its dissection from the neurovascular structures. Our paradigm of the skull base reconstruction technique experienced a substantial shift throughout the time span concerned, moving from a multi-layer reconstruction with fascia lata, fat, possibly bone or cartilage, and a graft of mucoperiosteum to a similar technique but using a dural substitute (Biodesign®, Cook Medical LLC, Bloomington, IN, USA) instead of fascia lata, fat, possibly bone or cartilage, covered by a naso-septal pedicled flap.

All histopathological diagnoses were retrospectively reviewed by a boarded neuropathologist (S.A.) according to the 2022 5th edition of WHO Classification of Tumors of Endocrine Organs [30]. ENT evaluation to assess the healing and remucosalization of the nasal cavity was performed one month after the procedure and as required subsequently. Bio-humoral assays, ophthalmological and neurological examinations, and post-contrast MRI were repeated 3 months after surgery and then annually.

Tumor resection was defined as radical in case of no tumor remnant at MRI at 3 months or non-radical in case a remnant tumor was detected. Clinical outcomes were evaluated based on follow-up examinations as normalized/improved, unchanged or worsened. Recurrence or tumor progression were evaluated at follow-up, as well as any following adjuvant treatment.

Table 1. Morphological classification of the PAs suitable for the ETTA approach, adapted from Barazi et al. [21].

Type 1	Ectopic peduncular or supradiaphragmatic peri-infundibular PAs, including ectopic microadenomas of the pituitary stalk or purely supradiaphragmatic macroadenomas (mostly remnant or recurrence after previous partial surgeries). These tumors are not suitable for an EEA because they have no sellar infradiaphragmatic component.
Type 2	PAs with sub-frontal extension, including macroadenomas with a supra- or infradiaphragmatic sub-frontal extension. These tumors are not fully resectable with an EEA because of their sub-frontal component, which extends anteriorly with an unfavorable angle and direction for the trans-sphenoidal approach.
Type 3	PAs presenting with a major extrasellar component, including macroadenomas with suprasellar supradiaphragmatic component exceeding the sellar volume (i.e., air balloon PAs) unlikely to be delivered through the sella with an EEA, and macroadenomas with both a large intrasellar infradiaphragmatic part and a large suprasellar supradiaphragmatic portion connected through a narrow isthmus (i.e., snowman PAs), which impairs their resection through an EEA.

2.3. Data Sources and Variables Included

Clinical, neuroradiological and surgical data, derived from the previously described pre- and post-operative examinations, were prospectively included in a digital anonymized archive.

The primary endpoint of the study was represented by the EOR rate, and the secondary endpoint consisted of the determination of the complication rate and patient endocrinological and visual outcomes. The following parameters were retrospectively collected and compared according to the study endpoints: (1) age; (2) BMI; (3) previous surgical or radiation treatments; (4) patient referral symptom leading to diagnosis; (5) pre-operative pituitary functional status; (6) pre-operative visual function; (7) tumor maximal diameters (measured in anteroposterior, laterolateral and craniocaudal extensions); (8) lesion volume;

(8) maximal cranial extension of the lesion and morphology (up to suprasellar cistern, third ventricle or foramina of Monro); (9) tumor consistency; (10) vessel encasement/engulfment; (11) subarachnoid invasion; (12) type of surgical approach; (13) tumor morphology according to Barazi et al. (Table 1) [21]; (14) skull base reconstruction technique. The rate of CSF leak was also compared between the first and second half of this patient series to assess the impact of surgeon experience and of the introduction of the naso-septal flap for this complication.

Continuous variables are outlined as mean (±standard deviation). The qualitative radiological parameters were independently evaluated by three blinded researchers (A.C., M.Z., A.R.), and a discussion took place in case of disagreement. For the continuous data collected, the mean among the three measurements was calculated and considered for statistical purposes.

2.4. Statistical Analysis

Statistical univariate analysis was performed with IBM SPSS Statistics Version 29.0.0.0 (IBM Corp. Released 2022. IBM SPSS Statistics for Mac. Armonk, NY, USA: IBM Corp.).

Normal distribution was analyzed with the Shapiro–Wilk test. According to their normal or non-normal distribution, continuous variables (age, BMI, volume, maximal diameter) were compared using Student's t-test or the Mann–Whitney U-test. Similarly, all the other categorical variables were cataloged in contingency tables according to the analyzed outcomes and compared with a chi-squared test. Parameters with significant correlation with study outcomes based on univariate analysis were further compared with a multi-variate logistic regression.

The p-value was assumed to be statistically significant at ≤ 0.05.

3. Results

In the time span included, a total of 2351 endoscopic adenomectomies were performed at our institution. After extensive review and application of the inclusion and exclusion criteria, 57 (2.4% of our case series) procedures were included in this study. Thirty-five (61.4%) patients were male, and the mean age was 54.1 ± 13.5 years.

Twenty-six (45.6%) patients were naïve for previous surgical or radiation treatments, while, as reported in Table 2, among the thirty-one patients already operated, one of them also underwent external-beam radiotherapy. The most common symptoms leading to diagnosis were visual deficits (32, 56.1%), followed by endocrinological disturbances (15, 26.3%). Of note, in six (10.5%) cases, the tumor was an incidental finding.

Table 2. Pre-operative demographic, clinical and radiological features of the included cohort. EEA: extended endoscopic endonasal approach; EA: endoscopic endonasal approach; TCA: transcranial approach; DI: diabetes insipidus.

			N, % or SD
Sex		Male	35, 61.4
		Female	22, 38.6
	Age		54.1 ± 13.5
	BMI		27.8 ± 5.4
Previous treatment		Naïve	26, 45.6
		Previous surgery	30, 52.6
		Previous surgery and radiotherapy	1, 1.8

Table 2. Cont.

		N, % or SD
Previous surgical procedure	EEA	20, 64.5
	EA + TCA	2, 6.5
	TCA	5, 16.1
	Microsurgical trans-sphenoidal	4, 12.9
First clinical manifestation	Cognitive decline	3, 5.3
	Endocrinological hyperproduction	15, 26.3
	Visual disturbances	32, 56.1
	Incidental	6, 10.5
	Headache	1, 1.8
Endocrinological hypersecretion at admission	PRL	5, 8.8
	ACTH	4, 7
	GH	4, 7
	TSH	1, 1.8
	No	43, 75.4
Endocrinological impairment at admission	Anterior partial hypopituitarism	1, 1.8
	Anterior panhypopituitarism	14, 24.6
	DI	0, 0
	Anterior partial hypopituitarism and DI	1, 1.8
	Panhypopituitarism and DI	1, 1.8
	No	40, 70.2
Visual acuity impairment at admission	Yes	6, 10.5
	No	51, 89.5
Visual field impairment at admission	Yes	34, 59.6
	No	23, 40.4
Volume, cm^3		13.8 ± 16.8
Maximal diameter, mm		30.3 ± 12.8
Cranial extension	Foramina of Monro	11, 19.3
	Third ventricle	22, 38.6
	Suprasellar cistern	24, 42.1
Morphology according to Barazi et al. [21]	Type 1	16, 28.1
	Type 2	7, 12.3
	Type 3	34, 59.6

Most PAs were non-functioning (43, 75.4%), and the remaining PAs included five PRL-secreting adenomas, four ACTH-secreting adenomas, four GH-secreting adenomas and one TSH-secreting adenoma. Pre-operative endocrinological hypopituitarism was observed in 17 cases (29.8%) and DI in 2 cases (3.5%). Pre-operative visual acuity deficits were present in 6 cases (10.5%) and field deficits in 34 cases (59.6%). The mean maximal tumor diameter was 30.3 ± 12.8 mm, and the mean tumor volume was 11.3 cm^3 ± 16.8. Their cranial extension reached the suprasellar cistern in 24 cases (42.1%), third ventricle in 22 cases (38.6%) and foramina of Monro in 11 cases (19.3%). According to Barazi et al., they can be classified as type 1 in 16 cases (28.1%), as type 2 in 7 cases (12.3%) and as type 3 in 34 cases (59.7%). Intra-operatively, 12 tumors (21.1%) were firm; vascular encasement/engulfment was observed in 9 cases (15.8%) and subarachnoid infiltration in 37 cases (64.9%) (Table 3). In 22 cases (38.6%), closure was performed with fascia lata, fat, possibly bone or cartilage, and mucoperiosteal graft. In 32 cases (56.1%), closure was performed with Biodesign, fat, possibly bone or cartilage, and a naso-septal flap.

Table 3. Intra-operative surgical findings and features of the included cohort.

		N, %
Consistency	Soft	45, 78.9
	Firm	12, 21.1
Vessel encasement/engulfment	Yes	9, 15.8
	No	48, 84.2
Subarachnoid invasion	Yes	37, 64.9
	No	20, 35.1
Type of surgical approach	ETTA	55, 96.5
	ETTA + TCA (one step)	2, 3.5
Closure with fascia lata, fat, possibly bone and cartilage, and mucoperiosteal graft	Yes	22, 38.6
	No	35, 61.4
Closure with Biodesign, fat, possibly bone and cartilage, and naso-septal flap	Yes	32, 56.1
	No	25, 43.8

Radical resection was achieved in 33 cases (57.9%), and hypersecretion was resolved in 9 cases (64.3%) (Table 4). All cases of functioning PAs not in remission after surgery only underwent a specific medical therapy, and in four cases, also irradiation (either with conventional radiotherapy, radiosurgery or adrotherapy), bringing the hypersecretion under control in all cases at follow-up. The complications consisted of one case (1.8%) of post-operative epistaxis, one case (1.8%) of meningitis requiring antibiotic treatment, two cases (3.5%) of silent lacunal ischemia of the head of caudate nucleus or the temporal pole revealed by post-operative imaging, two (3.5%) cases of transient third cranial nerve palsy (resolved at discharge), one case (1.8%) of transient diabetes insipidus (DI) resolved at discharge, six (10.5%) cases of surgical field hematomas treated conservatively in three cases and requiring surgical treatment in the other three (two through an EEA and one through a TCA). Among those, one patient (1.7.%) experienced hydrocephalus, requiring ventricular-peritoneal shunt. One patient (1.7%) with severe cardiovascular comorbidities developed a multiple-organ disfunction syndrome not related to surgical complications and passed away in ICU one month after the procedure. No cases of mortality due to surgical complications were reported.

Table 4. Surgical outcome, hypersecretion resolution and complications observed in the included cohort.

		N, %
EOR	Radical	33, 57.9
	Non-radical	24, 42.1
Hypersecretion post-operative normalization	PRL	3, 60
	ACTH	4, 100
	GH	1, 25
	TSH	1, 100
	Residual hypersecretion	5, 35.7
Complications	CSF leak	5, 8.8
	Epistaxis	1, 1.8
	Meningitis	1, 1.8
	Asymptomatic brain ischemia	2, 3.5
	Transient third cranial nerve palsy	2, 3.5
	Transient DI	1, 1.8
	Hematoma	6, 10.5
	Hydrocephalus requiring VPS	1, 1.8

Visual acuity and field deficits resolved or improved, respectively, in 2 (33.3%) and 25 (73.5%) cases, while post-operative visual acuity or field worsening was demonstrated in 2 cases each (Table 5). Conversely, a worsening of the anterior pituitary function was observed in 17 (29.8%) cases, and 15 (26.3%) patients developed a DI.

Table 5. Endocrinological and visual clinical outcomes of the included cohort.

		Normalized/Improved	Unchanged	Worsened
		N, %	N, %	N, %
Endocrinological disturbances	Intact	0, 0	22, 55	18, 45
	Anterior partial hypopituitarism	0, 0	0, 0	1, 100
	Anterior panhypopituitarism	0, 0	10, 71.4	4, 28.6
	DI	0, 0	0, 0	0, 0
	Anterior partial hypopituitarism and DI	0, 0	1, 100	0, 0
	Panhypopituitarism and DI	0, 0	0, 0	1, 100
Visual acuity deficits	Intact	0, 0	49, 86	2, 4
	Present	2, 33.3	4, 66.7	0, 0
Visual field deficits	Intact	0, 0	23, 100	0, 0
	Present	25, 73.5	7, 20.6	2, 5.9

At follow-up (mean 42.5 ± 30.7 months), three cases (5.2%) presented a recurrence after GTR, and they were treated, respectively, with radiosurgery in one case, transcranial resection in another case and further endoscopic endonasal resection in the latter case. Progression of a remnant tumor was reported in six (10.5%) cases, which was treated with irradiation in five cases (two with conventional radiotherapy and three with radiosurgery) and further standard endoscopic endonasal resection in one case. Alongside the aforementioned patient who died from cardiovascular comorbidities in the ICU, another one died from unrelated causes during follow-up. All the other patients included (96.5%) were alive at follow-up.

Statistical Analysis

According to the univariate analysis, a partial EOR correlates with previous surgeries ($p = 0.033$) and the presence of vessel encasement/engulfment ($p < 0.001$).

As reported in Table 6, higher BMI was the only parameter reported to be significantly correlated with post-operative CSF leak after ETTA ($p = 0.038$). CSF leak incidence was not reported to be significantly correlated with the skull base reconstruction technique ($p = 0.647$ and $p = 0.618$) or to exhibit differences ($p = 0.669$) between the first half of the patients treated with the ETTA approach (7.14%) and the second half (10.34%).

Table 6. Univariate analysis showing correlations between the parameters included and study outcomes (p values).

Parameter	EOR	CSF Leak	New-Onset Anterior Pituitary Impairment	New-Onset DI	Visual Acuity Outcome	Visual Field Outcome
BMI *	0.177	*0.038*	0.307	0.314	0.089	0.220
Age §	0.615	0.331	0.235	0.659	0.366	0.467
Sex	0.885	0.647	*0.034*	0.269	0.780	0.695
Volume *	0.482	0.593	0.092	*0.048*	*0.027*	0.827
Maximal diameter §	0.188	0.301	0.128	*0.006*	*0.017*	0.387
Remnant/recurrence	*0.033*	0.362	*0.049*	0.057	0.523	*0.024*
Consistency	0.972	0.719	0.067	0.534	0.781	0.061
Vessel encasement	*<0.001*	0.591	0.802	*0.030*	0.213	0.116
Subarachnoid invasion	0.174	0.332	0.558	*0.040*	0.924	0.904
TCA	0.091	0.655	0.525	*0.016*	0.064	0.177
Third ventricle extension	0.116	0.385	0.206	0.423	0.645	0.373
Morphology according to Barazi et al. [21]	0.906	0.622	0.178	0.328	0.104	0.428
Closure with fascia lata	-	0.647	-	-	-	-
Closure with naso-septal flap	-	0.618	-	-	-	-

*: Mann–Whitney U-test. §: Student's t-test.

Post-operative anterior hypopituitarism correlates with male sex ($p = 0.034$) and previous surgeries ($p = 0.049$). Conversely, the development of post-operative DI correlates with higher tumor volume ($p = 0.048$) and maximal diameter ($p = 0.006$), vessel encasement/engulfment ($p = 0.030$), subarachnoid invasion ($p = 0.040$) and inclusion of the simultaneous transcranial approach ($p = 0.016$).

An unsatisfactory visual acuity outcome, with post-operative worsening or absence of any improvement in pre-operative deficits, correlates with higher tumor volume ($p = 0.027$) and maximal diameter ($p = 0.017$). Similarly, an unsatisfactory visual field outcome is reported to be linked to previous surgeries ($p = 0.024$).

The multi-variate analysis performed by means of a logistic regression did not disclose any significant correlation.

4. Discussion

In our study, we demonstrated on a large series of 57 patients with PAs operated through an ETTA that this approach can both represent a valid alternative and an effective complementary route for the TCA, with a radical resection rate of 57.9% (33 cases) and hypersecretion resolution in 64.3% of cases (9 out of 14). Indeed, the ETTA has proved not only to allow the surgeon to manage through a trans-sphenoidal route those adenomas not approachable with a standard EEA and otherwise requiring a TCA (for example, because of their purely supradiaphragmatic location or due to atypical irregular morphology); it was also proved that the ETTA can be combined with a TCA, as reported in two cases in our series, for those asymmetrical tumors whose lateral extension would represent a limit for the ETTA. This is, to our knowledge, the largest surgical case series focusing on ETTA, which includes and compares all the different types of PAs suitable for the approach and discusses their indications.

4.1. Classification, Surgical Indications and EOR

The indications for an ETTA for PAs have been controversial in clinical practice and in the dedicated literature, and few studies have specifically considered this topic [16,17,20,21]. While well established in clinical practice for complex anterior skull base neoplasms, the ETTA conflicts with some fundamental principles of pituitary surgery, such as avoidance of diaphragm violation, with the consequent intra-operative CSF leak, and selective tumor resection, with the sparing of the gland and stalk structures to preserve the endocrinological function. Moreover, in the vast majority of cases, PAs—also including large or giant tumors—arise inside the sella from the pituitary gland, and they usually extend toward the suprasellar space in a caudocranial direction, displacing the diaphragm upwards. Therefore, after central debulking of the intrasellar part, the dome progressively descends in a downward direction, increasing its likelihood of being delivered through a conventional endoscopic endonasal approach without any need for a supradiaphragmatic extension. It has been hypothesized that less than 10% of PAs have an unsuitable morphology for a conventional EEA, thus requiring an alternative route, such as the TCA [31,32]. In 2013, Barazi et al. proposed that for these rare and selected cases unsuitable for a standard EEA, the ETTA could be considered as an alternative to the TCA, combining the advantages of the trans-sphenoidal corridor with the possibility to resect supradiaphragmatic PAs (Figure 1). Our series confirms that only few cases require this extended approach, accounting for 2.4% in our series of 2351 endoscopic endonasal adenomectomies, which should be considered exclusively for those cases with peculiar features, which makes them unapproachable with an EEA, which remains the first choice for PAs. In particular, based on the tumor location and morphology, these authors identify three possible types of PAs potentially suitable for the ETTA.

Ectopic peduncular or supradiaphragmatic peri-stalk PAs (Type 1, Table 1, Figure 2) are uncommon occurrences, as represented in our series (16, 28.1%), mostly including 5 (31.3%) ectopic secreting microadenomas of the pituitary stalk and 11 (68.7%) remnants or recurrences after previous partial surgeries of purely supradiaphragmatic macroadenomas. These tumors are not suitable for a conventional EEA because of the lack of any sellar infradiaphragmatic component, thus requiring a complete supradiaphragmatic corridor.

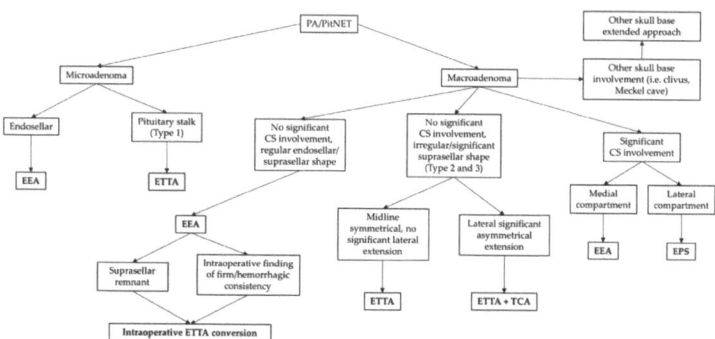

Figure 1. Illustrative flow chart of our general decisional algorithm for PA surgical management. Each approach should be tailored to the clinical–radiological features and intra-operative findings of the individual case. CS: cavernous sinus; EEA: standard endoscopic endonasal approach; EPS: ethmoidopterygosphenoidal approach [33]; ETTA: endoscopic endonasal transplanum–transtuberculum approach; TCA: transcranial approach.

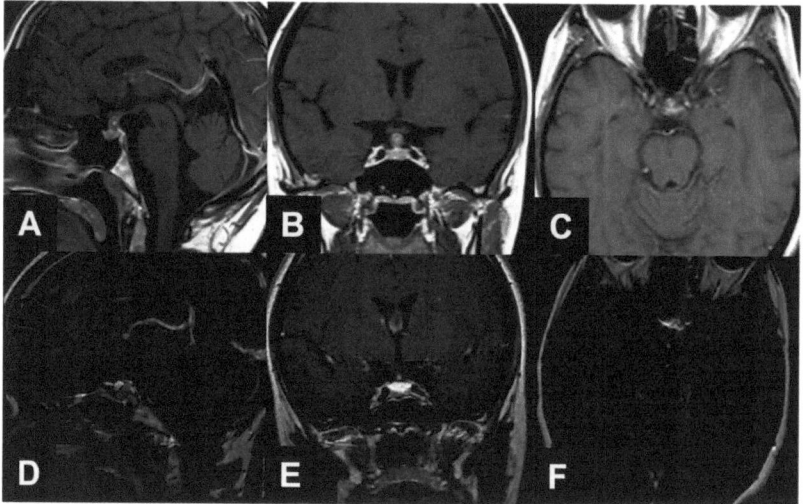

Figure 2. Illustrative case of a Type 1 sec. Barazi PA suitable for ETTA. (**A**–**C**) Midsagittal (**A**), coronal (**B**) and axial (**C**) pre-operative contrast-enhanced T1-weighted MR images of a 35-year-old female complaining of visual field disturbances, with a clinically manifest bitemporal hemianopsia. Imaging and laboratory exams reported a non-functioning supradiaphragmatic macroadenoma along the pituitary stalk, slightly compressing the optic chiasm. She underwent ETTA, which achieved radical resection with an unremarkable clinical course and a resolution of pre-operative symptomatology. (**D**–**F**) Midsagittal (**D**), coronal (**E**) and axial (**F**) post-operative contrast-enhanced T1-weighted MR images.

PAs with sub-frontal extension (Type 2, Table 1, Figure 3) are rare tumors (7, 12.3%) with a supra- or infradiaphragmatic sub-frontal extension, which extends rostrally up or beyond the tuberculum sellae, which prevents this portion from descending into the intrasellar cavity during tumor resection and which would require an unfavorable approach direction for a conventional EEA.

Finally, the most common indication for an ETTA was represented in our series by PAs presenting with a major extrasellar component (34, 59.6%) (Type 3, Table 1, Figure 4), such as macroadenomas with a suprasellar supradiaphragmatic component exceeding the sellar volume (i.e., air balloon PAs) unlikely to be delivered through the sella with an EEA, and macroadenomas with both a large intrasellar infradiaphragmatic part and a large suprasellar supradiaphragmatic portion connected through a narrow isthmus (i.e., snowman PAs), which impairs their resection through an EEA.

In some cases, a firm consistency may prevent the dome of the tumor from descending into the surgical cavity, and we primarily prefer to avoid extending the approach to these cases, instead using angled instruments and scopes to entirely remove the tumor. However, we noted that an increased consistency was reported in a significant number of PAs (21.1%), confirming that these tumors represent a challenge for the pituitary surgeon.

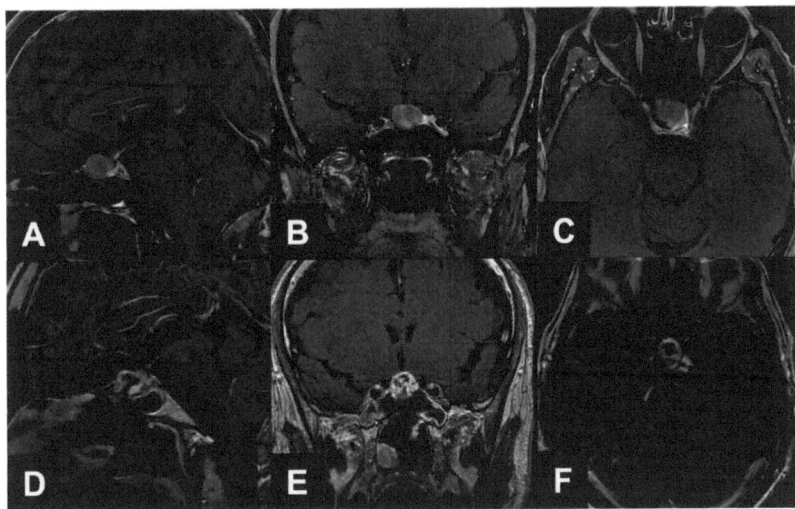

Figure 3. Illustrative case of a Type 2 sec. Barazi PA suitable for ETTA. (**A–C**) Midsagittal (**A**), coronal (**B**) and axial (**C**) pre-operative contrast-enhanced T1-weighted MR images of a 63-year-old male patient previously treated with a standard endoscopic endonasal approach for a non-functioning pituitary macroadenoma. Years later, a linearly progressing supradiaphragmatic recurrence with sub-frontal extension was observed. He underwent ETTA, which achieved near-radical resection (a small remnant was revealed with post-operative imaging posteriorly) with an unremarkable clinical course. (**D–F**) Midsagittal (**D**), coronal (**E**) and axial (**F**) post-operative contrast-enhanced T1-weighted MR images.

The flexibility of the approach, developed as an extension of the standard endoscopic endonasal route, also provides an opportunity for intra-operative conversion if required by the neoplasm features and surgical findings. Although in many cases, an ETTA is planned from the very beginning of the procedure (purely supradiaphragmatic neoplasms, major suprasellar extension), in other cases, where the standard endoscopic endonasal approach fails to achieve a satisfactory result (i.e., firm consistency of the neoplasm, non-descending diaphragm leading to suprasellar remnants), it can be intra-operatively extended to the ETTA to gain access to the supradiaphragmatic space. It is therefore our standard practice to preserve the septal mucosa during the first steps of every PA resection procedure, in case the harvesting of the naso-septal flap would later be unexpectedly necessary.

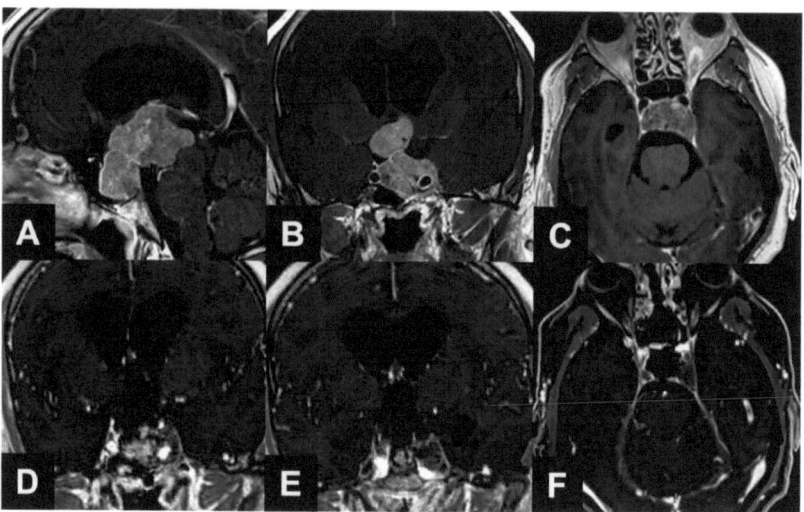

Figure 4. Illustrative case of a Type 3 sec. Barazi PA suitable for ETTA. (**A–C**) Midsagittal (**A**), coronal (**B**) and axial (**C**) pre-operative contrast-enhanced T1-weighted MR images of a 40-year-old male patient complaining of cognitive decline and urinary incontinence. Imaging and laboratory exams reported a non-functioning macroadenoma with a significant suprasellar portion, obliterating the third ventricle and causing hydrocephalus (Type 3). Visual examination revealed bitemporal hemianopsia. He underwent ETTA, which achieved near-radical resection (a small remnant was revealed with post-operative imaging near the left cavernous sinus). The patient experienced severe panhypopituitarism and diabetes insipidus, which required persistent complete substitution therapy; conversely, a complete resolution of pre-operative visual field deficit, as well as cognitive and urinary symptomatology was observed. (**D–F**) Coronal (**D,E**) and axial (**F**) post-operative contrast-enhanced T1-weighted MR images.

Radical resection was achieved in 57.9% of cases, in line with previous reports [17]. This result should be outlined in the context of a highly complex case series, encompassing very large lesions with atypical morphology, vessel encasement and a significant number of secondary treatments. Indeed, comparing these results with those reported for the TCA series, we can observe a comparable degree of resection [32,34–36]. In our study, surgery for remnants and recurrences was observed to be a predictor of PR ($p = 0.033$), probably due to the presence of adherences and scarring from previous approaches, precluding optimal and safe surgical maneuvers [37]. Moreover, a close vessel relationship was also a factor precluding GTR ($p < 0.001$), considering that surgical dissection around major cranial vessels is extremely challenging, even for experienced hands [38]. It is also conceivable that advanced intra-operative imaging tools, such as intra-operative MRI, although never used in our surgical series, could help the surgeon increase the EOR by means of locating small remnants in the surgical cavity not detected by the surgeon's eye, as reported in the literature [39,40]. Conversely, this could lengthen the duration of the procedure.

Although the ETTA represents an excellent extracranial approach for the suprasellar space, avoiding any brain retraction or vasculo-nervous manipulation, it poses an intrinsic drawback for the more lateral tumor extension than the carotid and the optic nerve planes. In these cases, the TCA could be proposed as a complementary approach to the ETTA (Figure 5) [41]. The lateral growing pattern of the neoplasm usually provides a "natural" surgical corridor for the TCA, while the ETTA helps the surgeon resect and debulk the median and paramedian part of the lesion, addressing the deepest intra- and suprasellar portion abutting the chiasm or the third ventricle from the ventral corridor, allowing for the achievement of a greater EOR and reducing the risk of recurrence [42]. However, it should be remarked that in our series, we noted that the combination of an ETTA with a TCA would add significant morbidity, namely increasing the risk of post-operative DI ($p = 0.018$) [43]. Therefore, the choice of a combined TCA–ETTA approach should be balanced in an optimal risk–benefit assessment.

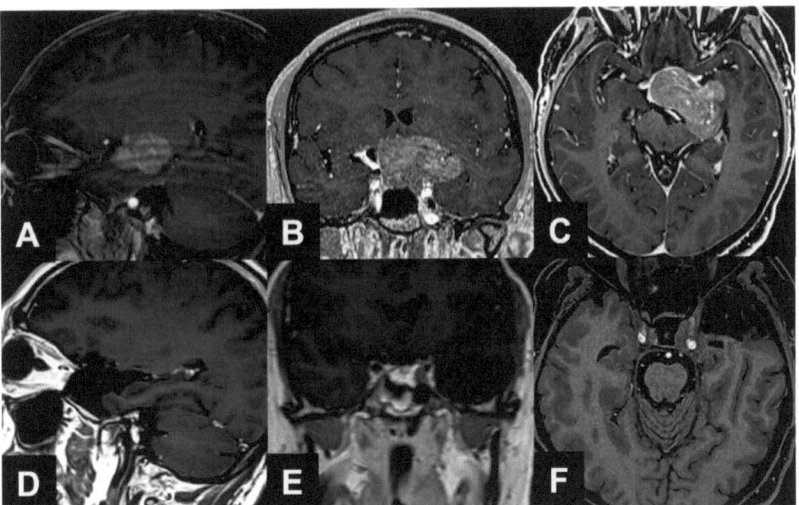

Figure 5. Illustrative case of a large PA suitable for combined ETTA–TCA. (**A**–**C**) Parasagittal (**A**), coronal (**B**) and axial (**C**) pre-operative contrast-enhanced T1-weighted MR images of a 55-year-old male patient complaining of visual disturbances, with a clinically manifest bitemporal hemianopsia and left eye visual impairment consistent with second left cranial nerve involvement. Imaging and laboratory exams reported a non-functioning macroadenoma with a significant left lateral extension, invading and obliterating the ipsilateral basal cisterns. He underwent ETTA with a left TCA in the same surgical session, which achieved near-radical resection. Two millimetric remnants were revealed with post-operative imaging at the level of left cavernous sinus and interpeduncular cistern. The patient experienced a clinically silent left temporal pole ischemia, severe post-operative panhypopituitarism and diabetes insipidus, which required persistent complete substitution therapy; conversely, a complete resolution of pre-operative visual acuity and field deficits was observed. (**D**–**F**) Parasagittal (**D**), coronal (**E**) and axial (**F**) post-operative contrast-enhanced T1-weighted MR images.

4.2. Surgical Complications

The incidence of post-operative CSF leak in our case series was 8.7% (five cases). All of them underwent a prompt endoscopic endonasal revision, and none of them developed meningitis. These results are in line with those reported by Khan et al., who assessed a pooled CSF leak incidence of 9% in a recent systematic review of extended endonasal approaches [44]. Indubitably, this rate is higher than those reported for conventional EEA, and this represents the main disadvantage of this approach. Throughout the years, the developing surgical experience and skills and the introduction of innovative repair techniques for large osteo-dural defects, such as the naso-septal flap, have led to an evolution in our techniques for skull base reconstruction. In our series, we observed no significant difference in CSF leak rates when comparing patients who underwent reconstruction with different techniques, as well as between the first and the second half of the case series. The only predictor of CSF leak was represented by higher BMI, which was also recognized as a negative prognostic factor in other series of endoscopic endonasal skull base cases [45–47]. Moreover, a careful management of post-operative nasal care, with periodic saline irrigation and ENT evaluations, allows the patients to preserve an acceptable quality of life during the uncomfortable phase of crusting and nasal remucosalization, quantified over three months [21,48,49].

Other complications were represented by the following incidences of 1.8% of post-operative epistaxis, 1.8% of meningitis requiring antibiotic treatment, 3.5% of asymptomatic brain ischemia, 3.5% of transient third cranial nerve palsy and 10.5% of surgical field hematomas, which required surgical treatment in 50% of cases. Analyzing the non-negligible incidence of surgical field hematomas, the remnant tumor apoplexy could be hypothesized as a strong risk factor for this occurrence. Unexpectedly, in only three cases (out of a total of six experiencing post-operative hemorrhages) was a non-radical resection performed. It is our opinion that, despite tumor remnant apoplexy being a crucial issue very well known to pituitary surgeons, the suprasellar, subarachnoid extension of our approach could slightly increase per se the risk factor for post-operative bleeding, unavoidably manipulating small capillaries and branches of hypophyseal arteries, which could bleed in a large emptied post-operative surgical cavity. Conversely, a resection as extensive as permitted, respecting vascular anatomy, should be the primary concern for the pituitary surgeon to also decrease the occurrence of swelling and bleeding of the remnant (especially in those cases, where a gross total resection is not amenable), whose risk, although reducible, could never be zero. The incidence of these complications represents a consequence of the expansion of the surgical approach into the supradiaphragmatic space. Comparing our complication rates with other ETTA series, we observe a similar incidence [21,50,51], and it is important to remark that they are in line with the overall complication rates of the TCA approaches, confirming that, although the ETTA has a higher complication rate compared to the EAA, it is not more unfavorable than the TCA [32].

4.3. Clinical Outcome

The most significant advantage of the ETTA is represented by the favorable clinical outcome. Full or partial regression of pre-operative visual acuity and field symptoms was observed in, respectively, 33.3% and 73.5% of cases. As reported by many authors, early decompression of the optic structures and vessel-preserving dissection enabled by the ETTA are the key features determining such positive results, which are significantly superior to the TCA for sellar and suprasellar pathologies [50,52,53]. Similarly, our endocrinological outcome, with 26.3% of new-onset DI and 29.8% of anterior pituitary function worsening, seems not to be inferior to the TCA [54].

In the context of an optimal multi-disciplinary management, the individuation of the predictors of visual and endocrinological post-operative impairment is crucial. In our cohort, the major predictors of post-operative DI were the volume ($p = 0.048$), maximal diameter ($p = 0.006$), vessel encasement ($p = 0.030$), subarachnoid invasion ($p = 0.040$) and inclusion of the TCA ($p = 0.016$). Neurohypophysis and pituitary stalk are delicate structures, which are strongly affected when performing the ETTA. If in smaller lesions, namely Type 1 and 2, the stalk can be visualized, dissected and preserved early, in larger invasive lesions, it is displaced, and it can be inadvertently harmed after surgical maneuvers and dissection [55]. Similarly, lesions with vessel encasement and subarachnoid invasion require prolonged surgical maneuvering, increasing the risk of meningo-hypophysial artery damage with consequent pituitary function deficits. Similarly, the neurovascular manipulation and dissection unavoidable in transcranial approaches represents a negative prognostic predictor of post-operative DI development. The predictors of unsatisfactory visual outcomes were larger lesion volume ($p = 0.027$), diameter ($p = 0.017$) and re-do surgery ($p = 0.024$) for comparable reasons with the involvement of optic nerves, chiasm and tracts.

4.4. Strengths and Limitations

The main strength of this study is that all the patients were treated and managed in the same referral center by a highly specialized multi-disciplinary team according to the same established surgical core principles (with expected improvements and implementations throughout the years), with adequate homogeneity. Moreover, despite its observational retrospective design, no patients were excluded from the study for lacking essential data. Conversely, the cohort size (even in a large referral center for pituitary neoplasms) precludes us from performing an effective advanced statistical analysis, such as a multi-variate analysis, limiting the generalizability of our findings, especially in a heterogenous cohort. Moreover, a thorough analysis of the post-operative endocrinological management of hypersecreting adenomas, progression-free survival for remnants and adjuvant treatments is beyond the scope of this paper.

5. Conclusions

In our study, we observed and highlighted in a large cohort that the ETTA can also play a significant role in PAs surgery, and it should be part of the pituitary surgeons' armamentarium. Indeed, it has both an alternative and complementary role with the TCA, expanding the indications of the endoscopic trans-sphenoidal approach to complex PAs unsuitable for the EEA, and it can also be combined with a TCA for tumors with significant lateral extension. Without the ETTA, the only surgical option for the management of those PAs would have been the transcranial route—either standalone or combined with a standard endoscopic endonasal approach—with major invasivity.

However, it should be considered that the ETTA presents a higher rate of complications— particularly the post-operative CSF leak—than the standard EEA, suggesting that it should be reserved for the few selected cases with strict indications. For these tumors, such morbidity is balanced by the advantages afforded by the EEA, with a favorable patient outcome and with particularly satisfactory visual and endocrinological results.

The identification of pre-operative factors predicting complications and unsuccessful outcomes (mainly re-do surgeries for recurrences, larger lesions, higher BMI, subarachnoid invasion and strict vessel relationship) is crucial for providing an accurate patient-tailored treatment and an optimal post-operative management. Further, multi-centric studies are warranted for a better characterization of those features.

Author Contributions: Conceptualization, A.C., M.Z. and D.M.; Methodology, M.Z. and D.M.; Validation, A.C.; Formal Analysis, A.C. and M.Z.; Investigation, A.C., M.Z., A.R. and S.A.; Resources, F.G., S.A., M.F.-F., E.P. and D.M.; Data Curation, A.C.; Writing—Original Draft Preparation, A.C. and M.Z.; Writing—Review and Editing, F.G., G.S., A.R., S.A., M.F.-F., E.P. and D.M.; Visualization, A.C. and M.Z.; Supervision, D.M.; Project Administration, D.M. All authors have read and agreed to the published version of the manuscript.

Funding: The authors declare that no funds, grants or other support was received.

Institutional Review Board Statement: The authors declare that the study was conducted according to the guidelines of the Declaration of Helsinki, and institutional review board approval for this study was waived because of its retrospective observational design.

Informed Consent Statement: The authors declare that informed consent for this study was waived because of its retrospective observational design.

Data Availability Statement: The authors declare that the gathered data included and used for the analysis outline are available in the manuscript. Further datasets are available upon reasonable request from the corresponding author.

Conflicts of Interest: The authors declare that they have no conflict of interest.

References

1. Weiss, M.H. Transnasal transsphenoidal approach. In *Surgery of the Third Ventricle*; Williams & Wilkins: Baltimore, MA, USA, 1987; pp. 476–494.
2. Couldwell, W.T.; Weiss, M.H.; Rabb, C.; Liu, J.K.; Apfelbaum, R.I.; Fukushima, T. Variations on the standard transsphenoidal approach to the sellar region, with emphasis on the extended approaches and parasellar approaches: Surgical experience in 105 cases. *Neurosurgery* **2004**, *55*, 539–547. [CrossRef]
3. Fatemi, N.; Dusick, J.R.; de Paiva Neto, M.A.; Kelly, D.F. The endonasal microscopic approach for pituitary adenomas and other parasellar tumors: A 10-year experience. *Neurosurgery* **2008**, *63*, 244–256. [CrossRef] [PubMed]

4. Hashimoto, N.; Handa, H.; Yamagami, T. Transsphenoidal extracapsular approach to pituitary tumors. *J. Neurosurg.* **1986**, *64*, 16–20. [CrossRef] [PubMed]
5. Kato, T.; Sawamura, Y.; Abe, H.; Nagashima, M. Transsphenoidal-transtuberculum sellae approach for supradiaphragmatic tumours: Technical note. *Acta Neurochir.* **1998**, *140*, 715–718. [CrossRef]
6. Kouri, J.G.; Chen, M.Y.; Watson, J.C.; Oldfield, E.H. Resection of suprasellar tumors by using a modified transsphenoidal approach. Report of four cases. *J. Neurosurg.* **2000**, *92*, 1028–1035. [CrossRef]
7. Maira, G.; Anile, C.; Rossi, G.F.; Colosimo, C. Surgical treatment of craniopharyngiomas: An evaluation of the transsphenoidal and pterional approaches. *Neurosurgery* **1995**, *36*, 715–724. [CrossRef] [PubMed]
8. Mason, R.B.; Nieman, L.K.; Doppman, J.L.; Oldfield, E.H. Selective excision of adenomas originating in or extending into the pituitary stalk with preservation of pituitary function. *J. Neurosurg.* **1997**, *87*, 343–351. [CrossRef]
9. Jho, H.D.; Carrau, R.L. Endoscopic endonasal transsphenoidal surgery: Experience with 50 patients. *J. Neurosurg.* **1997**, *87*, 44–51. [CrossRef]
10. Cappabianca, P.; Frank, G.; Pasquini, E.; de Divitiis, O.; Calbucci, F. Extended endoscopic endonasal transsphenoidal approaches to the suprasellar region, planum sphenoidale & clivus. In *Endoscopic Endonasal Transsphenoidal Surgery*; de Divitiis, E., Cappabianca, P., Eds.; Springer: Vienna, Austria, 2003; pp. 176–187. [CrossRef]
11. de Divitiis, E.; Cappabianca, P.; Cavallo, L.M.; Esposito, F.; de Divitiis, O.; Messina, A. Extended endoscopic transsphenoidal approach for extrasellar craniopharyngiomas. *Neurosurgery* **2007**, *61*, 219–227. [CrossRef]
12. de Divitiis, E.; Cavallo, L.M.; Cappabianca, P.; Esposito, F. Extended endoscopic endonasal transsphenoidal approach for the removal of suprasellar tumors: Part 2. *Neurosurgery* **2007**, *60*, 46–58. [CrossRef]
13. de Divitiis, E.; Cavallo, L.M.; Esposito, F.; Stella, L.; Messina, A. Extended endoscopic transsphenoidal approach for tuberculum sellae meningiomas. *Neurosurgery* **2008**, *62*, 1192–1201. [CrossRef] [PubMed]
14. Giammattei, L.; Starnoni, D.; Cossu, G.; Bruneau, M.; Cavallo, L.M.; Cappabianca, P.; Meling, T.R.; Jouanneau, E.; Schaller, K.; Benes, V.; et al. Surgical management of Tuberculum sellae Meningiomas: Myths. facts, and controversies. *Acta Neurochir.* **2020**, *162*, 631–640. [CrossRef] [PubMed]
15. Kulwin, C.; Schwartz, T.H.; Cohen-Gadol, A.A. Endoscopic extended transsphenoidal resection of tuberculum sellae meningiomas: Nuances of neurosurgical technique. *Neurosurg. Focus* **2013**, *35*, E6. [CrossRef] [PubMed]
16. Chibbaro, S.; Signorelli, F.; Milani, D.; Cebula, H.; Scibilia, A.; Bozzi, M.T.; Messina, R.; Zaed, I.; Todeschi, J.; Ollivier, I.; et al. Primary Endoscopic Endonasal Management of Giant Pituitary Adenomas: Outcome and Pitfalls from a Large Prospective Multicenter Experience. *Cancers* **2021**, *13*, 3603. [CrossRef]
17. Di Maio, S.; Cavallo, L.M.; Esposito, F.; Stagno, V.; Corriero, O.V.; Cappabianca, P. Extended endoscopic endonasal approach for selected pituitary adenomas: Early experience. *J. Neurosurg.* **2011**, *114*, 345–353. [CrossRef]
18. Mascarenhas, L.; Moshel, Y.A.; Bayad, F.; Szentirmai, O.; Salek, A.A.; Leng, L.Z.; Hofstetter, C.P.; Placantonakis, D.G.; Tsiouris, A.J.; Anand, V.K.; et al. The Transplanum Transtuberculum Approaches for Suprasellar and Sellar-Suprasellar Lesions: Avoidance of Cerebrospinal Fluid Leak and Lessons Learned. *World Neurosurg.* **2014**, *82*, 186–195. [CrossRef]
19. Mazzatenta, D.; Zoli, M.; Frank, G.; Pasquini, E. Transnasal Endoscopic Transplanum/Transtuberculum Approach in Pituitary Adenomas. In *Endoscopic Sinus Surgery: Anatomy, Three-Dimensional Reconstruction, and Surgical Technique*, 4th ed.; Thieme: Stuttgart, Germany, 2017.
20. Solari, D.; D'Avella, E.; Bove, I.; Cappabianca, P.; Cavallo, L.M. Extended endonasal approaches for pituitary adenomas. *J. Neurosurg. Sci.* **2021**, *65*, 160–168. [CrossRef]
21. Barazi, S.A.; Pasquini, E.; D'Urso, P.I.; Zoli, M.; Mazzatenta, D.; Sciarretta, V.; Frank, G. Extended endoscopic transplanum-transtuberculum approach for pituitary adenomas. *Br. J. Neurosurg.* **2013**, *27*, 374–382. [CrossRef]
22. Cavallo, L.M.; Messina, A.; Esposito, F.; de Divitiis, O.; Fabbro, M.D.; de Divitiis, E.; Cappabianca, P. Skull base reconstruction in the extended endoscopic transsphenoidal approach for suprasellar lesions. *J. Neurosurg.* **2007**, *107*, 713–720. [CrossRef]
23. Cavallo, L.M.; Solari, D.; Somma, T.; Cappabianca, P. The 3F (Fat, Flap, and Flash) Technique for Skull Base Reconstruction After Endoscopic Endonasal Suprasellar Approach. *World Neurosurg.* **2019**, *126*, 439–446. [CrossRef]
24. Eloy, J.A.; Choudhry, O.J.; Shukla, P.A.; Kuperan, A.B.; Friedel, M.E.; Liu, J.K. Nasoseptal flap repair after endoscopic transsellar versus expanded endonasal approaches: Is there an increased risk of postoperative cerebrospinal fluid leak? *Laryngoscope* **2012**, *122*, 1219–1225. [CrossRef] [PubMed]
25. Eloy, J.A.; Shukla, P.A.; Choudhry, O.J.; Singh, R.; Liu, J.K. Challenges and surgical nuances in reconstruction of large planum sphenoidale tuberculum sellae defects after endoscopic endonasal resection of parasellar skull base tumors. *Laryngoscope* **2013**, *123*, 1353–1360. [CrossRef] [PubMed]
26. Jin, B.; Wang, X.-S.; Huo, G.; Mou, J.-M.; Yang, G. Reconstruction of skull base bone defects using an in situ bone flap after endoscopic endonasal transplanum-transtuberculum approaches. *Eur. Arch. Otorhinolaryngol.* **2020**, *277*, 2071–2080. [CrossRef]
27. Liu, J.K.; Schmidt, R.F.; Choudhry, O.J.; Shukla, P.A.; Eloy, J.A. Surgical nuances for nasoseptal flap reconstruction of cranial base defects with high-flow cerebrospinal fluid leaks after endoscopic skull base surgery. *Neurosurg. Focus* **2012**, *32*, E7. [CrossRef] [PubMed]
28. Tosaka, M.; Prevedello, D.M.; Yamaguchi, R.; Fukuhara, N.; Miyagishima, T.; Tanaka, Y.; Aihara, M.; Shimizu, T.; Yoshimoto, Y. Single-Layer Fascia Patchwork Closure for the Extended Endoscopic Transsphenoidal Transtuberculum Transplanum Approach: Deep Suturing Technique and Preliminary Results. *World Neurosurg.* **2021**, *155*, e271–e284. [CrossRef]

29. Frank, G.; Pasquini, E.; Doglietto, F.; Mazzatenta, D.; Sciarretta, V.; Farneti, G.; Calbucci, F. The endoscopic extended transsphenoidal approach for craniopharyngiomas. *Neurosurgery* 2006, *59*, ONS75-83. [CrossRef]
30. WHO Classification of Tumours Online. Available online: https://tumourclassification.iarc.who.int/welcome/# (accessed on 11 June 2023).
31. Zhu, J.; Wang, Z.; Zhang, Y.; Liu, J.; Li, X.; Deng, K.; Lu, L.; Yao, Y. Suprasellar pituitary adenomas: A 10-year experience in a single tertiary medical center and a literature review. *Pituitary* 2020, *23*, 367–380. [CrossRef]
32. Buchfelder, M.; Kreutzer, J. Transcranial surgery for pituitary adenomas. *Pituitary* 2008, *11*, 375–384. [CrossRef]
33. Frank, G.; Pasquini, E. Endoscopic endonasal approaches to the cavernous sinus: Surgical approaches. *Neurosurgery* 2002, *50*, 675. [CrossRef]
34. Guan, X.; Wang, Y.; Zhang, C.; Ma, S.; Zhou, W.; Jia, G.; Jia, W. Surgical Experience of Transcranial Approaches to Large-to-Giant Pituitary Adenomas in Knosp Grade 4. *Front. Endocrinol.* 2022, *13*, 857314. [CrossRef]
35. Yaşargil, M.G. Transcranial Surgery for Large Pituitary Adenomas. In *Microneurosurgery*, 4th ed.; Thieme: New York, NY, USA, 1996; pp. 200–204.
36. Guidetti, B.; Fraioli, B.; Cantore, G.P. Results of surgical management of 319 pituitary adenomas. *Acta Neurochir.* 1987, *85*, 117–124. [CrossRef] [PubMed]
37. Pérez-López, C.; Palpán, A.J.; Saez-Alegre, M.; Zamarrón, Á.; Alfonso, C.; Álvarez-Escola, C.; Isla, A. Volumetric Study of Nonfunctioning Pituitary Adenomas: Predictors of Gross Total Resection. *World Neurosurg.* 2021, *147*, e206–e214. [CrossRef]
38. Gellner, V.; Tomazic, P.V. Limits of the endoscopic transnasal transtubercular approach. *J. Neurosurg. Sci.* 2018, *62*, 297–300. [CrossRef] [PubMed]
39. Serra, C.; Burkhardt, J.-K.; Esposito, G.; Bozinov, O.; Pangalu, A.; Valavanis, A.; Holzmann, D.; Schmid, C.; Regli, L. Pituitary surgery and volumetric assessment of extent of resection: A paradigm shift in the use of intraoperative magnetic resonance imaging. *Neurosurg. Focus* 2016, *40*, E17. [CrossRef]
40. Staartjes, V.E.; Togni-Pogliorini, A.; Stumpo, V.; Serra, C.; Regli, L. Impact of intraoperative magnetic resonance imaging on gross total resection, extent of resection, and residual tumor volume in pituitary surgery: Systematic review and meta-analysis. *Pituitary* 2021, *24*, 644–656. [CrossRef]
41. Cossu, G.; Jouanneau, E.; Cavallo, L.M.; Froelich, S.; Starnoni, D.; Giammattei, L.; Harel, E.; Mazzatenta, D.; Bruneau, M.; Meling, T.R.; et al. Surgical management of giant pituitary neuroendocrine tumors: Meta-analysis and consensus statement on behalf of the EANS skull base section. *Brain Spine* 2022, *2*, 100878. [CrossRef]
42. Lee, M.H.; Lee, J.H.; Seol, H.J.; Lee, J.-I.; Kim, J.H.; Kong, D.-S.; Nam, D.-H. Clinical Concerns about Recurrence of Non-Functioning Pituitary Adenoma. *Brain Tumor Res Treat.* 2016, *4*, 1–7. [CrossRef]
43. Wang, S.; Li, D.; Ni, M.; Jia, W.; Zhang, Q.; He, J.; Jia, G. Clinical Predictors of Diabetes Insipidus After Transcranial Surgery for Pituitary Adenoma. *World Neurosurg.* 2017, *101*, 1–10. [CrossRef] [PubMed]
44. Khan, D.Z.; Ali, A.M.S.; Koh, C.H.; Dorward, N.L.; Grieve, J.; Horsfall, H.L.; Muirhead, W.; Santarius, T.; Van Furth, W.R.; Najafabadi, A.H.Z.; et al. Skull base repair following endonasal pituitary and skull base tumour resection: A systematic review. *Pituitary* 2021, *24*, 698–713. [CrossRef] [PubMed]
45. Dlouhy, B.J.; Madhavan, K.; Clinger, J.D.; Reddy, A.; Dawson, J.D.; O'Brien, E.K.; Chang, E.; Graham, S.M.; Greenlee, J.D.W. Elevated body mass index and risk of postoperative CSF leak following transsphenoidal surgery. *J. Neurosurg.* 2012, *116*, 1311–1317. [CrossRef]
46. Fraser, S.; Gardner, P.A.; Koutourousiou, M.; Kubik, M.; Fernandez-Miranda, J.C.; Snyderman, C.H.; Wang, E.W. Risk factors associated with postoperative cerebrospinal fluid leak after endoscopic endonasal skull base surgery. *J. Neurosurg.* 2018, *128*, 1066–1071. [CrossRef] [PubMed]
47. Ivan, M.E.; Iorgulescu, J.B.; El-Sayed, I.; McDermott, M.W.; Parsa, A.T.; Pletcher, S.D.; Jahangiri, A.; Wagner, J.; Aghi, M.K. Risk factors for postoperative cerebrospinal fluid leak and meningitis after expanded endoscopic endonasal surgery. *J Clin Neurosci.* 2015, *22*, 48–54. [CrossRef] [PubMed]
48. Schreiber, A.; Bertazzoni, G.; Ferrari, M.; Rampinelli, V.; Verri, P.; Mattavelli, D.; Fontanella, M.; Nicolai, P.; Doglietto, F. Nasal Morbidity and Quality of Life After Endoscopic Transsphenoidal Surgery: A Single-Center Prospective Study. *World Neurosurg.* 2019, *123*, e557–e565. [CrossRef] [PubMed]
49. Georgalas, C.; Badloe, R.; van Furth, W.; Reinartz, S.; Fokkens, W.J. Quality of life in extended endonasal approaches for skull base tumours. *Rhinology* 2012, *50*, 255–261. [CrossRef]
50. Cavallo, L.M.; Frank, G.; Cappabianca, P.; Solari, D.; Mazzatenta, D.; Villa, A.; Zoli, M.; D'Enza, A.I.; Esposito, F.; Pasquini, E. The endoscopic endonasal approach for the management of craniopharyngiomas: A series of 103 patients. *J. Neurosurg.* 2014, *121*, 100–113. [CrossRef]
51. Solari, D.; d'Avella, E.; Agresta, G.; Catapano, D.; D'Ecclesia, A.; Locatelli, D.; Massimi, L.; Mazzatenta, D.; Spena, G.; Tamburrini, G.; et al. Endoscopic endonasal approach for infradiaphragmatic craniopharyngiomas: A multicentric Italian study. *J. Neurosurg.* 2023, *138*, 522–532. [CrossRef]
52. Komotar, R.J.; Starke, R.M.; Raper, D.M.S.; Anand, V.K.; Schwartz, T.H. Endoscopic endonasal compared with microscopic transsphenoidal and open transcranial resection of giant pituitary adenomas. *Pituitary* 2012, *15*, 150–159. [CrossRef]
53. Müslüman, A.M.; Cansever, T.; Yılmaz, A.; Kanat, A.; Oba, E.; Çavuşoğlu, H.; Sirinoğlu, D.; Aydın, Y. Surgical results of large and giant pituitary adenomas with special consideration of ophthalmologic outcomes. *World Neurosurg.* 2011, *76*, 141–148. [CrossRef]

54. Graillon, T.; Castinetti, F.; Fuentes, S.; Gras, R.; Brue, T.; Dufour, H. Transcranial approach in giant pituitary adenomas: Results and outcome in a modern series. *J. Neurosurg. Sci.* **2020**, *64*, 25–36. [CrossRef]
55. Kinoshita, Y.; Taguchi, A.; Tominaga, A.; Sakoguchi, T.; Arita, K.; Yamasaki, F. Predictive factors of postoperative diabetes insipidus in 333 patients undergoing transsphenoidal surgery for non-functioning pituitary adenoma. *Pituitary* **2022**, *25*, 100–107. [CrossRef]

Disclaimer/Publisher's Note: The statements, opinions and data contained in all publications are solely those of the individual author(s) and contributor(s) and not of MDPI and/or the editor(s). MDPI and/or the editor(s) disclaim responsibility for any injury to people or property resulting from any ideas, methods, instructions or products referred to in the content.

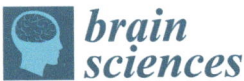

Article

Endoscopic Endonasal Approach in Craniopharyngiomas: Representative Cases and Technical Nuances for the Young Neurosurgeon

Jorge F. Aragón-Arreola, Ricardo Marian-Magaña, Rodolfo Villalobos-Diaz, Germán López-Valencia, Tania M. Jimenez-Molina, J. Tomás Moncada-Habib, Marcos V. Sangrador-Deitos and Juan L. Gómez-Amador *

Department of Neurosurgery at National Institute of Neurology and Neurosurgery "Manuel Velasco Suárez", Mexico City P.C. 14260, Mexico; jaragon@innn.edu.mx (J.F.A.-A.); ricardomarian@neurocirugia-innn.com (R.M.-M.); rvillalobos@innn.edu.mx (R.V.-D.); glopezv@innn.edu.mx (G.L.-V.); tjimenezmolina@innn.edu.mx (T.M.J.-M.); jmoncadahabib@innn.edu.mx (J.T.M.-H.); msangrador@innn.edu.mx (M.V.S.-D.)
* Correspondence: jlga@neurocirugia-innn.com; Tel.: +52-55-5416-5276

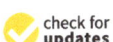

Citation: Aragón-Arreola, J.F.; Marian-Magaña, R.; Villalobos-Diaz, R.; López-Valencia, G.; Jimenez-Molina, T.M.; Moncada-Habib, J.T.; Sangrador-Deitos, M.V.; Gómez-Amador, J.L. Endoscopic Endonasal Approach in Craniopharyngiomas: Representative Cases and Technical Nuances for the Young Neurosurgeon. *Brain Sci.* **2023**, *13*, 735. https://doi.org/10.3390/brainsci13050735

Academic Editor: Miguel Lopez-Gonzalez

Received: 19 March 2023
Revised: 11 April 2023
Accepted: 12 April 2023
Published: 28 April 2023

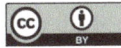

Copyright: © 2023 by the authors. Licensee MDPI, Basel, Switzerland. This article is an open access article distributed under the terms and conditions of the Creative Commons Attribution (CC BY) license (https://creativecommons.org/licenses/by/4.0/).

Abstract: Craniopharyngiomas (CPs) are Rathke's cleft-derived benign tumors originating most commonly in the dorsum sellae and representing 2% of intracranial neoplasms. CPs represent one of the more complex intracranial tumors due to their invasive nature, encasing neurovascular structures of the sellar and parasellar regions, making its resection a major challenge for the neurosurgeon with important postoperative morbidity. Nowadays, an endoscopic endonasal approach (EEA) provides an "easier" way for CPs resection allowing a direct route to the tumor with direct visualization of the surrounding structures, diminishing inadvertent injuries, and providing a better outcome for the patient. In this article, we include a comprehensive description of the EEA technique and nuances in CPs resection, including three illustrated clinical cases.

Keywords: craniopharyngioma; endoscopic; infundibulum

1. Introduction

Craniopharyngiomas (CPs) are benign intracranial extra-axial tumors (OMS grade I) that originate from remnants of the Rathke's cleft, representing 2% of all intracranial neoplasms, with an estimated incidence of 0.17 to 0.2 and prevalence of 4.78 per 100,000 [1].

Surgical management of CPs is challenging because of the vicinity to critical neurovascular structures, demanding a thorough understanding of the anatomy of the suprasellar region. The extension of the tumor in relation to the optic chiasm, pituitary gland and stalk, hypothalamus, carotid artery, and anterior cerebral artery complex is essential for surgical planning. Surgical options include transcranial and endonasal endoscopic approaches (EEA) [2].

EEA provides a direct route to the sellar region, with improved midline exposure without retraction of brain parenchyma and neurovascular structures, obtaining a better visualization. This approach is ideal for lesions without significant lateral growth and retrosellar CPs with suprasellar third ventricular extension [3,4].

The aim of this study is to familiarize young neurosurgeons with the anatomy of the sellar and suprasellar region, as well as the advantages of EEA in the resection of craniopharyngiomas. This remains paramount as endoscopic resection techniques have become an accessible option for all neurosurgeons, making it necessary to master dissection techniques to preserve critical neurovascular structures when facing CPs.

2. Materials and Methods

A comprehensive description of the surgical EEA in CPs is deeply analyzed by summarizing the technique and detailing a step-by-step approach based on the senior author's experience in our hospital. For its comprehensive description, the technique was divided into nasal, sphenoidal, sellar, and closure phases. Three illustrative clinical cases are included.

3. Results

3.1. Endoscopic Endonasal Approach

In the operative room, the patient is positioned supine with the head tilted 15 degrees away from the surgeon so the nasal fossae are facing the endoscope's trajectory. The trunk is elevated 20 to 30 degrees in order to aid venous return. The patient's head is in neutral position when our target is the sellar region, and extended 10 to 30 degrees or flexed 20 to 40 degrees when the target is located in the anterior fossa or the clival region, respectively. Perioperative steroids (100 mg hydrocortisone) are administered, as well as a single dose of broad-spectrum antibiotics. Topical nasal decongestant is employed in order to reduce nasal bleeding. It is important to consider preparing the abdominal wall and outer thigh in an antiseptic manner since abdominal fat and fascial graft may be used for reconstruction [5,6].

The EEA is divided into four phases: nasal, sphenoidal, sellar/parasellar, and closure.

3.1.1. Nasal Phase

A 0-degree endoscope is introduced into one nostril to identify the relevant anatomy (superior, middle, and inferior turbinates laterally, nasal septum medially, and the choana posteroinferiorly) [7]. The superior and middle turbinates are landmarks to identify the sphenoid ostium and both turbinates are coagulated and lateralized with blunt dissection, avoiding mucosal injury. The sphenoid ostium is identified 1.5 cm above the choana. A nasoseptal flap is harvested, as described elsewhere [8], if needed. The flap can be harvested at the beginning of the procedure, or after tumor resection in case of cerebrospinal fluid (CSF) leak, and should be tucked into the choana for protection during the operation [9]. The next step is to expose the sphenoidal rostrum, removing the mucosa in order to detach the nasal septum and vomer with a dissector. About 1.0 to 1.5 cm of the posterior nasal septum is removed for simultaneous access to the sphenoid sinus through both nasal nostrils.

3.1.2. Sphenoidal Phase

The anterior wall of the sphenoid sinus is enlarged circumferentially, preserving the sphenopalatine artery which is located inferolaterally [2]. The sphenoid rostrum is removed using Kerrison rongeurs and high-speed drills. It is imperative to know the anatomy of the sphenoid sinus and its variants: "sellar", "pre-sellar", and "conchal" types (Figure). Pre-sellar and conchal variantes are not absolute contraindications to perform an EEA and, in these cases, the bone is removed through careful drilling and employing neuronavigation. Mucosa within the sphenoid sinus is removed to reduce the risk of postoperative mucocele [10]. There are septations inside the sphenoid sinus that must be removed carefully, being aware that 20% of septations lead to a cavernous carotid protuberance [7].

3.1.3. Sellar Phase

A 4 mm diamond burr is preferred to make an initial opening of the pituitary fossa, as the sellar floor can be thin and partially dehiscent because of chronic remodeling by a large intrasellar mass. The durotomy is usually carried out with a sickle or retractable knife in a cruciate fashion, starting in the middle sector and extending it with angled microscissors in a cruciform fashion. After the dura is opened and hemostasis is achieved, exploration of the intrasellar mass depends on the nature of the pathologic process. For a large mass, as CPs, with a cystic and solid component, resection begins in the inferior and lateral portions of the tumor to allow the superior aspect to descend into the surgical field at last. If the superior portion is delivered first, diaphragmatic descent will obscure the operative field. If the tumor has a suprasellar component, the diaphragm can be sharply dissected and incised. Most CPs are soft in consistency and the resection is usually performed with a variety of microdissectors, ringed curettes, and suction cannulas. On the other hand, if the tumor has a harder consistency, it can be removed with the aid of an ultrasonic aspirator. After tumor removal, exploration of the surgical field with the 0-degree or 30-degree endoscope is mandatory to look for any residual tumor [11].

3.1.4. Closure

In case of a CSF leak, there are two well-described techniques: the gasket seal and the multilayered technique. The gasket seal method consists in placing a piece of allograft dural substitute over the bony defect so that its dimensions exceed that of the defect by at least 1 cm circumferentially. A rigid implant cut to fit the opening is then placed over the dural substitute and counter-sunk within the bony defect [12,13]. The multilayered reconstruction consists of placing layers in apposition to one another, the first being an inlay dural substitute, followed by an onlay fascia lata graft, thereby potentially obviating the need for a rigid buttress [13]. The nasoseptal flap is placed over the preferred method so that the flap is in direct contact with the surrounding bony skull base and is subsequently held in place with fibrin glue. In cases with no evident CSF leak, a free mucosal graft from the middle turbinate or nasal floor can be placed alone over the surgical cavity and held in place with absorbable nasal packing [14].

3.2. Representative Clinical Cases

3.2.1. Case 1

A 24-year-old man with a previous history of incomplete transcranial resection of a CP was admitted to the emergency department with a 3-month history of progressive visual loss, nausea, and vomiting. Neurological examination revealed a Glasgow Coma Scale of 14, pupils of 4 mm with poor light response, and no motor or peripheral sensory deficits. Endocrinological examination was relevant only for central hypothyroidism. An MRI was performed (Figure 1), revealing a T1 hypointense and T2 hyperintense large sellar and suprasellar cystic, lobulated lesion, with significant upward displacement of the third ventricular floor. An EEA was performed on this patient, using the technique described previously (Figure 2 and Video S1). Following a dural opening, the cyst wall was punctured, releasing a motor-oil-like liquid content. After cyst drainage, meticulous debulking of the solid component of the tumor with ringed curettes was performed. Finally, the sellar floor was reconstructed in a multilayered fashion. Postoperative CT showed no evident residual tumor. Postoperatively, the patient developed transient diabetes insipidus (DI), which was satisfactorily managed with oral desmopressin, and he was discharged from the hospital on the fifth postoperative day.

3.2.2. Case 2

A 34-year-old woman with complaints of headache and bilateral loss of visual acuity in the last year, presented to our emergency department due to acute onset of gait disturbance and sleepiness. Upon arrival, an urgent CT scan was performed, revealing an isodense mass in the sellar and suprasellar region with calcifications, conditioning obstructive hydrocephalus. An emergent ventriculoperitoneal shunt was placed. Endocrinological testing revealed low levels of thyroid-stimulating hormone, cortisol, and free thyroxine, so hormonal replacement therapy was initiated before surgical treatment was deemed safe. Brain MRI revealed a hypo and hyper-intense lesion on T1 and T2-weighted MRI, respectively, compatible with a cystic lesion located in the sellar region and extending upward into the third ventricle with brainstem displacement (Figure 3). The patient underwent resection of the lesion by an endoscopic extended transplanum–transtuberculum approach as shown in Figure 4 and Video S2. The patient developed DI postoperatively and received subcutaneous desmopressin. No cerebrospinal fluid leakage was observed postoperatively. A vision assessment 6 months postoperatively showed no changes in visual acuity.

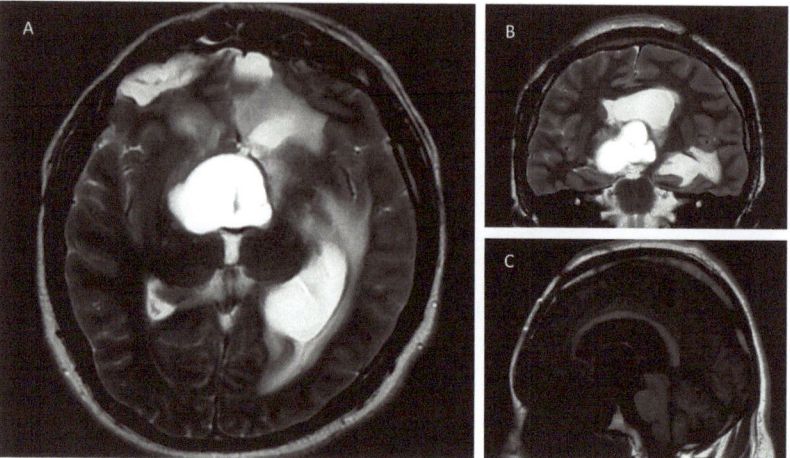

Figure 1. Axial (**A**) and coronal (**B**) T2-weighted MRI demonstrates a sellar lesion with suprasellar extension composed predominantly of a T2 hyperintense cystic component. Image (**A**) also shows dilatation of the left temporal horn of the lateral ventricle and postsurgical changes in both frontal lobules. In Image (**B**) the cystic and lobulated features of the lesion are seen. (**C**): Sagittal T1 weighted MRI image shows a hypointense cystic sellar lesion with upward displacement of the third ventricle.

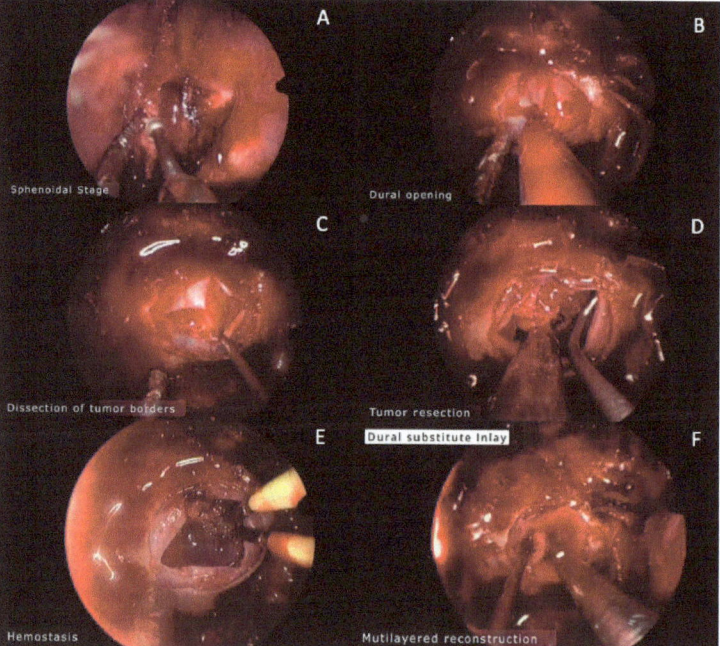

Figure 2. Intraoperative images. (**A**) Drilling the sphenoidal rostrum. (**B**) Dural opening in cruciform fashion using no. 11 blade. (**C**) Dissection of the tumor borders away from the dura mater using a fine microdissector. (**D**) Tumor resection begins from the inferior and lateral components in order to avoid the superior component of the tumor that obstructs the surgeon's view. (**E**) Hemostasis. (**F**) Multilayered reconstruction.

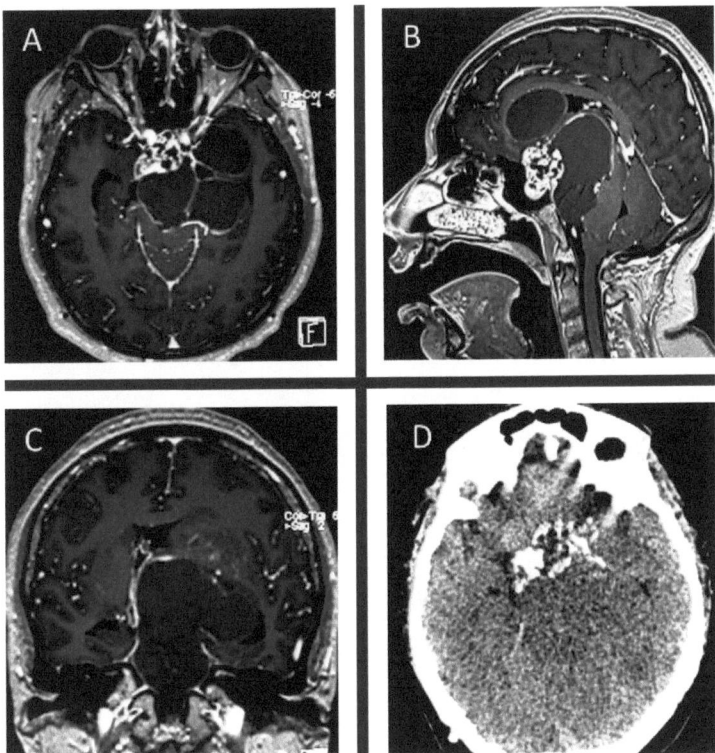

Figure 3. Axial (**A**), sagittal (**B**), and coronal (**C**) T1-post contrast MRI images show a mixed cystic-solid mass with a solid sellar, heterogeneously enhancing component, associated with a massive suprasellar and parasellar cystic, peripherally enhancing component extending upward into the third ventricle and displacing backwardly the brainstem. Axial, non-contrast CT (**D**) shows a hypodense sellar mass associated with massive peripheral calcifications.

3.2.3. Case 3

A 19-year-old man was referred to our hospital for endocrinological evaluation due to delayed pubertal development. Hormonal tests were performed revealing low testosterone, thyroxine, and cortisol levels. The patient reported a 2-month history of asthenia, polyuria, polydipsia, and blurred vision. Neurological examination was relevant for decreased bilateral visual acuity and bitemporal hemianopsia. Brain MRI revealed a sellar and suprasellar hypointense lesion on T1W, mixed iso and hyperintense lesion on T2W and FLAIR, and heterogeneous enhancement on postcontrast sequence, suggestive of a cystic lesion with a solid sellar component (Figure 5). The patient underwent transsphenoidal endoscopic resection of the lesion wranssellarsellar approach as shown in Figure 6 and Video S3. After opening the cyst wall, the solid component of the lesion was drained, which had a greenish and muddy appearance, but was otherwise easily aspirable. The solid intratumoral content was removed using ringed curettes and suction, followed by capsule mobilization and sharp extracapsular dissection employing pituitary rongeurs and microscissors. Finally, a multilayered reconstruction of the sellar floor was performed. The patient had an uneventful postoperative course and, during the follow-up appointment, he reported significant vision improvement. Histopathologic evaluation reported an adamantinomatous CP and the patient was referred to radiosurgery for adjuvant treatment.

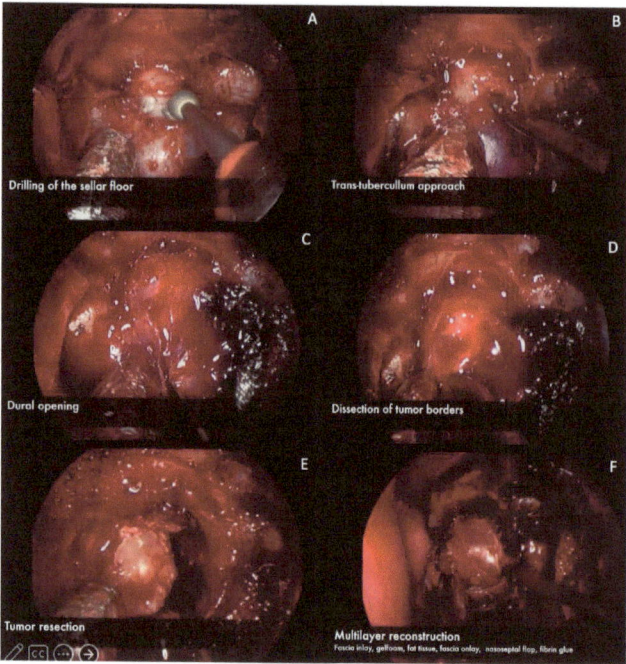

Figure 4. Intraoperative images. (**A**) Drilling of the sellar floor using a diamond drill. (**B**) In this case it was necessary to remove the tuberculum sellae because of the tumor size, using a diamond drill and rongeurs. (**C**) Dural opening in a cruciform manner. (**D**) Dissection of tumor borders away from the durI (**E**) Tumor resection. (**F**) Multilayer reconstruction (In-lay fascia, gelfoam, fat tissue, On-lay fascia, nasoseptal flap, and fibrin glue).

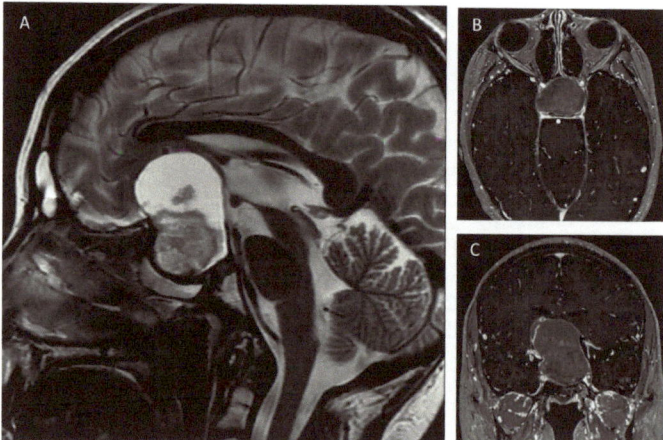

Figure 5. Sagittal T2-weighted MRI image (**A**) shows a large sellar and suprasellar mass with components of different signal characteristics. An isointense component relative to brain parenchyma is located predominantly in the sellar region, which is associated with an hyperintense cystic component in its superior aspect. Axial (**B**) and coronal (**C**) T1-post contrast MRI image reveals a sellar and suprasellar mass, with areas of peripheral and central enhancement. In image (**C**), a constriction of the mass at the level of the diaphragma sellae is seen.

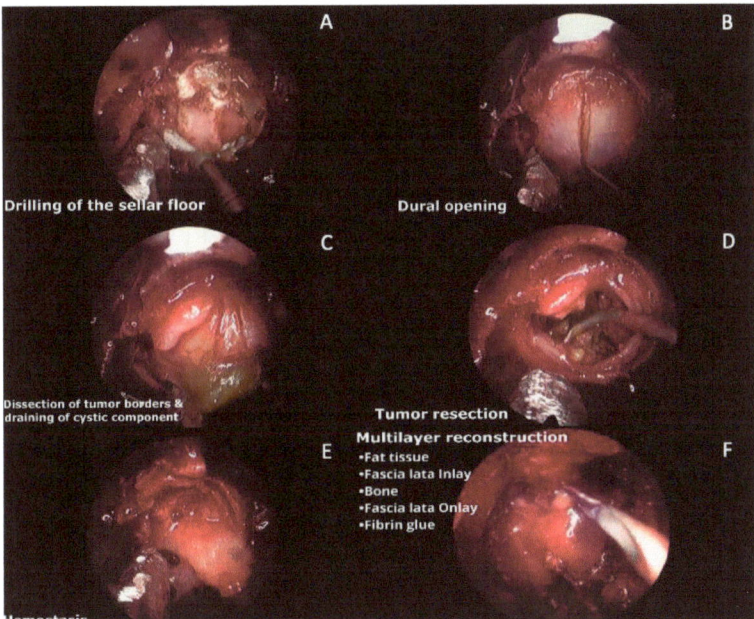

Figure 6. Intraoperative images. (**A**) Drilling of the sellar floor with a diamond drill. (**B**) Dural opening in a cruciform manner using a no. 11 blade. (**C**). Dissection of the tumor borders away from the dura, and, in this case, the cystic component was opened and suctioned. (**D**) Tumor resection of the lateral and superior parts until identification of the arachnoid layer Ip. (**E**) Hemostasis. (**F**) Multilayer reconstruction (fat tissue inside the sella, in-lay fascia lata, bone (gasket technique), on-lay fascia lata, and fibrin glue).

4. Discussion

CPs represent quite challenging lesions that require multidisciplinary management. What has been theorized and later proven to be the advantage of the extended endonasal endoscopic approach (EEEA) for resection of CPs is that gross total resection (GTR) is more achievable with this technique, having ranges of up to 70% in some series [3,15,16]. One of the key factors to determine whether an EEEA is feasible is preoperative evaluation of the lesion, with many details to pay attention to. However, many authors have consistently described the most important characteristics as the position of the optic chiasm (OC), the pituitary stalk (PS), and the invasion of the lateral compartments [2,17,18]. Many classifications have been suggested for surgical approach decisions, being one of the most iconic the one proposed by Kassam and the Pittsburgh group in 2008, dividing these lesions into four categories, according to the relation to pituitary stalk and naming grade IV the lesions that are exclusively in the third ventricle [17]. These grade IV lesions have been suggested to be better reached through transcranial approaches. Although some authors are exploring the capability of doing it purely endonasal in a safe manner, this remains one of the limitations of an EEEA for the treatment of purely intraventricular CPs [17]. Recent publications affirm that retrochiasmatic CPs with extension to the third ventricle can be successful reached via EEA; however, as we previously mentioned, this statement should be taken carefully. From this perspective, the European Association of Neurosurgical Societies still recommends the transcranial approach for intraventricular CPs [19–21].

One of the key considerations for surgeons in their learning curve is to divide the invasion of the tumor into infra and supra diaphragmatic compartments. Originally, only tumors in the infradiaphragmatic compartment were removed with the EEA but, as more experience was obtained, the supradiaphragmatic lesions started to be treated this way [22]. Doing a thorough analysis of the preoperative MRI is key to making the most optimal decision for the approach.

Understanding each stage during the endonasal approach is essential for the young neurosurgeon. The nasal stage is usually performed by an ENT surgeon in most centers, although the anatomical knowledge and technique mastering is a great ability to achieve as a neurosurgeon. CSF leak is one of the most prevalent complications of these approaches and, historically, the use of nasoseptal flap (NSF) had proven to reduce CSF leak rates in all kinds of endonasal approaches [8,23].

For lesions extending to the suprasellar compartment, we must try to harvest an NSF from the beginning of the nasal step. This NSF is usually harvested from the side which will undergo less manipulation depending on the lateral invasion of the tumor. As we mentioned, the NSF is a crucial step in the prevention of CSF leak and meningitis hence for its correct realization technique must be well understood and dominated by the surgeon [23,24].

During the sphenoidal phase, widening the opening on the sphenoid rostrum is an advisable behavior with the goal to attain freedom of movement in the field with the tools. This will strongly depend on the sinus pneumatization but should not be a limitation to accomplishing a sufficient opening and a comfortable setup. Anatomical knowledge plays a crucial role and landmark identification will consist the main goal of the sinus stage in which the visualization of the sella turcica, tuberculum sellae, planum sphenoidale, and other landmarks, gives the surgeon the confidence and safety needed to continue with the approach [25]. Some less pneumatized sinuses will offer a harder challenge for less experienced surgeons. In these cases, neuronavigation may come as a very useful tool.

In the sellar stage, opening the sella turcica is usually done with a high-speed drill to thin the bone and after making a small opening, the use of angled dissectors may constitute a safe way to continue with the already thinned bone removal. Approaching the lateral limits of the boney opening, rongeurs are usually used taking special care to remove these portions with small bites avoiding the use of excessive force, further drilling may be used to thin the bone and see through the structures behind these lateral portions of the bone removal. The visualization of the anterior compartment of the cavernous sinus should be the goal permitting early coagulation but this can be tailored for each specific tumor invasion [3].

The goal is to find a safe and direct route to the tumor. Usually, the tumor is not adherent in its whole circumference and classical CPs show most adherent parts in the hypothalamus, which is to be expected when taking into consideration the origin of the lesion. Even when preoperative hypothalamic disfunction exists by tumor compression, this part of the lesion should be always evaluated with direct sight of the adherences, and should be dissected when possible, either bluntly or preferably sharply, since sharp dissection needs the least amount of traction to bring the lesion into the field. Sometimes, it is preferable to leave a small tumor capsule cuff when none of these techniques can be performed in a safe manner. This point can be debatable as some authors prefer to reach GTR if any preoperative sign of hypothalamic involvement exists [26].

Retracting or manipulating the tumor is thought to be a risky maneuver but it is nonetheless unavoidable in some instances, when this situation is presented, it is advisable to never pull the tumor without pushing the tissue you are trying to separate it from. This creates a pivot point that is usually in the field and on sight, rather than a blind spot that can be an important structure (i.e., carotid or hypothalamus). We usually call this maneuver traction–countertraction.

It has been proposed in the literature a useful classification for endoscopic endonasal surgery according to the degree of technical complexity, taking into account two main factors: the affected compartment (for example, pituitary fossa or cavernous sinus) and the pathology in question, as shown in Table 1 [27,28]. As can be seen, although craniopharyngiomas are classified in grade II of technical complexity when they are limited to the pituitary fossa, their invasive nature could classify them in a higher grade when they extend to the interpeduncular cistern. This classification must be known and used by young neurosurgeons in the planning of resection of these complex tumors, permitting them to visualize the anatomical corridors and associated structures compromised by the tumor and prepare the necessary endoscopic equipment for the procedure.

Table 1. CSF. Cerebrospinal fluid, ACo. Anterior communicating artery.

Level	Compartment	Pathology
	Modified Level of Complexity in Endoscopic Endonasal Surgery	
I	Extradural	CSF leak Chordoma Carcinoma
II	Pituitary fossa	Pituitary adenoma Craniopharyngioma Meningioma
III	Anterior skull base floor	Esthesioneuroblastoma Fibrous displasia
IV	Orbit Pterygo-pallatine fossa Maxillary sinus	Trigeminal Schwannoma
V	Cisterns Interpeduncular fossa Clivus	Craniopharyngioma Chordoma Pituitary adenoma
VI	Cavernous sinus	Pituitary adenoma Hemangioblastoma Meningioma
VII	Vascular	Paraclinoid aneurysm ACo aneurysm Basilar aneurysm Vertebral aneurysm
VIII	Intrinsic	Cavernoma Metastasis Glioma

Accordingly, young neurosurgeons must keep in mind that these approaches require a steep learning curve, which may be associated with an increase in complication rates as the surgeon obtains experience. Therefore, to minimize surgical morbidity, it is highly advised to acquire surgical experience and technical competency from less complex pathologies in a step-by-step fashion before proceeding to the most technically demanding ones [27,28]. As previously noted, the technical complexity and degree of expertise needed for endoscopic resection of craniopharyngiomas are highly variable depending on the tumor location, extension, and relationships with neurovascular structures [3,16,20]. Consequently, we have found it useful to divide the endoscopic endonasal approaches for craniopharyngiomas into different categories of progressive technical complexity and expertise required, as initially proposed by Baldauf et al. [3] and subsequently modified in the present article Table 2.

A suggested strategy is to first acquire experience with intrasellar and intra-suprasellar lesions before moving to more complex procedures such as suprasellar craniopharyngiomas (Category C), often requiring an extended approach, intradural tumor dissection and exposure of neurovascular structures. Additionally, the importance of laboratory training with anatomical models and cadaveric dissections cannot be over-emphasized, as well as assisting/observing experienced surgeons before attempting these procedures. Finally, it is essential for young neurosurgeons to recognize their limitations and to not hesitate in performing a transcranial approach when the case complexity is beyond their endoscopic capabilities [27,28].

Table 2. Modified from Baldauf et al. [3]. References [16,17,20,22,27–30].

Category	Tumor Location/Extension	Technical Nuances
A	Intrasellar/infradiaphragmatic	Anatomic relationships similar to that of pituitary adenomas. The sellar floor is enlarged providing enough space for resection and, thus, facilitating the approach.
B	Intra-suprasellar/infradiaphragmatic	Neurovascular structures in the suprasellar side of the tumor protected by the diaphragm. Sufficient space between pituitary gland and the optic chiasm for tumor resection.
C	Suprasellar/preinfundibular or transinfundibular	An extended endoscopic endonasal approach is required. Size of the sella is often normal or reduced, resulting in a narrower approach due to closeness of the two intracavernous carotids. Arteries of the circle of Willis are often displaced by the suprasellar mass.
D	Suprasellar/retroinfundibular	Requires a more posterior approach. Stretch relationship with important neurovascular structures such as the mammillary bodies and basilar apex. Requires a pituitary transposition, increasing the technical complexity of the approach.
E	Arising or extending into the third ventricle	Risk of injury to the hypothalamus, brainstem, and other important neurovascular structures. Increased risk for CSF fistula due to communication of the ventricular cavity with the sphenoid sinus.

5. Conclusions

CPs continue to be a high-complexity intracranial pathology despite advances in neurosurgery, nevertheless as EEAs evolve this technique offers greater advantages over the conventional transcranial approaches, allowing a better visualization of the tumor and its relationships with neurovascular structures surrounding it, thus contributing to achieve a GTR whenever possible. A comprehensive knowledge of this technique and its nuances, in conjunction with intensive laboratory training, is fundamental for young neurosurgeons who aim to perform these approaches. Finally, it should be noted that these approaches require a long learning curve, hence, the acquisition of surgical skills and experience from less complex cases is imperative before moving to the most challenging ones, and should be recognized that some cases may be better managed transcranially if the surgeon feels more comfortable and experienced with this approach.

Supplementary Materials: The following supporting information can be downloaded at: https://www.mdpi.com/article/10.3390/brainsci13050735/s1, Video S1: Caso 1; Video S2: Caso 2; Video S3: Caso 3.

Author Contributions: Conceptualization, J.F.A.-A., R.M.-M., and J.L.G.-A.; methodology J.T.M.-H. and G.L.-V.; software, R.V.-D.; validation, J.L.G.-A. and R.M.-M.; formal analysis, R.M.-M., R.V.-D. and J.F.A.-A.; investigation, J.F.A.-A.; resources, M.V.S.-D.; data curation, R.V.-D. and R.M.-M.; writing—original draft preparation, J.L.G.-A., J.F.A.-A., R.M.-M., R.V.-D. and T.M.J.-M.; writing—review and editing, M.V.S.-D.; visualization, J.L.G.-A.; supervision, J.L.G.-A. All authors have read and agreed to the published version of the manuscript.

Funding: This research received no external funding.

Institutional Review Board Statement: Not applicable.

Informed Consent Statement: Informed consent was obtained from all subjects involved in the study. Written informed consent has been obtained from the patients to publish this paper.

Data Availability Statement: Not applicable.

Conflicts of Interest: The authors declare no conflict of interest.

References

1. Al-Dahmani, K.; Mohammad, S.; Imran, F.; Theriault, C.; Doucette, S.; Zwicker, D.; Yip, C.E.; Clarke, D.B.; Imran, S.A. Sellar Masses: An Epidemiological Study. *Can. J. Neurol. Sci.* **2016**, *43*, 291–297. [CrossRef]
2. Cavallo, L.M.; Somma, T.; Solari, D.; Iannuzzo, G.; Frio, F.; Baiano, C.; Cappabianca, P. Endoscopic Endonasal Transsphenoidal Surgery: History and Evolution. *World Neurosurg.* **2019**, *127*, 686–694. [CrossRef]
3. Baldauf, J.; Hosemann, W.; Schroeder, H.W.S. Endoscopic Endonasal Approach for Craniopharyngiomas. *Neurosurg. Clin. N. Am.* **2015**, *26*, 363–375. [CrossRef]
4. Liu, J.K.; Sevak, I.A.; Carmel, P.W.; Eloy, J.A. Microscopic versus endoscopic approaches for craniopharyngiomas: Choosing the optimal surgical corridor for maximizing extent of resection and complication avoidance using a personalized, tailored approach. *Neurosurg. Focus* **2016**, *41*, E5. [CrossRef]
5. Jho, H.-D. Endoscopic transsphenoidal surgery. *J. Neuro-Oncol.* **2001**, *54*, 187–195. [CrossRef]
6. Zador, Z.; Gnanalingham, K. Endoscopic Transnasal Approach to the Pituitary—Operative Technique and Nuances. *Br. J. Neurosurg.* **2013**, *27*, 718–726. [CrossRef]
7. Youmans, J.R. *Youmans and Winn Neurological Surgery*; Winn, H.R., Ed.; Elsevier: Amsterdam, The Netherlands, 2022.
8. Hadad, G.; Bassagasteguy, L.; Carrau, R.L.; Mataza, J.C.; Kassam, A.; Snyderman, C.H.; Mintz, A. A Novel Reconstructive Technique after Endoscopic Expanded Endonasal Approaches: Vascular Pedicle Nasoseptal Flap. *Laryngoscope* **2006**, *116*, 1882–1886. [CrossRef]
9. Kulwin, C.; Schwartz, T.H.; Cohen-Gadol, A.A. Endoscopic extended transsphenoidal resection of tuberculum sellae meningiomas: Nuances of neurosurgical technique. *Neurosurg. Focus* **2013**, *35*, E6. [CrossRef]
10. Conger, A.R.; Lucas, J.; Zada, G.; Schwartz, T.H.; Cohen-Gadol, A.A. Endoscopic extended transsphenoidal resection of craniopharyngiomas: Nuances of neurosurgical technique. *Neurosurg. Focus* **2014**, *37*, E10. [CrossRef]
11. Santos, R.D.P.; Zymberg, S.T.; Filho, J.Z.A.; Gregório, L.C.; Weckx, L.L.M. Endoscopic Transnasal Approach to Sellar Tumors. *Braz. J. Otorhinolaryngol.* **2007**, *73*, 463–475. [CrossRef]
12. Leng, L.Z.; Brown, S.; Anand, V.K.; Schwartz, T.H. "Gasket-Seal" Watertight Closure in Minimal-Access Endoscopic Cranial Base Surgery. *Oper. Neurosurg.* **2008**, *62*, ONSE342–ONSE343. [CrossRef]
13. Navarro, V.G.; Anand, V.K.; Schwartz, T.H. Gasket Seal Closure for Extended Endonasal Endoscopic Skull Base Surgery: Efficacy in a Large Case Series. *World Neurosurg.* **2013**, *80*, 563–568. [CrossRef]
14. Scagnelli, R.J.; Patel, V.; Peris-Celda, M.; Kenning, T.J.; Pinheiro-Neto, C.D. Implementation of Free Mucosal Graft Technique for Sellar Reconstruction after Pituitary Surgery: Outcomes of 158 Consecutive Patients. *World Neurosurg.* **2019**, *122*, e506–e511. [CrossRef]
15. Komotar, R.J.; Starke, R.M.; Raper, D.M.; Anand, V.K.; Schwartz, T.H. Endoscopic Endonasal Compared with Microscopic Transsphenoidal and Open Transcranial Resection of Craniopharyngiomas. *World Neurosurg.* **2012**, *77*, 329–341. [CrossRef]
16. Cavallo, L.M.; Prevedello, D.M.; Solari, D.; Gardner, P.A.; Esposito, F.; Snyderman, C.H.; Carrau, R.L.; Kassam, A.B.; Cappabianca, P. Extended endoscopic endonasal transsphenoidal approach for residual or recurrent craniopharyngiomas. *J. Neurosurg.* **2009**, *111*, 578–589. [CrossRef]
17. Kassam, A.B.; Gardner, P.A.; Snyderman, C.H.; Carrau, R.L.; Mintz, A.H.; Prevedello, D.M. Expanded endonasal approach, a fully endoscopic transnasal approach for the resection of midline suprasellar craniopharyngiomas: A new classification based on the infundibulum. *J. Neurosurg.* **2008**, *108*, 715–728. [CrossRef]
18. Tang, B.; Xie, S.H.; Xiao, L.M.; Huang, G.L.; Wang, Z.G.; Yang, L.; Yang, X.Y.; Xu, S.; Chen, Y.Y.; Ji, Y.Q.; et al. A Novel Endoscopic Classification for Craniopharyngioma Based on Its Origin. *Sci. Rep.* **2018**, *8*, 10215. [CrossRef]
19. Na, M.K.; Jang, B.; Choi, K.S.; Lim, T.H.; Kim, W.; Cho, Y.; Shin, H.G.; Ahn, C.; Kim, J.G.; Lee, J.; et al. Craniopharyngioma resection by endoscopic endonasal approach versus transcranial approach: A systematic review and meta-analysis of comparative studies. *Front. Oncol.* **2022**, *12*, 1058329. [CrossRef]
20. Lei, C.; Chuzhong, L.; Chunhui, L.; Peng, Z.; Jiwei, B.; Xinsheng, W.; Yazhuo, Z.; Songbai, G. Approach selection and outcomes of craniopharyngioma resection: A single-institute study. *Neurosurg. Rev.* **2021**, *44*, 1737–1746. [CrossRef]
21. Liu, J.K.; Eloy, J.A. Endoscopic endonasal transplanum transtuberculum approach for resection of retrochiasmatic craniopharyngioma. *Neurosurg. Focus* **2012**, *32*, E3. [CrossRef]
22. de Divitiis, E.; Cavallo, L.M.; Cappabianca, P.; Esposito, F. Extended endoscopic endonasal transsphenoidal approach for the removal of suprasellar tumors: Part 2. *Neurosurgery* **2007**, *60*, 46–59. [CrossRef]
23. Hannan, C.J.; Almhanedi, H.; Al-Mahfoudh, R.; Bhojak, M.; Looby, S.; Javadpour, M. Predicting post-operative cerebrospinal fluid (CSF) leak following endoscopic transnasal pituitary and anterior skull base surgery: A multivariate analysis. *Acta Neurochir.* **2020**, *162*, 1309–1315. [CrossRef]
24. Soudry, E.; Turner, J.H.; Nayak, J.V.; Hwang, P.H. Endoscopic reconstruction of surgically created skull base defects: A systematic review. *Otolaryngol. Head Neck Surg.* **2014**, *150*, 730–738. [CrossRef]
25. Azab, W.A.; Abdelnabi, E.A.; Mostafa, K.H.; Burhamah, T.A.; Alhaj, A.K.H.; Khalil, A.M.B.; Yousef, W.; Nasim, K. Effect of Sphenoid Sinus Pneumatization on the Surgical Windows for Extended Endoscopic Endonasal Transsphenoidal Surgery. *World Neurosurg.* **2020**, *133*, e695–e701. [CrossRef]

26. Nie, C.; Ye, Y.; Wu, J.; Zhao, H.; Jiang, X.; Wang, H. Clinical Outcomes of Transcranial and Endoscopic Endonasal Surgery for Craniopharyngiomas: A Single-Institution Experience. *Front. Oncol.* **2022**, *12*, 755342. [CrossRef]
27. Snyderman, C.; Kassam, A.; Carrau, R.; Mintz, A.; Gardner, P.; Prevedello, D.M. Acquisition of surgical skills for endonasal skull base surgery: A training program. *Laryngoscope* **2007**, *117*, 699–705. [CrossRef]
28. Lavigne, P.; Faden, D.; Gardner, P.A.; Fernandez-Miranda, J.C.; Wang, E.W.; Snyderman, C.H. Validation of training levels in endoscopic endonasal surgery of the skull base. *Laryngoscope* **2019**, *129*, 2253–2257. [CrossRef]
29. Cavallo, L.M.; Solari, D.; Esposito, F.; Cappabianca, P. The endoscopic endonasal approach for the management of craniopharyngiomas involving the third ventricle. *Neurosurg. Rev.* **2013**, *36*, 27–38. [CrossRef]
30. Kassam, A.B.; Prevedello, D.M.; Carrau, R.L.; Snyderman, C.H.; Thomas, A.; Gardner, P.; Zanation, A.; Duz, B.; Stefko, S.T.; Byers, K.; et al. Endoscopic endonasal skull base surgery: Analysis of complications in the authors' initial 800 patients. *J. Neurosurg.* **2011**, *114*, 1544–1568. [CrossRef]

Disclaimer/Publisher's Note: The statements, opinions and data contained in all publications are solely those of the individual author(s) and contributor(s) and not of MDPI and/or the editor(s). MDPI and/or the editor(s) disclaim responsibility for any injury to people or property resulting from any ideas, methods, instructions or products referred to in the content.

Article

Postoperative Cerebral Venous Sinus Thrombosis Following a Retrosigmoid Craniotomy—A Clinical and Radiological Analysis

Lukasz Przepiorka [1], Katarzyna Wójtowicz [1,*], Katarzyna Camlet [1], Jan Jankowski [1], Sławomir Kujawski [2], Laretta Grabowska-Derlatka [3], Andrzej Marchel [1] and Przemysław Kunert [1]

1. Department of Neurosurgery, Medical University of Warsaw, 02-097 Warsaw, Poland
2. Department of Exercise Physiology and Functional Anatomy, Ludwik Rydygier Collegium Medicum in Bydgoszcz Nicolaus Copernicus University in Toruń, 85-077 Bydgoszcz, Poland
3. Second Department of Radiology, Medical University of Warsaw, 02-097 Warsaw, Poland
* Correspondence: kasia-wojtowicz@wp.pl; Tel.: +48-(22)-599-25-75

Abstract: Postoperative cerebral venous sinus thrombosis (CVST) is a rare complication of the retrosigmoid approach. To address the lack of literature, we performed a retrospective analysis. The thromboses were divided into those demonstrating radiological (rCVST) and clinical (cCVST) features, the latter diagnosed during hospitalization. We identified the former by a lack of contrast in the sigmoid (SS) or transverse sinuses (TS), and evaluated the closest distance from the craniotomy to quantify sinus exposure. We included 130 patients (males: 52, females: 78) with a median age of 46.0. They had rCVST in 46.9% of cases, most often in the TS (65.6%), and cCVST in 3.1% of cases. Distances to the sinuses were not different regarding the presence of cCVST ($p = 0.32$ and $p = 0.72$). The distance to the SS was not different regarding rCVST ($p = 0.13$). However, lower exposure of the TS correlated with a lower incidence of rCVST ($p = 0.009$). When surgery was performed on the side of the dominant sinuses, rCVSTs were more frequent ($p = 0.042$). None of the other examined factors were related to rCVST or cCVST. Surgery on the side of the dominant sinus, and the exposing of them, seems to be related with rCVST. Further prospective studies are needed to identify the risk factors and determine the best management.

Keywords: dural; sinus; thrombosis; craniotomy; cerebellopontine; tumor

1. Introduction

The retrosigmoid approach (RSA) is one of the most common neurosurgical approaches to the posterolateral skull base [1–3]. It provides exposure of the cerebellopontine angle region (CPA) and its surroundings, from Meckel's cave to the jugular foramen [4–6]. Postoperative cerebral venous sinus thrombosis (CVST) is a rare but known complication following RSA [7].

There is a paucity of literature regarding CVSTs. Postoperative CVSTs have a wide range of presentation, from asymptomatic to death, and management is difficult. Treatment is inferred from a spontaneously occurring CVST, after which aggressive anticoagulation is immediately initiated [8]. Such management in the early postoperative period may increase the risk of an intracranial hemorrhage. Further, it is unclear whether any treatment should be started in asymptomatic thrombosis.

To address the above, we performed radiological and clinical analyses to report our experience with CVSTs after RSA. We started with categorizing the CVSTs. In the radiological part of the study, we looked for the radiologic features of CVSTs and evaluated the extent of the bony opening in relation to the sinuses. In the clinical part, we looked for the risk factors for, and clinical manifestations of, CVSTs (cCVSTs).

The aim of our study was to assess the frequency of radiologic features of CVSTs and cCVSTS. We assessed the relationships between clinical symptoms and the radiologic features of CVSTs. We looked for CVST risk factors, with particular emphasis on evaluating the relevance of transverse and sigmoid sinus exposures during bony openings.

2. Materials and Methods

2.1. Study Design

We designed this study as a retrospective, single-center evaluation of radiological and clinical data. Radiological data consisted of contrast-enhanced computed tomographic head scans performed routinely after elective RSAs, usually between postoperative days 3 and 7. Clinical data incorporated medical charts from RSA hospitalization.

We included adults undergoing elective RSAs, from 2016 to 2021, for which postoperative CT and medical charts were available. We could not reconstruct and evaluate studies prior to 2016 because of their insufficient quality. A CVST prior to surgery was an exclusion criterion. Patients were identified by reviewing all operative reports in our institution during the study period.

2.2. CVST Classification

CVSTs were divided into those demonstrating radiological features of CVSTs (rCVSTs, recognized retrospectively, as described in detail below) and cCVSTs, for which a clinical diagnosis of CVST had been established during hospitalization.

2.3. Radiological Analysis

CT studies were reviewed by two teams, consisting of two neurosurgeons (attending and resident) and two medical students, all of whom were previously instructed by the attending neuroradiologist. We performed evaluations with GE software on radiological stations with diagnostic monitors. CT scans were evaluated for features of rCVST in the sigmoid sinus, transverse sinus, and their junction (each treated as a separate entity) on the ipsilateral side to the RSA. Recognizing rCVSTs required the visualization of a lack of contrast in the sinuses in postoperative CT scans. We considered intraluminal thrombi that partially or completely filled the sinuses as rCVST. Arachnoid (Pacchionian) granulations [9,10] were distinguished from rCVSTs by their distinctive, regular shape, in contrast to rCVSTs, which are irregular and often larger. We analyzed CT scans without any previous knowledge of the medical history of a patient or radiological report. We then reviewed the radiological reports of patients with rCVSTs, if these included descriptions of sinus thromboses. In addition, we evaluated the closest distance from the edge of the craniotomy to the sinuses on postoperative CT scans. It was measured and presented so that a positive value expressed the closest distance between the edge of the craniotomy and the sinus, whereas a negative value represented the magnitude of overlap of the craniotomy with the sinus (Figure 1). We performed such measurements for sigmoid and transverse sinus using axial and coronal scans, respectively. These continuous measurements were subsequently translated into qualitative evaluations of sinus exposure (which corresponded to all nonnegative measurements) and non-exposure of the sinus.

Furthermore, we evaluated the dominant side of the transverse-sigmoid sinuses, presence of intraparenchymal hematoma, and other cerebral sinus thrombosis (e.g., superior sagittal sinus).

2.4. Clinical Analysis

We reviewed the medical charts of analyzed patients to evaluate perioperative-, tumor-, procedure- and patient-related factors. Other venous thromboses (deep venous thrombosis, pulmonary embolism, etc.) were not studied.

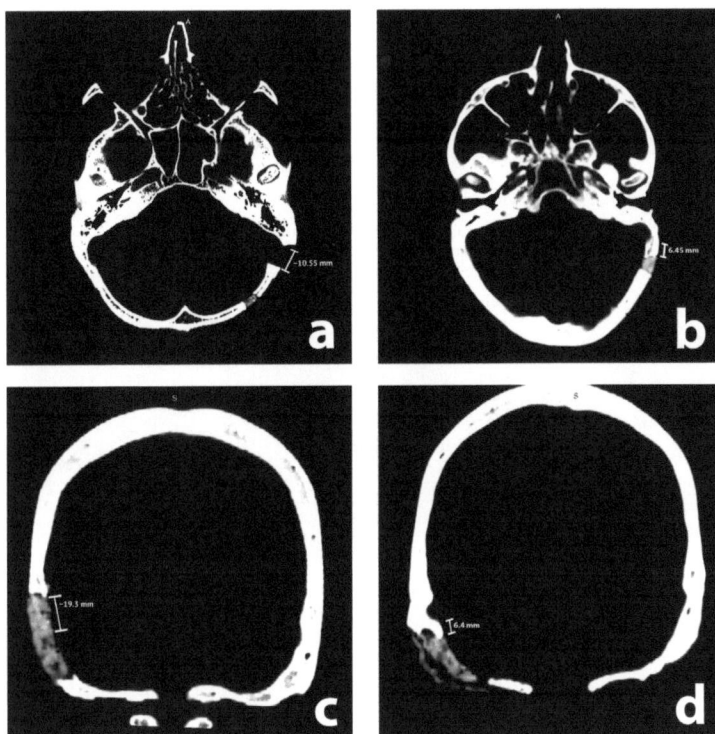

Figure 1. Illustrative radiological axial (**a**,**b**) and coronal (**c**,**d**) contrast enhanced postoperative computed tomography scans with measurements. Sigmoid and transverse sinuses are exposed in (**a**,**c**), while unexposed in (**b**,**d**), respectively.

2.5. Statistical Analysis

We used the means of two measurements for continuous variables (e.g., distance to the sinus). In case of any disagreement over qualitative variables (e.g., the presence of a rCVST), a final decision was made after discussion with a senior neuroradiologist. We additionally tried to find a threshold for the distance from the craniotomy to the sinus (Figure 1) in which the risk of CVST rises significantly. We examined the association between qualitative variables using the chi-squared test or Fisher's exact test. The Kendall rank correlation coefficient was used to examine the relationship between ordinal and qualitative variables. Between-group differences in quantitative variables were examined using an independent samples t-test, Welch's *t*-test, or Mann–Whitney U test, depending on whether the assumptions were met. ROC analysis was performed using the "MaxSpSe" method in the R package 'OptimalCutpoints' (R packages retrieved from MRAN snapshot 1 January 2022) [11,12].

3. Results

3.1. Patient Demographics

We included 130 patients (males: 52, females: 78) with a median age of 46.0 (Supplementary Table S1). Table 1 presents the radiological analysis and Table 2 presents the clinical analysis.

Table 1. Radiological analysis. CVST—cerebral venous sinus thrombosis, N/A—not applicable.

Data	Measurement	p-Value
Distance to the sigmoid sinus (mm)		
median (range)	−1.75 (−10.55, 7.45)	N/A
1st, 3rd quartile	−5.23, 0.95	
Exposure of the sigmoid sinus		
exposed	79 (60.77%)	0.01
hidden	51 (39.23%)	
Distance to the transverse sinus (mm)		
median (range)	−6.60 (−23.15, 9.2)	N/A
1st, 3rd quartile	−10.13, −2.76	
Exposure of the transverse sinus		
exposed	108 (83.1%)	<0.0001
hidden	22 (16.9%)	
Radiologic features of CVST		
present	61 (46.9%)	0.48
none	69 (53.1%)	
Transverse sinus thrombosis		
present	40 (30.8%)	0.01
absent	21 (16.2%)	
Sigmoid sinus thrombosis		
present	37 (28.5%)	0.1
absent	24 (18.5%)	
Junctions of sinuses thrombosis		
present	32 (24.6%)	0.7
absent	29 (22.3%)	
Intraparenchymal hemorrhage		
present	2 (1.5%)	<0.0001
absent	128 (98.5%)	
Sinus dominance		
right	94 (72.3%)	
left	32 (24.6%)	<0.0001
none	4 (3.1%)	

Table 2. Clinical results of analysis. CVST—cerebral venous sinus thrombosis.

Data	Measurement
Clinical diagnosis of CVST	
present	4 (3.1%)
absent	126 (96.9%)
Intraoperative injuries of the sinuses	
present	6 (4.6%)
absent	124 (95.4%)
Clinical risk factors	
Overweight/obesity	23 (17.7%)
Oncologic past medical history	10 (7.7%)
Deep venous thrombosis	2 (1.5%)
Chronic venous insufficiency	3 (2.3%)
Other	14 (10.8%)
Length of stay (days)	
median (range)	11 (8–48)
1st, 3rd quartile	10, 14
Postoperative headaches refractory to regular medical treatment	
present	12 (9.2%)
absent	115 (88.5%)
not applicable/patient unconscious	1 (0.8%)
no data	2 (1.5%)
Exposure of the transverse sinus	
exposed	108 (83.1%)
hidden	22 (16.9%)

3.2. Radiological and Clinical Results

We recognized rCVSTs in 46.9% (61/130) of the study population, and most often in the transverse sinus.

3.3. Patients with cCVST

In our study group ($n = 130$) there were 4 cases of cCVSTs (Supplementary Table S2).

One of the four patients with a cCVST died: a 41-year-old female was discharged home after RSA in a good condition. She was readmitted in a critical condition two days after discharge with a superior sagittal sinus thrombosis. She underwent unsuccessful endovascular treatment before dying in the intensive care unit. Of note, we did not recognize rCVST in the transverse or sigmoid sinus in this patient in our retrospective radiological analysis.

The second patient, a 46-year-old female, reported headaches on postoperative day six, before suddenly deteriorating neurologically. Her CT scan revealed a CVST with an intraparenchymal hematoma in the temporal lobe; she underwent an emergency craniotomy with hematoma removal and temporal lobe resection. Immediately after the surgery, she started improving and was discharged home, able to walk unassisted.

A 66-year-old male was diagnosed with a small intraparenchymal hemorrhage in the basal part of the temporal lobe, in his routine contrast-enhanced CT scan. A CVST diagnosis was confirmed using MRI, and this was followed by medical treatment. The patient was subsequently transferred to the neurology department for rehabilitation.

The fourth patient, a 42-year-old female, presented with aphasia on postoperative day two. After confirming a CVST with MRI, she was treated medically, then her symptoms resolved.

Half (2/4) of patients with cCVST had documented postoperative headaches refractory to regular medical treatment. However, severe postoperative headaches developed 9.2% of the whole study group (12/130). A comparison of patients with and without rCVST revealed no significant difference in postoperative headache frequencies (6/61, 9.8% and 6/69, 8.7%, respectively).

In our retrospective radiologic studies, we identified 3 rCVSTs in 4 cases of cCVSTs. The remaining patient had superior sagittal sinus thrombosis, but no rCVST in their transverse/sigmoid sinus—which was defined as a rCVST in our study.

3.4. Radiological and Clinical Analysis

For the whole study population, median distances to the sigmoid and transverse sinuses were -1.75 mm and -6.60 mm, respectively; 60.77% of the sigmoid sinuses and 83.1% of the transverse sinuses were at least partially exposed. The right-sided sinuses were dominant in 72.3% of the cases.

Distances to the sigmoid and transverse sinuses were not significantly different between patients with and without cCVST ($p = 0.340$ and $p = 0.707$, respectively, Student's t-test). The distance to the sigmoid sinus was not significantly different in the group with rCVST in comparison to the group without rCVST ($p = 0.125$, Mann–Whitney U test). However, reduced exposure of the transverse sinus correlated with reduced frequency of rCVST ($p = 0.028$, Student's t-test).

When we analyzed the distance to the sigmoid sinus and rCVST in the sigmoid sinus only, there was a significant difference: a rCVST in the sigmoid sinus was related to significantly larger exposure of the sigmoid sinus ($p = 0.04$, Mann–Whitney U test).

A similar analysis for the transverse sinus did not reveal such a correlation ($p = 0.209$, Welch's test). A receiver operating characteristic curve analysis for the discrimination threshold for rCVST presence revealed that exposing a transverse sinus by over 6.55 mm increases the risk of rCVST (sensitivity 39%, specificity 41%, positive predictive value 37%, negative predictive value 43%, area under curve 0.367 (95% confidence interval = 0.269; 0.464), Figure 2).

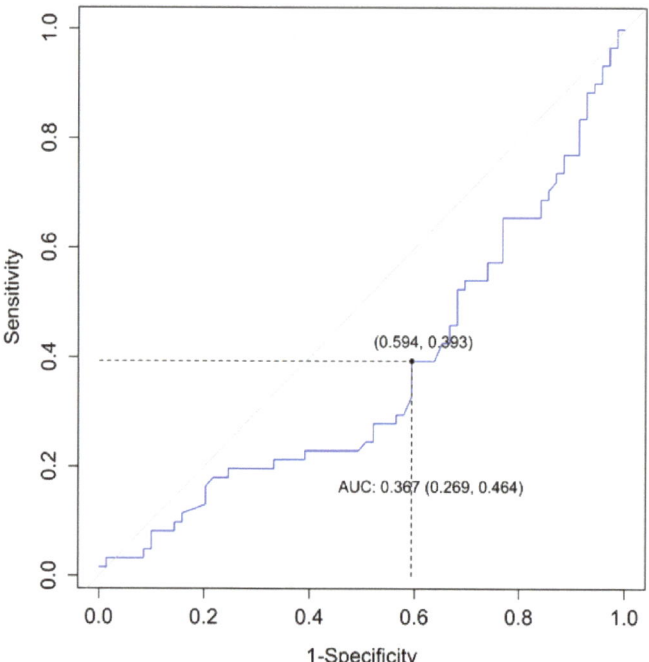

Figure 2. A receiver operating characteristic (ROC) curve analysis shows that exposing a transverse sinus by over 6.55 mm increases the risk of radiologic features of cerebral venous sinus thrombosis (rCVST). ROC curve is shown in blue color, reference line is shown in grey, an optimal cut-point according to the MaxSpSe method is shown in black dashed lines.

We compared the exposing of each of the sinuses in a qualitative manner (exposed versus not exposed), and it correlated neither with rCVST nor cCVST (both $p = 1$, Fisher's exact test for exposing sigmoid and transverse sinus and cCVST; and $p = 0.16$ χ^2 test and $p = 0.35$, Fisher's exact test for exposing sigmoid and transverse sinus and rCVST). Similarly, exposing both sinuses did not correlate with rCVST or cCVST ($p = 0.460$ and $p = 0.1$, Fisher's exact test, respectively).

The side of sinus dominance did not correlate with cCVST or rCVST. However, when the surgery was on the side of the dominant sinus, a rCVST occurred more frequently ($p = 0.042$, χ^2 test). We did not find such a correlation for cCVST ($p = 0.631$, Fisher's exact test).

None of the remaining examined factors correlated with cCVST or rCVST, except for an oncologic past medical history being more frequent among the cCVST group ($p = 0.03$, Fisher's exact test). In binary analyses, the presence of any risk factor (compared to none) did not correlate with cCVST ($p = 0.609$, Fisher's exact test), nor with rCVST ($p = 0.486$, χ^2 test). In addition, when the number of risk factors was treated as an ordinal variable, there was no correlation with cCVST ($p = 0.233$, Kendall rank correlation coefficient) or with rCVST ($p = 0.437$, Kendall rank correlation coefficient).

Intraoperative injuries of the sinuses did not correlate with rCVST or cCVST ($p = 0.705$, Fisher's exact test; $p = 1$, Fisher's exact test, respectively). Analysis of the radiological and clinical risk factors is summarized in Table 3.

Table 3. Selected analyzed radiological and clinical factors and their correlation with any type of radiological features of cerebral venous sinus thrombosis (rCVST).

Analyzed Factor	Value	rCVST Present	rCVST Absent	p-Value
Sex	male	19 (37.3%)	32 (62.7%)	0.076
	female	42 (53.2%)	37 (46.8%)	
Age (years)	median (range)	48 (22–76)	43 (20–82)	0.774
	1st, 3rd quartile	40, 58	33, 57	
Side	right	26 (40.6%)	38 (59.4%)	0.157
	left	35 (53.0%)	31 (47.0%)	
Tumor maximal size (mm)	median (range)	31 (12–50)	32 (9–57)	0.810
	1st, 3rd quartile	24, 39	22, 38	
Tumor volume (cm^3)	median (range)	11 (0.26–41.89)	11.73 (0.18–59.9)	0.493
	1st, 3rd quartile	3.78, 18.25	3.94, 18.38	
Distance to the sigmoid sinus (quantitative)	median (range)	−2.67 (−9.4–6.2)	−1.6 (−10.6–7.5)	0.04
	1st, 3rd quartile	−5.6, 0	−4.75, 1.95	
Exposure of the sigmoid sinus (qualitative)	exposed	41 (51.9%)	38 (48.1%)	1
	hidden	20 (39.2%)	31 (60.8%)	
Distance to the transverse sinus (quantitative)	median (range)	−7.3 (−21.5–9.2)	−4.9 (−23.15–7.8)	0.028
	1st, 3rd quartile	−11.4, −5.15	−7.95, −2.5	
Exposure of the transverse sinus (qualitative)	exposed	53 (49.1%)	55 (50.9%)	1
	hidden	8 (36.4%)	14 (63.6%)	
Exposure of both sinuses (qualitative)	both exposed	38 (52.1%)	35 (47.9%)	0.46
	one exposed or none	23 (40.4%)	34 (59.6%)	
Exposure of at least one sinus (qualitative)	one or two sinuses exposed	56 (49.1%)	58 (50.9%)	0.180
	none exposed	5 (31.3%)	11 (68.8%)	
Sinus dominance	right	42 (44.7%)	52 (55.3%)	0.46
	left	18 (56.3%)	14 (43.8%)	
	none	1 (25%)	3 (75%)	
Overweight/obesity	present	12 (52.2%)	11 (47.8%)	0.578
	absent	49 (45.8%)	58 (54.2%)	
Oncologic past medical history	present	6 (60%)	4 (40%)	0.514
	absent	55 (45.8%)	65 (54.2%)	
Deep venous thrombosis	present	1 (50%)	1 (50%)	1
	absent	60 (49.6%)	68 (53.1%)	
Chronic venous insufficiency	present	2 (66.7%)	1 (33.3%)	0.600
	absent	59 (46.5%)	68 (53.5%)	
Other clinical risk factors	present	7 (50%)	7 (50%)	0.807
	absent	54 (46.6%)	62 (53.4%)	
Postoperative headaches refractory to regular medical treatment	present	6 (50%)	6 (50%)	0.546
	absent	53 (46.1%)	62 53.9%)	
	not applicable/patient unconscious	1 (100%)	0	
	no data	1 (50%)	1 (50%)	
Surgery on the side of dominant sinus	yes	21 (36.8%)	36 (63.2%)	0.042
	no	40 (54.8%)	33 (45.2%)	
Intraoperative injuries of the sinus	yes	4 (57.1%)	3 (42.9%)	0.705
	no	57 (46.3%)	66 (53.7%)	

4. Discussion

In this study, we retrospectively analyzed CVST after RSA. To our great surprise, an rCVST occurred after nearly every second (46.9%) surgery. Yet only a small portion of these cases (4.9%) bore clinical significance. Except for the occurrence, there is a handful of other topics arising from the results that will be explored below.

4.1. Mechanisms and Risk Factors

Possible risk factors of CVST after RSA have already been discussed in the literature [13,14], which can be divided into patient- and surgery-related. Patients at an increased risk of CVST (e.g., with the factor V Leiden mutation) should be identified prior to surgery. Outside of medical conditions, Gerges et al., in an anatomic study, found that acute petrous angle and shorter IAC to sinus distance were associated with CVST [15]. CVST prevention is yet to be explored, but clinicians might consider perioperative IV fluids and early anticoagulation postoperatively. In our series, only oncological past medical history correlated with cCVST, but this may be a statistical error caused by a small sample size, given the statistical test's low power.

We should also recognize surgery-related risk factors for CVST, and tailor our surgical approaches to avoid them. Intraoperative maneuvers that are speculated to increase the risk of CVST include direct and indirect sinus injuries, along with the migration of bone wax used on emissary veins [13]. Interestingly, an intraoperative injury of the sinus in our material was not associated with any type of CVST, as reported by Apra et al. [16]. The importance of the surgical position for RSA is yet to be evaluated; we routinely choose a supine position with the head turned and fixed in a skull clamp.

In our institution, the craniotomy technique is focused on minimal (ideally no) exposure of the sigmoid and transverse sinuses. For this, we evaluate preoperative CT scans, use anatomical landmarks, and place the initial burr hole just below the expected junction of the sinuses [1]. As a rule, we do not use neuronavigation for RSA [17].

In case of a sinus injury, our strategy is tailored to the extent of bleeding. Just exposing the sinus, even partially, is followed by keeping it moist and applying a layer of an absorbable hemostat (e.g., Surigcel®) on the surface or just the patties. Minor bleedings are dealt with similarly. More serious bleedings are most often successfully stopped with a fibrin sealant patch (e.g., TachoSil®). A direct sinus injury is sutured.

When designing our study, we conjectured that exposing sinuses—even partially—may cause CVSTs. To some degree, this has been confirmed, but this requires analysis with a larger sample size in a prospective manner. Apra et al. found that exposure of the sinus was a risk factor for rCVST [16]. It is worth mentioning that all patients with cCVST had at least the transverse sinus exposed.

Noteworthily, we found that rCVSTs occurred more frequently when the surgery was performed on the dominant sinus side. Our findings differ from the results of Guazzo et al., who discovered an association between CVSTs and surgery on the side of non-dominant sinus. However, they evaluated only the translabyrinthine approach, which may make direct comparisons inappropriate [18].

4.2. Diagnosis and Presentation

A CVST diagnosis is hard to establish, particularly when symptoms are mild. Headaches associated with CVST are unspecific, and their absence cannot rule out CVST [19]. Importantly, patients might have neurologic deficits—or headaches—after retrosigmoid craniotomy, even without CVST. On the other hand, it may be possible that some postoperative neurological deteriorations are in fact caused by CVSTs that are undiagnosed. Still, most CVSTs are clinically silent. The reason for wide spectrum of CVST clinical presentation may be attributed—to some degree—to different venous drainage patterns [20]. The relevant collateral circulations consist of torcular Herophili, contralateral transverse and sigmoid sinuses, the occipital sinus, the vein of Labbe, and the superficial middle cerebral vein. Most studies report CT venography or MR venography as a study of choice for CVSTs [21–23].

It is a tenet in our institution that diagnosing a CVST is primarily clinical. We are watchful for alarming headaches in the postoperative period that do not respond to the usual painkillers. In such cases, a contrast enhanced thin-sliced CT scan is an auxiliary diagnostic tool. Yet, the most burning question remains: should only the presence of radiological features of CVST necessitate aggressive pharmacologic treatment?

4.3. Medical Treatment

Prospective studies suggest conservative management [14,18]. Guazzo et al. suggested no anticoagulation in incidental rCVSTs [18]. Benjamin et al. chose observation in 23 out of 24 asymptomatic patients with rCVST (the remaining patient was hydrated with IV fluids) [14]. Interestingly, both these studies reported increased CSF leak rates in patients with rCVST, as did Shew et al. in a retrospective cohort study [24]. Orlev et al. reported that most cases resolve without anticoagulation treatment [25]. Kow et al. suggested anticoagulation treatment for symptomatic cases, or those in which rCVST occurs on the dominant sinus side [26]. On the other hand, Moore et al. radically recommended 6 months of anticoagulants in patients with CVST [13]. We suggest aggressive pharmacologic treatment—enoxaparin, mannitol, dexamethasone, IV fluids—only in symptomatic cases. This is because there were no readmissions or any other complications for asymptomatic rCVST cases (which constituted the majority of rCVST sample: 95.1%, 58/61). That said, we believe that asymptomatic rCVST patients should be instructed before discharge about possible cCVST.

4.4. Interventional Treatment

Outside of medical treatment, certain cases may require intervention. A large intracerebral hemorrhage may be removed surgically, as described herein. Similarly, endovascular venous thrombectomies have been reported, as unsuccessfully attempted in our fatal cCVST case. The first successful endovascular treatment of CVST after translabyrinthine vestibular schwannoma resection was reported by Manzoor et al. in 2016 [27]. Since then, endovascular treatment of postoperative CVST has not been described in the literature.

4.5. Comparison with Other Studies

Supplementary Table S3 presents case series and case reports describing postoperative CVSTs. Prospective and retrospective studies vary markedly in the presented incidence rates—the former report rates in the range of 32.4% to 38.9% (median 35.7%), while the latter report rates in the range of 0.8% to 22.4% (median 9.1%). Our results are comparable with prospective studies, which may be attributed to the meticulous radiological analysis we performed. Nevertheless, the incidence in clinical practice remains to be evaluated, bearing in mind a broad category of posterior fossa tumors and a narrower category of cerebellopontine angle tumors and specifically vestibular schwannomas. Some authors suggested increased CVST rate after meningioma surgery.

We found that less than 5% of rCVSTs were symptomatic, which is similar to the results of Shew et al., who reported 1 symptomatic patient out of 22 (4.5%) in a study with a similar design to ours [24].

4.6. Pediatric Population

This paper focuses exclusively on adult patients. Noteworthily, there is a lack of studies describing CVST in a pediatric population after skull base surgery. Teping et al. described a 7.1% rate of intraoperative sinus bleeding after posterior fossa surgery in the semisitting position in the pediatric population [28]. Petrov et al. reported sinus exposure and injury as potential risk factors for CVST; however, their study included any type of cranial surgery [29].

4.7. Approach Selection in CPA Surgery

Currently available reports suggest higher frequencies of CVST after a translabyrinthine approach when compared to using the RSA [13], possibly due to the wide exposure of the sigmoid sinus necessary during such an approach. This remains to be objectively evaluated, and hopefully will be in future prospective studies. It may become an additional factor to consider in choosing the best surgical approach to a given CPA pathology.

4.8. Rare Case Reports

A CVST distant to the operative field is a rare event, described in the literature on a case-report basis. There are few case reports in the literature, and one case in our series ended in death [27,30–32].

4.9. Limitations and Future Studies

Though this study has a larger sample size than similar studies (Supplementary Table S3), this is still a limiting factor along with its retrospective nature. This may be a reason why, in our study, there were no significant differences in headache occurrences among patients with and without rCVST. This may also be a cause of lack of correlation between the sinus exposure and cCVST. That said, oncologic past medical history was found more frequently among cCVST patients with significance. Finally, we measured only the width of the exposure of each of the sinuses. Additional measurements of the length (or, ideally, the area of surface) of the exposure would improve theoretical accuracy. Unfortunately, in practice, these were impossible to perform reliably. Future prospective studies are needed to evaluate CVST incidence and management, and, in particular, the necessity of prophylactic treatment of asymptomatic patients with rCVST.

5. Conclusions

Although it rarely becomes symptomatic, rCVST is a common, underreported consequence of RSA. Surgery on the side of the dominant sinus seems to be related to rCVST. Exposing the sinuses during craniotomy may contribute to rCVST, but it requires more analysis. Otherwise, we did not find any other risk factors associated with either cCVST or rCVST, in particular intraoperative sinus injury. Further, prospective studies are needed to identify risk factors.

Supplementary Materials: The following supporting information can be downloaded at: https://www.mdpi.com/article/10.3390/brainsci13071039/s1, Supplementary Table S1: Surgical and postoperative characteristics of 130 patients included in the study; Supplementary Table S2: Characteristics of patients diagnosed with clinical cerebral venous sinus thrombosis; Supplementary Table S3: Literature review on the cerebral venous sinus thrombosis after cerebellopontine angle surgery [33–36]; Supplementary Figure S1: Radiologic images of patients diagnosed with clinical cerebral venous sinus thrombosis.

Author Contributions: Conceptualization, L.P., K.W. and P.K.; methodology, L.P., K.W., P.K. and L.G.-D.; software, L.G.-D. and S.K.; validation, A.M., P.K. and L.G.-D.; formal analysis, L.P., S.K. and L.G.-D.; investigation, K.C., J.J., L.P. and K.W.; resources, K.C. and J.J.; data curation, K.C. and J.J.; writing—original draft preparation, K.W. and L.P.; writing—review and editing, L.P. and P.K.; visualization, S.K.; supervision, A.M.; project administration, A.M. All authors have read and agreed to the published version of the manuscript.

Funding: This research received no external funding.

Institutional Review Board Statement: The study was conducted in accordance with the Declaration of Helsinki, and approved by The Bioethics Committee of the Medical University of Warsaw.

Informed Consent Statement: Patient consent was waived by The Bioethics Committee of the Medical University of Warsaw due to retrospective character of a study and participants anonymity.

Data Availability Statement: The data presented in this study are available on request from the corresponding author after acceptance of all the co-authors.

Acknowledgments: The authors would like to thank Andrew Tuson for his language editing help in preparing the manuscript.

Conflicts of Interest: The authors declare no conflict of interest.

References

1. Zhou, C.; Evins, A.I.; Boschi, A.; Tang, Y.; Li, S.; Przepiorka, L.; Sadhwani, S.; Stieg, P.E.; Xu, T.; Bernardo, A. Preoperative identification of the initial burr hole site in retrosigmoid craniotomies: A teaching and technical note. *Int. J. Med. Robot.* **2019**, *15*, e1987. [CrossRef]
2. Przepiórka, Ł.; Kunert, P.; Rutkowska, W.; Dziedzic, T.; Marchel, A. Surgery After Surgery for Vestibular Schwannoma: A Case Series. *Front. Oncol.* **2020**, *10*, 588260. [CrossRef] [PubMed]
3. You, W.; Meng, J.; Yang, X.; Zhang, J.; Jiang, G.; Yan, Z.; Gu, F.; Tao, X.; Chen, Z.; Wang, Z.; et al. Microsurgical Management of Posterior Circulation Aneurysms: A Retrospective Study on Epidemiology, Outcomes, and Surgical Approaches. *Brain Sci.* **2022**, *12*, 1066. [CrossRef] [PubMed]
4. Peris-Celda, M.; Graffeo, C.S.; Perry, A.; Carlstrom, L.P.; Link, M.J. Trigeminal Nerve Schwannoma of the Cerebellopontine Angle. *J. Neurol. Surg. B Skull Base.* **2018**, *79* (Suppl. S5), S389–S390. [CrossRef] [PubMed]
5. Matsushima, K.; Kohno, M.; Komune, N.; Miki, K.; Matsushima, T.; Rhoton, A.L. Suprajugular extension of the retrosigmoid approach: Microsurgical anatomy. *J. Neurosurg.* **2014**, *121*, 397–407. [CrossRef]
6. Li, Q.; Yu, Y.; Zhang, L.; Liu, J.; Ren, H.; Zhen, X. Staged Surgery for Intra-Extracranial Communicating Jugular Foramen Paraganglioma: A Case Report and Systematic Review. *Brain Sci.* **2022**, *12*, 1257. [CrossRef] [PubMed]
7. Abou-Al-Shaar, H.; Gozal, Y.M.; Alzhrani, G.; Karsy, M.; Shelton, C.; Couldwell, W.T. Cerebral venous sinus thrombosis after vestibular schwannoma surgery: A call for evidence-based management guidelines. *Neurosurg. Focus.* **2018**, *45*, E4. [CrossRef]
8. Gogu, A.E.; Jianu, D.C.; Dumitrascu, V.; Ples, H.; Stroe, A.Z.; Axelerad, D. MTHFR Gene Polymorphisms and Cardiovascular Risk Factors, Clinical-Imagistic Features and Outcome in Cerebral Venous Sinus Thrombosis. *Brain Sci.* **2020**, *11*, 23. [CrossRef]
9. Pacchioni, A. *Dissertatio Epistolaris de Glandulis Conglobatis Durae Meningis Humanae, Indeque Ortis Lymphaticis ad Piam Meningem Productis*; Buagni: Rome, Italy, 1705.
10. Brunori, A.; Vagnozzi, R.; Giuffrè, R. Antonio Pacchioni (1665–1726): Early studies of the dura mater. *J. Neurosurg.* **1993**, *78*, 515–518. [CrossRef]
11. López-Ratón, M.; Rodríguez-Álvarez, M.X.; Cadarso-Suárez, C.; Gude-Sampedro, F. OptimalCutpoints: An R Package for Selecting Optimal Cutpoints in Diagnostic Tests. *J. Stat. Softw.* **2014**, *61*, 1–36. [CrossRef]
12. R Core Team. R: A Language and Environment for Statistical Computing [Internet]. Vienna, Austria: R Foundation for Statistical Computing. 2021. Available online: https://www.R-project.org/ (accessed on 10 September 2022).
13. Moore, J.; Thomas, P.; Cousins, V.; Rosenfeld, J.V. Diagnosis and Management of Dural Sinus Thrombosis following Resection of Cerebellopontine Angle Tumors. *J. Neurol. Surg. B Skull Base.* **2014**, *75*, 402–408. [PubMed]
14. Benjamin, C.G.; Sen, R.D.; Golfinos, J.G.; Sen, C.; Roland, J.T.; McMenomey, S.; Pacione, D. Postoperative cerebral venous sinus thrombosis in the setting of surgery adjacent to the major dural venous sinuses. *J. Neurosurg.* **2018**, *1*, 1–7. [CrossRef] [PubMed]
15. Gerges, C.; Malloy, P.; Rabah, N.; Defta, D.; Duan, Y.; Wright, C.H.; van Keulen, M.; Wright, J.; Mowry, S.; Megerian, C.A.; et al. Functional Outcomes and Postoperative Cerebral Venous Sinus Thrombosis after Translabyrinthine Approach for Vestibular Schwannoma Resection: A Radiographic Demonstration of Anatomic Predictors. *J. Neurol. Surg. B Skull Base.* **2022**, *83* (Suppl. 2), e89–e95. [CrossRef] [PubMed]
16. Apra, C.; Kotbi, O.; Turc, G.; Corns, R.; Pagès, M.; Souillard-Scémama, R.; Dezamis, E.; Parraga, E.; Meder, J.-F.; Sauvageon, X. Presentation and management of lateral sinus thrombosis following posterior fossa surgery. *J. Neurosurg.* **2017**, *126*, 8–16. [CrossRef] [PubMed]
17. Izzo, A.; Stifano, V.; Della Pepa, G.M.; Di Domenico, M.; D'Alessandris, Q.G.; Menna, G.; D'Ercole, M.; Lauretti, L.; Olivi, A.; Montano, N. Tailored Approach and Multimodal Intraoperative Neuromonitoring in Cerebellopontine Angle Surgery. *Brain Sci.* **2022**, *12*, 1167. [CrossRef]
18. Guazzo, E.; Panizza, B.; Lomas, A.; Wood, M.; Amato, D.; Alalade, A.; Gandhi, M.; Bowman, J. Cerebral Venous Sinus Thrombosis After Translabyrinthine Vestibular Schwannoma-A Prospective Study and Suggested Management Paradigm. *Otol. Neurotol.* **2020**, *41*, e273–e279. [CrossRef] [PubMed]
19. Aliprandi, A.; Borelli, P.; Polonia, V.; Salmaggi, A. Headache in cerebral venous thrombosis. *Neurol. Sci.* **2020**, *41* (Suppl. S2), 401–406. [CrossRef]
20. Ohata, K.; Haque, M.; Morino, M.; Nagai, K.; Nishio, A.; Nishijima, Y.; Hakuba, A. Occlusion of the sigmoid sinus after surgery via the presigmoidal-transpetrosal approach. *J. Neurosurg.* **1998**, *89*, 575–584. [CrossRef]
21. Vogl, T.J.; Bergman, C.; Villringer, A.; Einhäupl, K.; Lissner, J.; Felix, R. Dural sinus thrombosis: Value of venous MR angiography for diagnosis and follow-up. *AJR Am. J. Roentgenol.* **1994**, *162*, 1191–1198. [CrossRef]
22. Rodallec, M.H.; Krainik, A.; Feydy, A.; Hélias, A.; Colombani, J.M.; Jullès, M.C.; Marteau, V.; Zins, M. Cerebral venous thrombosis and multidetector CT angiography: Tips and tricks. *Radiographics* **2006**, *26* (Suppl. S1), S5–S18; discussion S42–S43. [CrossRef]
23. Salgado-Lopez, L.; Custozzo, A.; Raviv, N.; Abdelhak, T.; Peris-Celda, M. Cerebral sinus thrombosis as an initial symptom of acute promyelocytic leukemia: Case report and literature review. *Surg. Neurol. Int.* **2022**, *13*, 89. [CrossRef]
24. Shew, M.; Kavookjian, H.; Dahlstrom, K.; Muelleman, T.; Lin, J.; Camarata, P.; Ledbetter, L.; Staecker, H. Incidence and Risk Factors for Sigmoid Venous Thrombosis Following CPA Tumor Resection. *Otol. Neurotol.* **2018**, *39*, e376–e380. [CrossRef] [PubMed]
25. Orlev, A.; Jackson, C.M.; Luksik, A.; Garzon-Muvdi, T.; Yang, W.; Chien, W.; Harnof, S.; Tamargo, R.J. Natural History of Untreated Transverse/Sigmoid Sinus Thrombosis Following Posterior Fossa Surgery: Case Series and Literature Review. *Oper. Neurosurg.* **2020**, *19*, 109–116. [CrossRef] [PubMed]

26. Kow, C.Y.; Caldwell, J.; Mchugh, F.; Sillars, H.; Bok, A. Dural venous sinus thrombosis after cerebellopontine angle surgery: Should it be treated? *J. Clin. Neurosci.* **2020**, *75*, 157–162. [CrossRef] [PubMed]
27. Manzoor, N.F.; Ray, A.; Singer, J.; Nord, R.; Sunshine, J.; Megerian, C.A.; Bambakidis, N.C.; Semaan, M.T. Successful endovascular management of venous sinus thrombosis complicating trans-labyrinthine removal of vestibular schwanomma. *Am. J. Otolaryngol.* **2016**, *37*, 379–382. [CrossRef]
28. Teping, F.; Linsler, S.; Zemlin, M.; Oertel, J. The semisitting position in pediatric neurosurgery: Pearls and pitfalls of a 10-year experience. *J. Neurosurg. Pediatr.* **2021**, *28*, 724–733. [CrossRef]
29. Petrov, D.; Uohara, M.Y.; Ichord, R.; Ali, Z.; Jastrzab, L.; Lang, S.S.; Billinghurst, L. Pediatric cerebral sinovenous thrombosis following cranial surgery. *Childs Nerv. Syst.* **2017**, *33*, 491–497. [CrossRef]
30. Sawarkar, D.P.; Verma, S.K.; Singh, P.K.; Doddamani, R.; Kumar, A.; Sharma, B.S. Fatal Superior Sagittal Sinus and Torcular Thrombosis After Vestibular Schwannoma Surgery: Report of a Rare Complication and Review of the Literature. *World Neurosurg.* **2016**, *96*, e19–e607. [CrossRef]
31. Nadkarni, T.D.; Dindorkar, K.S.; Desai, K.; Goel, A. Cavernous sinus thrombosis and air embolism following surgery for acoustic neurinoma: A case report. *Neurol. India.* **2002**, *50*, 201–203.
32. Wong, A.K.; Wong, R.H. Successful treatment of superior sagittal sinus thrombosis after translabyrinthine resection of metastatic neuroendocrine tumor: A case report and review of literature. *Surg. Neurol. Int.* **2020**, *11*, 410. [CrossRef]
33. Keiper, G.L.; Sherman, J.D.; Tomsick, T.A.; Tew, J.M. Dural sinus thrombosis and pseudotumor cerebri: Unexpected complications of suboccipital craniotomy and translabyrinthine craniectomy. *J. Neurosurg.* **1999**, *91*, 192–197. [CrossRef] [PubMed]
34. Jean, W.C.; Felbaum, D.R.; Stemer, A.B.; Hoa, M.; Kim, H.J. Venous sinus compromise after pre-sigmoid, transpetrosal approach for skull base tumors: A study on the asymptomatic incidence and report of a rare dural arteriovenous fistula as symptomatic manifestation. *J. Clin. Neurosci.* **2017**, *39*, 114–117. [CrossRef] [PubMed]
35. Ziegler, A.; El-Kouri, N.; Dymon, Z.; Serrano, D.; Bashir, M.; Anderson, D.; Leonetti, J. Sigmoid Sinus Patency following Vestibular Schwannoma Resection via Retrosigmoid versus Translabyrinthine Approach. *J. Neurol. Surg. B Skull Base.* **2021**, *82*, 461–465. [CrossRef] [PubMed]
36. Krystkiewicz, K.; Wrona, D.; Tosik, M.; Birski, M.; Szylberg, Ł.; Morawska, A.; Furtak, J.; Wałęsa, C.; Stopa, K.; Harat, M. Dural sinus thrombosis after resection of vestibular schwannoma using suboccipital retrosigmoid approach-thrombosis classification and management proposal. *Neurosurg. Rev.* **2022**, *45*, 2211–2219. [CrossRef] [PubMed]

Disclaimer/Publisher's Note: The statements, opinions and data contained in all publications are solely those of the individual author(s) and contributor(s) and not of MDPI and/or the editor(s). MDPI and/or the editor(s) disclaim responsibility for any injury to people or property resulting from any ideas, methods, instructions or products referred to in the content.

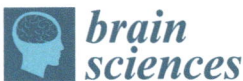

Article

A New Finding on Magnetic Resonance Imaging for Diagnosis of Hemifacial Spasm with High Accuracy and Interobserver Correlation

Guilherme Finger [1], Kyle C. Wu [1], Joshua Vignolles-Jeong [2], Saniya S. Godil [1], Ben G. McGahan [1], Daniel Kreatsoulas [1], Mohammad T. Shujaat [3], Luciano M. Prevedello [3] and Daniel M. Prevedello [1,*]

1. Department of Neurosurgery, The Ohio State University College of Medicine, Columbus, OH 43210, USA; guilhermefingermd@gmail.com (G.F.); kyle.wu@osumc.edu (K.C.W.); daniel.kreatsoulas@osumc.edu (D.K.)
2. College of Medicine, The Ohio State University College of Medicine, Columbus, OH 43210, USA; joshua.vignolles-jeong@osumc.edu
3. Department of Radiology, The Ohio State University College of Medicine, Columbus, OH 43210, USA; luciano.prevedello@osumc.edu (L.M.P.)
* Correspondence: daniel.prevedello@osumc.edu

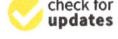

Citation: Finger, G.; Wu, K.C.; Vignolles-Jeong, J.; Godil, S.S.; McGahan, B.G.; Kreatsoulas, D.; Shujaat, M.T.; Prevedello, L.M.; Prevedello, D.M. A New Finding on Magnetic Resonance Imaging for Diagnosis of Hemifacial Spasm with High Accuracy and Interobserver Correlation. Brain Sci. 2023, 13, 1434. https://doi.org/10.3390/brainsci13101434

Academic Editor: Miguel Lopez-Gonzalez

Received: 30 August 2023
Revised: 27 September 2023
Accepted: 7 October 2023
Published: 9 October 2023

Copyright: © 2023 by the authors. Licensee MDPI, Basel, Switzerland. This article is an open access article distributed under the terms and conditions of the Creative Commons Attribution (CC BY) license (https://creativecommons.org/licenses/by/4.0/).

Abstract: Among patients with clinical hemifacial spasm (HFS), imaging exams aim to identify the neurovascular conflict (NVC) location. It has been proven that the identification in the preoperative exam increases the rate of surgical success. Despite the description of specific magnetic resonance image (MRI) acquisitions, the site of neurovascular compression is not always visualized. The authors describe a new MRI finding that helps in the diagnosis of HFS, and evaluate the sensitivity, specificity, and interobserver correlation of the described sign. A cross-sectional study including cases of hemifacial spasm treated surgically from 1 August 2011 to 31 July 2021 was performed. The MRIs of the cases were independently evaluated by two experienced neuroradiologists, who were blinded regarding the side of the symptom. The neuroradiologists were assigned to evaluate the MRIs in two separate moments. Primarily, they evaluated whether there was a neurovascular conflict based on the standard technique. Following this initial analysis, the neuroradiologists received a file with the description of the novel sign, named Prevedello Sign (PS). In a second moment, the same neuroradiologists were asked to identify the presence of the PS and, if it was present, to report on which side. A total of 35 patients were included, mostly females (65.7%) with a mean age of 59.02 (+0.48). Since the 35 cases were independently evaluated by two neuroradiologists, a total of 70 reports were included in the analysis. The PS was present in 66 patients (sensitivity of 94.2%, specificity of 91.4% and positive predictive value of 90.9%). When both analyses were performed in parallel (standard plus PS), the sensitivity increased to 99.2%. Based on the findings of this study, the authors conclude that PS is helpful in determining the neurovascular conflict location in patients with HFS. Its presence, combined with the standard evaluation, increases the sensitivity of the MRI to over 99%, without increasing risks of harm to patients or resulting in additional costs.

Keywords: hemifacial spasm; diagnosis; facial nerve disorders; facial nerve disease; magnetic resonance imaging

1. Introduction

Hemifacial spasm is characterized by unilateral involuntary spasms of the facial musculature [1] with an annual incidence of 1/100,000 [2] and a prevalence ranging from 9.8 to 11 cases per 100,000 [2,3].

Neurovascular conflict is the main cause of HFS. Identification and evaluation of the NVC via preoperative imaging are critical to guide surgical procedure and technique [4]. The main goal of the preoperative image exam is to identify the point at which the facial nerve is being compressed by a vascular structure. If this NVC is identified preoperatively, surgical treatment has a higher chance of success due to the surgeon's more comprehensive understanding of the anatomy surrounding the NVC that must be navigated through to release the nerve.

The aim of MRI investigation is to identify the facial nerve and to search for any vascular attachment or compression. The combination of high-resolution 3D T2-weighted imaging with 3D time-of-flight angiography and 3D T1-weighted gadolinium-enhanced sequences is considered the standard for the investigation of primary NVC [5–8]. However, MRI exploration has limitations. The nature of the conflicting vessel(s) is sometimes difficult to assess, particularly if the area explored by thin sections does not capture the vessel or nerve's origin. Other reasons described that diminish the efficacy of the MRI are very small caliber of the involved vessel, patients with "small posterior fossa", or crowded cisternal contents [8]. Therefore, the description of a new image pattern to diagnose the NVC among patients with HFS is valid and helpful to increase the sensibility and accuracy of MRI as the ideal image exam to achieve preoperative diagnoses in these patients.

The authors conducted a study in order to describe a new MRI finding for the diagnosis of HFS and to evaluate its sensitivity, specificity, prevalence ratio, and interobserver identification correlation.

2. Materials and Methods

2.1. Definition

When the trajectory of the vessel is evaluated in the coronal view, it may be possible to visualize the vessel forming a loop superior and medial (towards the exit of the facial nerve) (Figure 1). When the MRI is visualized in the axial view, at the highest level of the loop in the coronal section, the proximity of the vascular structures to the pons may be seen in the axial view as if the artery was located inside of the brainstem, surrounded by the pons parenchyma (Figure 2).

The Prevedello Sign is the identification of an arterial loop enfolded by the pons near the exit of the facial nerve, in the brainstem. This finding is best visualized in T1WI with contrast and in FIESTA acquisitions of MRI sequences (Figure 3).

2.2. Study Design

The study was conducted at the Department of Neurosurgery, Skull Base section, at the Ohio State University and approved by the Ethics Review Board under the number 2022E0740.

The authors conducted a cross-sectional study evaluating all cases of hemifacial spasm treated surgically from 1 August 2011 to 31 July 2021. A retrospective chart review of the surgical records of the hospital's database was performed in order to identify all patients diagnosed with hemifacial spasm and had been treated surgically.

Two experienced neuroradiologists evaluated all cases independently. They were aware that the patients were clinically diagnosed with HFS, but they were blinded from knowing the symptomatic side. They evaluated each case two different times. Primarily, they were asked to analyze the MRI in order to evaluate whether there was a neurovascular conflict based on the gold standard technique which consists of identifying the facial nerve and accurately evaluating its entire path from the pontomedullary transition to the internal acoustic canal and to search for any vascular attachment or compression. Once they had finished this initial analysis, the neuroradiologists received a file with the description of the PS. In a second instance, the same neuroradiologists were asked to reassess the same MRI list, looking to identify the presence of this novel sign and to determine on which side it was present.

Once the authors received the reports from both neuroradiologists, we analyzed the accuracy of the diagnosis based on the standard evaluation (percentage of diagnosis in the symptomatic sign) and also the presence of the PS and its accuracy (to calculate sensibility). The authors utilized the contralateral side (asymptomatic side) as the control to calculate the specificity.

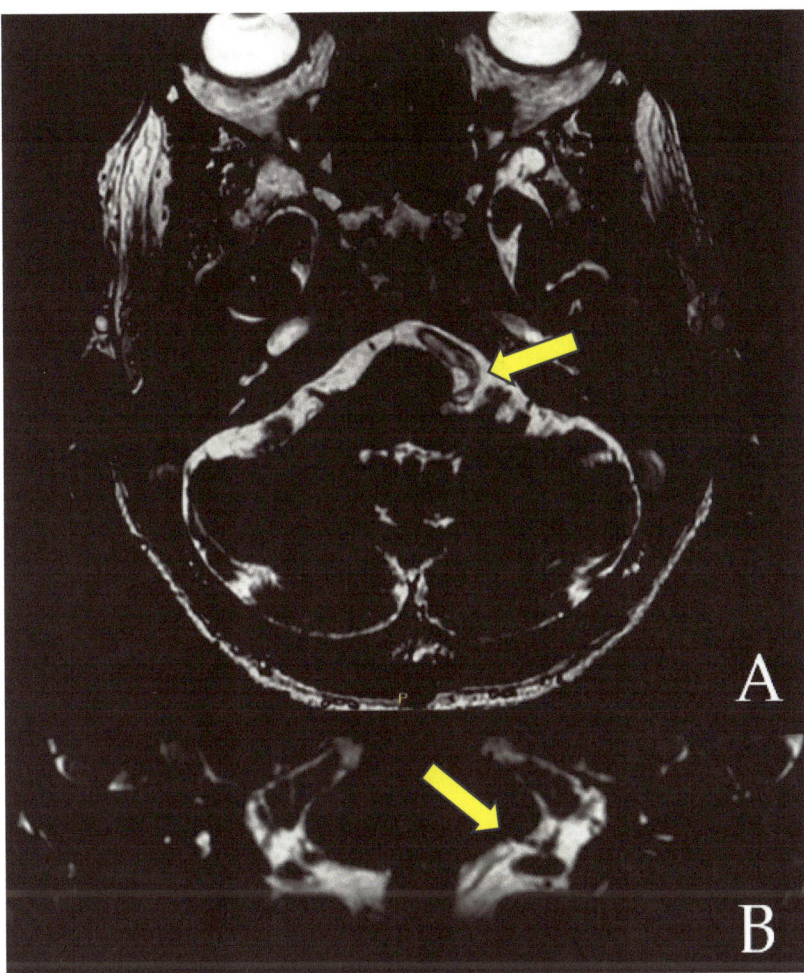

Figure 1. The axial view gives the false impression that the artery is located inside the pons (**A**). However, the coronal view clearly demonstrates that the vessel does not enter the brainstem (**B**). The yellow arrows point to the local of the NVC.

2.3. Image Study

The MRI examinations were performed on a 3 T MR scanner. The MRIs were performed using our cranial nerve protocol, which were sagittal, and axial T2-heavily weighted images (T2WI) in thin-sliced acquisitions; axial, sagittal, and coronal T1 weighted images (T1WI) with contrast of the whole brain and also a thin-slice sequence of the posterior fossa; and axial fluid-attenuated inversion recovery (FLAIR) and diffusion-weighted imaging (DWI) sequences.

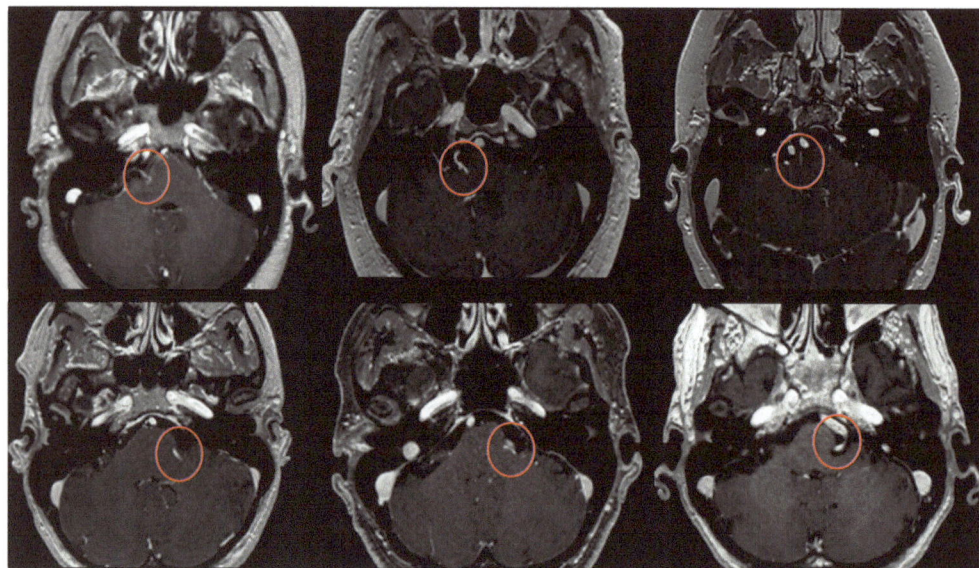

Figure 2. Six examples of the PS identified (inside the red circles) in T1WI with gadolinium axial images.

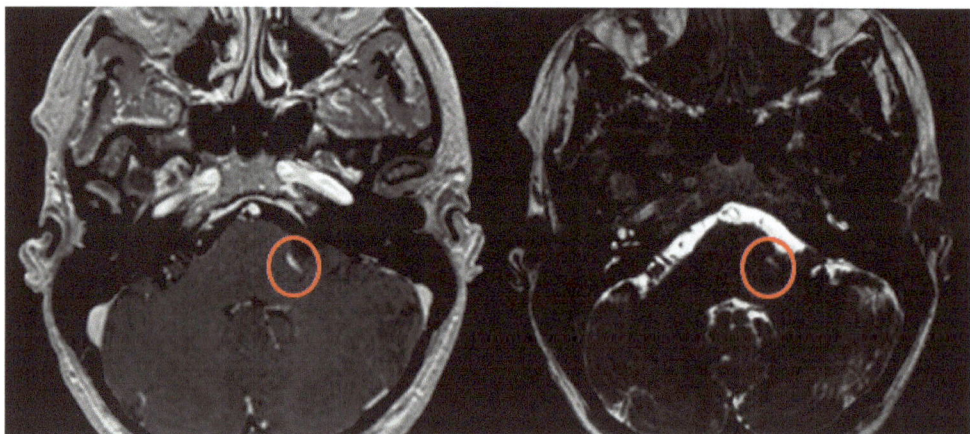

Figure 3. Axial view of MRI in T1WI with gadolinium and FIESTA sequences demonstrating the presence of the Prevedello sign (an arterial loop attached to the pons near the exit of the facial nerve), highlighted by the red circles.

The image sequences were obtained in 0.3 to 0.4 mm slice thickness and a multiplanar oblique reconstructions were obtained in axial, sagittal, and coronal views, following the course of the facial nerve.

2.4. Variables

The variables analyzed included radiological, clinical, and demographic-related variables. The radiological related variables included the presence of the NVC according to the standard criteria established in the medical literature, the presence or absence of the PS, and the side on which it was identified. The clinical variables analyzed included the side of the symptom and the vessel responsible for the NVC. The possible arteries involved in the NVC were the vertebral artery (VA), posterior inferior cerebellar artery (PICA), and anterior inferior cerebellar artery (AICA). When the compression involved more than one artery, all of the arteries were described as contributing to the NVC (i.e., AICA and VA, PICA, and AICA). The demographic data evaluated was the age and gender of the patients.

2.5. Patient Eligibility

Patients admitted at The Ohio State University Wexner Medical Center between 1 August 2011 and 31 July 2021, who were diagnosed with HFS and submitted to microsurgical neurovascular decompression were included.

2.6. Statistical Analysis

Data were collected using Microsoft Excel 2019 software. Statistical analysis was performed using the Statistical Package for the Social Sciences (IBM SPSS Statistics for Windows, Version 22.0. Armonk, NY, USA: IBM Corp.). Numerical variables parametricity were tested and parametric distributed variables were presented as mean and standard deviation. Categorical variables were presented in absolute numbers and proportion. The sensitivity, specificity, and Cohen's Kappa Index were calculated for the analyses based on the results of the standard evaluation and the presence of the PS.

The prevalence ratio of the PS was calculated according to the formula: percentage of PS in the symptomatic sign divided by the percentage of PS in the asymptomatic sign.

Parallel combined sensitivity was calculated using the following formula: sensitivity of standard method + sensitivity of PS − [sensitivity of standard method × sensitivity of PS].

Parallel combined specificity was calculated according to the formula: specificity of standard method × specificity of PS.

3. Results

During the study period, a total of 35 patients were surgically treated for HFS. The majority of patients were females (65.7%) with a mean age of 59.02 (+0.48). According to the symptoms, the right side was involved in 13 cases (37.14%) and the left side in 22 cases (62.85%). There were no cases of bilateral hemifacial spasm in this sample (Table 1).

Table 1. Epidemiological and clinical results.

Age	59.02 (±0.48) *
Gender	
Female	23 (65.7%) °
Male	12 (34.2%) °
Symptomatic side	
Right	13 (37.14%) °
Left	22 (62.85%) °
Artery involved	
PICA	11 (31.42%) °
AICA	8 (22.85%) °
VA	4 (11.42%) °
AICA + PICA	6 (17.14%) °
PICA + VA	5 (14.28%) °

* Mean (±standard deviation), ° Absolute number (percentage).

The intraoperative vascular compression was identified in all cases, but in one case the vessel was not specified. The PICA was solely responsible for the NVC in 11 cases (31.42%), combined PICA and AICA arteries were responsible for NVC in 6 cases (17.14%), solely AICA in 8 cases (22.85%), combined PICA and VA in 5 cases (14.28%), and the VA alone was responsible for 4 cases (11.42%) of NVC in this sample.

Since two different neuroradiologists evaluated the 35 cases searching for the presence of neurovascular compression on both sides, a total of 140 evaluations were performed.

Since all patients presented symptoms unilaterally and both neuroradiologists independently evaluated each case but they were blinded from the symptomatic side, they were forced to evaluate both sides in every patient; this totaled 140 reports that were included in the analysis (35 cases × 2 sides evaluated × 2 neuroradiologists).

Based on MRI analysis using the standard technique, 66 neurovascular compressions were identified on the symptomatic side (sensitivity of 94.2%, specificity of 97.1%, PPV of 97.05% and NPV of 94.4%). The PS was present in 66 analyses (sensitivity of 94.2%) and among the 70 analyses of the asymptomatic side, 64 did not have the PS (specificity 91.4%). Among the patients in whom the PS was present, 90.9% of the time it was identified on the symptomatic side (PPV 90.9%) (Table 2). The calculated prevalence ratio was 1.41.

Table 2. Test analysis results.

	Sensitivity	Specificity	PPV	NPV	Cohen Kappa Index
Standard MRI evaluation	94.2%	97.1%	97.05%	94.4%	0.714
Prevedello sign	94.2%	91.4%	90.9%		0.82
Tests in parallel	99.2%	88.7%			

PPV: positive predictive value, NPV: negative predictive value.

When both analyses were performed in parallel (standard plus PV), the sensitivity increased to 99.2%.

The correlation Cohen Kappa index was performed for both analyses, demonstrating an index of 0.714 for the gold standard evaluation and 0.542 for the Prevedello sign.

4. Discussion

Primary HFS is triggered by neurovascular conflict (NVC), whereas secondary HFS comprises all other causes that may compress the facial nerve, such as posterior fossa tumors, arteriovenous malformation, Paget's disease, and Chiari malformation [7].

The facial nerve exits the brain stem as a single entity forming the cisternal segment extending towards the internal acoustic meatus with a mean length of 17.93 mm (range, 14.8–20.9 mm) [9]. Along its path, the facial nerve runs close to vascular structures. If these structures are in contact with the nerve, an NVC may occur. According to the literature, the AICA is the most common vessel causing NVC (corresponding for 43% of the cases), followed by the PICA (31%) and VA (23%) [3,10]. In our series, the PICA was the most frequently involved artery solely responsible for NVC and was involved in additional instances in conjunction with the AICA or the VA. The AICA alone and the VA alone were responsible for one third of the cases.

In the majority of cases, the location of the neurovascular compression is in the first few millimeters from the brainstem. The facial nerve emerges in the brainstem surface from the pontomedullary sulcus at the upper edge of the supraolivary fossette and strongly adheres to the surface of the pons for 8–10 mm before separating from the brainstem [10]. Once separated from the brainstem, the first 1.9 to 2.86 mm of the facial nerve is a segment characterized by the transition of cells responsible for myelination of the nerve (from oligodendrocytes to the Schwann cells) [3,11], and is anatomically known as root exit/entry zone of cranial nerve [12]. Histologically, this specific area of the nerve is defined as Obersteiner–Redlich transition zone (TZ). Since this zone lacks an epineurium, the nerve is protected by an arachnoid membrane only, which makes it vulnerable to mechanical compression caused by vessel's pulsation [13]. Pressure applied in this region may trigger action potentials from the demyelinated segment of the nerve, leading to symptoms [14].

Regular MRI sequences are essential in determining secondary causes of HFS [7,15]. Post-contrast T1 sequences (to evaluate cerebellopontine angle solid tumors), T2-weighted sequence (to evaluate intra-axial lesions in the brainstem, i.e.: demyelinating disease), and diffusion-weighted imaging (to evaluate for the presence of cystic disease, i.e., differentiating epidermoid cysts from arachnoid) are useful for the differential diagnosis.

In the context of primary NVC, since it mainly occurs at the REZ, this segment should be carefully explored [8]. Image slice thickness should optimally be between 0.3 to 0.4mm [7,16], especially in the arterial phase [17,18].

Multiplanar oblique reconstructions should be obtained following the course of the facial nerve. A variety of high-resolution 3D heavily T2WI sequences are currently available, depending on the manufacturer, and may be helpful during investigation. These sequences include constructive interference in steady-state (CISS), steady-state-free precession (SSFP), T2WI-driven equilibrium radio frequency reset pulse (DRIVE), three-dimensional fast imaging employing steady-state acquisition (FIESTA), and sampling perfection with application-optimized contrasts by using different flip angle evolutions (SPACE) [7,19]. Additionally, 3D T2WI sequences provide "cisterno-graphic" images of cranial nerves and vessels surrounded by cerebrospinal fluid, with high spatial resolution [7,16].

Despite the various imaging modalities described above, in some patients the NVC is not visualized. According to this sample analysis, 6 patients out of a 100 will not have the diagnosis of the NVC using the standard MRI method. This scenario puts the neurosurgeon in a challenging situation, since not indicating surgical intervention will prolong the patient's symptomatology and increase their morbidity when it could be resolved surgically (this would represent an error type 1/alpha, due to the limitation of the diagnosis method). On the other hand, indicating surgery without preoperative visualization of an NVC on image exams increases the risk of surgery misindication or surgical failure.

An interesting paper published by Ahmad et al. [20], investigated the relationship between practice setting of radiologist interpreting MRI scans and reported detection of NVC in patients with trigeminal neuralgia (TN), whose neurovascular compression was confirmed intraoperatively. According to their results, blinded academic neuroradiologists are more likely to detect neurovascular compression when compared with community radiologists. Although this paper included only TN cases, the physiopathology, investigative methods, and treatment of TN are similar to HFS; therefore, we can assume that the variability reported in papers related to TN may also occur in the evaluation of HFS [21,22].

The advent of a second independent method to determine the NVC is helpful to increase the diagnosis rate. Even though the PS used independently had a lower sensitivity and specificity when compared to the standard criteria, the use of both diagnostic methods in conjunction increased the sensitivity to 99%.

This new MRI criteria is helpful for the diagnosis of NVC in patients with HFS, not in terms of being a substitute of the standard pattern, but as a complementary diagnostic method.

This paper has several limitations that should be highlighted. The sample size of this study was determined by the number of patients meeting the inclusion criteria rather than based on sample size calculation. The sample size of 35 patients may influence the sensitivity of the MRI evaluation, and a higher number of patients would better approximate the epidemiologic values calculated in this study. A single center study may bias the evaluation of the MRI and also the agreement between the neuroradiologists (even though they evaluated the cases independently, the proximity and weekly radiological discussion of skull base cases may interfere in the evaluation). The patients were not submitted to a 3D time-of-flight magnetic resonance angiography, which was recently described as having the better diagnostic performance for detecting NVC in patients with trigeminal neuralgia or HSF [23]. On the other hand, the interpretation of the exams by neuroradiologists focused on skull base pathologies may overestimate the sensitivity of the standard MRI evaluation. The moderate correlation index for the PS may be due to the low familiarity of the neuroradiologists with this sign, but also may represent variable interpretation of the sign. Finally, the purpose of the study was to describe a new MRI finding for HFS and to analyze its frequency patterns. The MRI images were retrospectively assessed; therefore, the presence of the PS was not used as a criterion for surgery indication in the cases included in this sample. However, it is important to emphasize that the senior author has been using this sign as an easy method of corroboration with the patient's symptomatology, which is the most important factor to indicate surgery. In addition, the study's design (cross-section) is not ideal for evaluating outcomes. To determine if the presence of the PS helps to achieve a better surgical result, it is necessary to perform a longitudinal study (either prospective or retrospective, which are cohort and case-control, respectively).

Despite the limitations discussed above, the main strength of this paper is to describe an MRI sign that is helpful in the diagnosis of NVC for HFS in cases where the standard diagnosis is doubtful or not visualized. Additionally, the evaluation of the PS is performed with regular MRI protocols and does not require any additional or different image acquisitions (it does not increase the cost of the exam, extra gadolinium infusion is not necessary, and it does not present any increased risk for the patients). The only additional work required to evaluate the presence of the PS is a supplementary examination of the T1WI and FIESTA axial acquisitions by the radiologists to evaluate for the presence of the PS.

5. Conclusions

The PS is helpful in determining the neurovascular conflict point for diagnosis in patients with HFS. The presence of this sign, combined with the standard evaluation, increases the sensitivity of the MRI to over 99%, without increasing risk of harm to patients or resulting in additional costs.

Author Contributions: Conceptualization, G.F., L.M.P. and D.M.P.; methodology, G.F., K.C.W., L.M.P. and D.M.P.; software, S.S.G., B.G.M., D.K., M.T.S. and L.M.P.; validation, K.C.W. and J.V.-J.; formal analysis, G.F., K.C.W. and J.V.-J.; investigation, B.G.M., D.K., L.M.P. and M.T.S.; data curation, G.F. and D.M.P.; writing—original draft preparation, G.F., K.C.W. and J.V.-J.; writing—review and editing, B.G.M., D.K., L.M.P. and D.M.P.; visualization, L.M.P. and D.M.P.; supervision, D.M.P.; project administration, L.M.P. All authors have read and agreed to the published version of the manuscript.

Funding: This research received no external funding.

Institutional Review Board Statement: The study was conducted at the Department of Neurosurgery, Skull Base section, at the Ohio State University and approved by the institutional Ethics Review Board under the number 2022E0740.

Informed Consent Statement: Patient consented was waived by the IRB due to the retrospective design of the study.

Data Availability Statement: The data for this study is unavailable due to privacy or ethical restrictions in concordance to the institutional HIPAA's policy.

Conflicts of Interest: Daniel M. Prevedello is a consultant for Stryker Corp., Medtronic Corp., BK Medical and Integra; he has received an honorarium from Mizuho and royalties from Mizuho, KLS-Martin and ACE Medical. The other authors have no personal, financial, or institutional interest in any of the drugs, materials, or devices described in this article.

Previous Presentations: The authors included the following paragraph to the manuscript: This study was presented as oral presentation at the North American Skull Base Society 32nd Annual Meeting in Tampa/FL, 2023.

References

1. Tan, N.-C.; Chan, L.L.; Tan, E.K. Hemifacial spasm and involuntary facial movements. *Qjm Int. J. Med.* **2002**, *95*, 493–500. [CrossRef] [PubMed]
2. Auger, R.G.; Whisnant, J.P. Hemifacial Spasm in Rochester and Olmsted County, Minnesota, 1960 to 1984. *Arch. Neurol.* **1990**, *47*, 1233–1234. [CrossRef] [PubMed]
3. Chaudhry, N.; Srivastava, A.; Joshi, L. Hemifacial spasm: The past, present and future. *J. Neurol. Sci.* **2015**, *356*, 27–31. [CrossRef] [PubMed]
4. McGahan, B.G.; Albonette-Felicio, T.; Kreatsoulas, D.C.; Magill, S.T.; Hardesty, D.A.; Prevedello, D.M. Simultaneous Endoscopic and Microscopic Visualization in Microvascular Decompression for Hemifacial Spasm. *Oper. Neurosurg.* **2021**, *21*, 540–548. [CrossRef] [PubMed]
5. Yousry, I.; Moriggl, B.; Holtmannspoetter, M.; Schmid, U.D.; Naidich, T.P.; Yousry, T.A. Detailed anatomy of the motor and sensory roots of the trigeminal nerve and their neurovascular relationships: A magnetic resonance imaging study. *J. Neurosurg.* **2004**, *101*, 427–434. [CrossRef]
6. Leal, P.R.L.; Hermier, M.; Souza, M.A.; Cristino-Filho, G.; Froment, J.C.; Sindou, M. Visualization of Vascular Compression of the Trigeminal Nerve With High-Resolution 3T MRI: A Prospective Study Comparing Preoperative Imaging Analysis to Surgical Findings in 40 Consecutive Patients Who Underwent Microvascular Decompression for Trigeminal Neuralgia. *Neurosurgery* **2011**, *69*, 15–26.
7. Haller, S.; Etienne, L.; Kövari, E.; Varoquaux, A.D.; Urbach, H.; Becker, M. Imaging of neurovascular compression syndromes: Trigeminal neuralgia, Hemifacial spasm, vestibular Paroxysmia, and Glossopharyngeal neuralgia. *Am. J. Neuroradiol.* **2016**, *37*, 1384–1392. [CrossRef]
8. Hermier, M. Imaging of hemifacial spasm. *Neurochirurgie* **2018**, *64*, 117–123. [CrossRef]
9. Guclu, B.; Sindou, M.; Meyronet, D.; Streichenberger, N.; Simon, E.; Mertens, P. Cranial nerve vascular compression syndromes of the trigeminal, facial and vago-glossopharyngeal nerves: Comparative anatomical study of the central myelin portion and transitional zone—Correlations with incidences of corresponding hyperactive dysfunction. *Acta Neurochir.* **2011**, *153*, 2365–2375. [CrossRef]
10. Campos-Benitez, M.; Kaufmann, A.M. Neurovascular compression findings in hemifacial spasm. *J. Neurosurg.* **2008**, *109*, 416–420. [CrossRef]
11. Tarlov, I. Structure of the nerve root, I: Nature of the junction between the central and the peripheral nervous system. *Arch. Neur.-Psych.* **1937**, *37*, 555–583. [CrossRef]
12. Nielsen, V.K. Electrophysiology of the facial nerve in hemifacial spasm: Ectopic/ephaptic excitation. *Muscle Nerve* **1985**, *8*, 545–555. [CrossRef] [PubMed]
13. Peker, S.; Kurtkaya, O.; Üzün, I.; Pamir, M.N. Microanatomy of the Central Myelin-Peripheral Myelin Transition Zone of the Trigeminal Nerve. *Neurosurgery* **2006**, *59*, 354–359. [CrossRef] [PubMed]
14. Sindou, M.; Keravel, Y. Neurosurgical treatment of primary hemifacial spasm with microvascular decompression. *Neuro-Chirurgie* **2009**, *55*, 236–247. [CrossRef] [PubMed]
15. Donahue, J.H.; Ornan, D.A.; Mukherjee, S. Imaging of Vascular Compression Syndromes. *Radiol. Clin. N. Am.* **2017**, *55*, 123–138. [CrossRef]
16. Ohta, M.; Kobayashi, M.; Wakiya, K.; Takamizawa, S.; Niitsu, M.; Fujimaki, T. Preoperative assessment of hemifacial spasm by the coronal heavilyT2-weighted MR cisternography. *Acta Neurochir.* **2014**, *156*, 565–569. [CrossRef]
17. Hughes, M.A.; Traylor, K.S.; Branstetter, I.V.B.F.; Eubanks, K.P.; Chang, Y.-F.; Sekula, R.F., Jr. Imaging predictors of successful surgical treatment of hemifacial spasm. *Brain Commun.* **2021**, *3*, fcab146. [CrossRef]
18. Tash, R.; DeMerritt, J.; Sze, G.; Leslie, D. Hemifacial spasm: MR imaging features. *AJNR Am. J. Neuroradiol.* **1991**, *12*, 839–842.
19. Hughes, M.; Branstetter, B.; Taylor, C.; Fakhran, S.; Delfyett, W.; Frederickson, A.; Sekula, R. MRI Findings in Patients with a History of Failed Prior Microvascular Decompression for Hemifacial Spasm: How to Image and Where to Look. *Am. J. Neuroradiol.* **2014**, *36*, 768–773. [CrossRef]
20. Ahmad, H.S.; Blue, R.; Ajmera, S.; Heman-Ackah, S.; Spadola, M.; Lazor, J.W.; Lee, J.Y. The Influence of Radiologist Practice Setting on Identification of Vascular Compression from Magnetic Resonance Imaging in Trigeminal Neuralgia. *World Neurosurg.* **2023**, *171*, e398–e403. [CrossRef]
21. Anderson, V.; Berryhill, P.; Sandquist, M.; Ciaverella, D.; Nesbit, G.; Burchiel, K.J. High-resolution three-dimensional magnetic resonance angiography and three-dimensional spoiled gradient-recalled imaging in the evaluation of neurovascular compression in patients with trigeminal neuralgia: A double-blind pilot study. *Neurosurgery* **2006**, *58*, 666–673. [CrossRef] [PubMed]
22. Miller, J.P.; Acar, F.; Hamilton, B.E.; Burchiel, K.J. Radiographic evaluation of trigeminal neurovascular compression in patients with and without trigeminal neuralgia. *J. Neurosurg.* **2009**, *110*, 627–632. [CrossRef] [PubMed]
23. Liang, C.; Yang, L.; Reichardt, W.; Zhang, B.; Li, R. Different MRI-based methods for the diagnosis of neurovascular compression in trigeminal neuralgia or hemifacial spasm: A network meta-analysis. *J. Clin. Neurosci.* **2023**, *108*, 19–24. [CrossRef] [PubMed]

Disclaimer/Publisher's Note: The statements, opinions and data contained in all publications are solely those of the individual author(s) and contributor(s) and not of MDPI and/or the editor(s). MDPI and/or the editor(s) disclaim responsibility for any injury to people or property resulting from any ideas, methods, instructions or products referred to in the content.

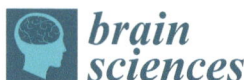

Article

Comparison of Surgeons' Assessment of the Extent of Vestibular Schwannoma Resection with Immediate Post Operative and Follow-Up Volumetric MRI Analysis

Hossein Mahboubi [1], William H. Slattery III [1], Mia E. Miller [1,2] and Gregory P. Lekovic [1,3,*]

1 House Institute, Los Angeles, CA 90057, USA
2 Cedars-Sinai Hospital, Los Angeles, CA 90048, USA
3 Department of Neurosurgery, David Geffen School of Medicine, University of California Los Angeles, Los Angeles, CA 90024, USA
* Correspondence: glekovic@mednet.ucla.edu; Tel.: +1-(310)-825-8111

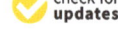

Citation: Mahboubi, H.; Slattery, W.H., III; Miller, M.E.; Lekovic, G.P. Comparison of Surgeons' Assessment of the Extent of Vestibular Schwannoma Resection with Immediate Post Operative and Follow-Up Volumetric MRI Analysis. *Brain Sci.* **2023**, *13*, 1490. https://doi.org/10.3390/brainsci13101490

Academic Editor: Miguel Lopez-Gonzalez

Received: 23 September 2023
Revised: 18 October 2023
Accepted: 20 October 2023
Published: 22 October 2023

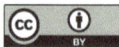

Copyright: © 2023 by the authors. Licensee MDPI, Basel, Switzerland. This article is an open access article distributed under the terms and conditions of the Creative Commons Attribution (CC BY) license (https://creativecommons.org/licenses/by/4.0/).

Abstract: (1) Background: Incomplete excision of vestibular schwannomas (VSs) is sometimes preferable for facial nerve preservation. On the other hand, subtotal resection may be associated with higher tumor recurrence. We evaluated the correlation between intra-operative assessment of residual tumor and early and follow-up imaging. (2) Methods: The charts of all patients undergoing primary surgery for sporadic vestibular schwannoma during the study period were retrospectively reviewed. Data regarding surgeons' assessments of the extent of resection, and the residual size of the tumor on post-operative day (POD) one and follow-up MRI were extracted. (3) Results: Of 109 vestibular schwannomas meeting inclusion criteria, gross-total resection (GTR) was achieved in eighty-four, near-total (NTR) and sub-total resection (STR) in twenty-two and three patients, respectively. On follow up imaging, volumetric analysis revealed that of twenty-two NTRs, eight were radiographic GTR and nine were radiographic STR (mean volume ratio 11.9%), while five remained NTR (mean volume ratio 1.8%). Of the three STRs, two were radiographic GTR while one remained STR. Therefore, of eighteen patients with available later follow up MRIs, radiographic classification of the degree of resection changed in six. (4) Conclusions: An early MRI (POD#1) establishes a baseline for the residual tumor that may be more accurate than the surgeon's intraoperative assessment and may provide a beneficial point of comparison for long-term surveillance.

Keywords: vestibular schwannoma; magnetic resonance imaging; residual tumor; gross total resection; near-total resection; subtotal resection

1. Introduction

Vestibular schwannoma is a slow growing benign neoplasm of the eighth cranial nerve, commonly referred to as acoustic neuroma. The tumors are rare (1:100,000 incidence) but are the most common tumor of the temporal bone. VS usually presents with hearing loss; less common presenting symptoms include vestibulopathy, facial numbness, headache, or other neurologic signs and symptoms.

Recent decades have been witness to significant changes in the management of vestibular schwannomas. Improvements in understanding the natural history of vestibular schwannomas and enhancements in magnetic resonance imaging (MRI) techniques along with favorable long-term outcomes of radiosurgery have transformed the vestibular schwannoma treatment algorithms [1–4]. While gross-total resection remains the goal in vestibular schwannoma surgery, incomplete resections have gained popularity where preservation of the integrity of the facial nerve and other structures is otherwise in jeopardy [5].

When incomplete resection is performed, the estimated residual size and shape is used as a baseline for long-term follow-up. The residual tumor is usually observed with serial MRIs for regrowth, which may necessitate treatment by radiosurgery or revision microsurgery. Surgeons' assessment of a near- or sub-total resection may not be consistent with how much tumor is actually left behind. This intra-operative assessment can be inaccurate as demonstrated in a previous published study [6] in which the authors found no correlation between intra-operative assessment of a near-total resection and post-operative MRI findings. Furthermore, post-surgical changes will occur at the surgical bed over time, which may impede the differentiation of residual tumor from scar tissue. This can become especially problematic if the residual tumor noted on the delayed post-operative MRI is much larger than anticipated. In this situation, it would be challenging to determine whether a small residual tumor underwent significant growth, or a larger residual tumor was left at the initial surgery.

While practices among vestibular schwannoma surgeons vary, at our institution, an MRI is obtained on post-operative day one in all patients undergoing vestibular schwannoma resection. In this study, we aimed to assess the correlation between the intra-operative assessment of a residual tumor and early post-operative MRI findings by reviewing the data from our cohort of vestibular schwannomas. Furthermore, we compared the immediate and follow-up post-operative images to evaluate for changes in tumor shape and size with time. The results from this study can provide a better understanding of the differences between intra-operative assessment of residual size and post-operative MRI findings.

2. Materials and Methods

This study was approved by our local Institutional Review Board (IRB# SV-018-21). Upon approval, a retrospective chart review was performed on patients who underwent surgery for vestibular schwannomas between October 2017 and October 2019 at our tertiary referral center. Patients with neurofibromatosis type II, revision cases, and those without available pre- or post-operative MRIs were excluded. Data regarding patient demographics, surgical approach, extent of resection (EOR), and intra-operative assessment of residual size were extracted from the charts. Intra-operative degree of resection was reported as gross-total resection (GTR), near-total resection (NTR), or sub-total resection (STR). A GTR was determined when the surgeon was confident of complete tumor removal. NTR was determined when only a thin layer of the tumor capsule was left on the facial nerve or other structures, and this was estimated to be less than 5% of the original tumor volume. Other cases were considered STR. A surgical endoscope was routinely used in cases where the lateral border of the tumor could not be directly visualized (e.g., in the case of the tumor extending laterally to the transverse crest when approaching via the middle fossa).

Patients' pre- and post-operative MRIs were obtained and analyzed. Our institution's protocol is to obtain an MRI of the brain with and without contrast, including fat suppression, on post-operative day one. This post-operative MRI was used to evaluate for the presence of any radiographic residual tumor and then compared to the patient's last available follow up MRI. Horos DICOM image analysis software (v 3.3.5, www.horosproject.org, accessed on 1 October 2019) was used to compute the volume of the pre-operative tumor and those of any residual tumors if present. Volumetric analysis was performed on post-contrast, T1 weighted images. The presence of a residual tumor was confirmed by comparing these images to pre-contrast T1 and fluid-attenuated inversion recovery (FLAIR) as well as other available sequences to rule out hemorrhage or edema. The perimeter method was used to calculate the volumes [7]. The perimeters of tumor or residual tumor were outlined on consecutive images and then the volume of the region of interest (ROI) was calculated using the built-in function from the software.

Using this volumetric analysis, the degree of resection was defined as radiographic GTR (undetectable residual), radiographic NTR (residual $\leq$ 5% of the pre-operative tumor volume), or radiographic STR (residual > 5% of pre-operative tumor volume). The correlation between the radiographic and intra-operative assessments of the degree of resection were then compared. The shapes of the residual tumors were further analyzed and classified as linear or nodular. Statistical analysis was performed using SPSS 1.0 (IBM, Armonk,

NY, USA). Nonparametric tests were used given the skewed distribution of samples. A p value of 0.05 was considered as the threshold of statistical significance.

3. Results

A total of two hundred and three patients undergoing surgery for VSs during the study period were identified, excluding patients with neurofibromatosis type II, revision cases, and those with unavailable MRI images. A total of 109 cases of primary vestibular schwannoma surgeries were analyzed. The mean age was 52.7 years (range 19–79) and 35.8% were males.

3.1. Surgeon's Asssessment vs. Immediate and Follow Up MRI

3.1.1. Surgical Approach and Surgeon's Assessment of EOR

The surgical approach was translabyrinthine in sixty-nine (63.3%), middle fossa in thirty (27.5%), retrosigmoid in nine (8.3%), and transotic in one (0.9%). Based on the intra-operative assessments by the senior neurosurgeon, GTR was achieved in eighty-four (77.1%) while a residual was left behind in twenty-five cases (22.9%), consisting of twenty-two NTRs (20.2%) and three STRs (2.8%). The main reason for leaving a residual was severe adherence to the facial nerve in all cases. The intra-operative estimate of residual size varied from 1 to 10 mm.

3.1.2. Immediate Post-Operative MRI Evaluation of EOR

The average pre-operative volume was 3.23 cm^3 (range 0.02–24.97 cm^3). The tumors that underwent GTR had a significantly smaller volume (mean 1.93 cm^3, median 0.55 cm^3) than those with a residual (mean 7.26 cm^3, median 4.05 cm^3, $p < 0.001$). This difference was not statistically significant between tumors that underwent NTR and STR ($p = 0.9$). As detailed in Table 1, MRI confirmed no residual tumor in all cases when the neurosurgeon's assessment was GTR intra-operatively. Lack of a residual tumor was further confirmed during follow-up MRIs obtained at around 3 and/or 12 months post-operatively.

Table 1. Surgical resection based on intra-operative versus radiographic assessment.

Intra-Operative Assessment	Immediate Post-Operative MRI			
	Gross-Total	Near-Total	Sub-Total	Total
Gross-total	84 (100%)	0 (0%)	0 (0%)	84
Near-total	8 (36%)	5 (23%)	9 (41%)	22
Sub-total	2 (67%)	0 (0%)	1 (33%)	3
Total	94	5	10	

Volumetric analysis of residual tumors on the immediate post-operative MRI revealed that of twenty-two near-total cases, eight were radiographic GTR and nine were radiographic STR (mean volume ratio 11.9%), while five remained radiographic NTR (mean volume ratio 1.8%). Of the three sub-total cases, two were radiographic GTR while one remained radiographic STR. Of cases with a radiographic residual, seven had linear and eight had nodular residuals. Figure 1 demonstrate examples of these pre- and post-operative tumor images. Overall, radiographic assessment changed the degree of resection in nineteen cases (17.4% of all cases and 76% of cases with a residual).

A sub-analysis was performed on the pre-operative volumes of the tumors for which residual size was underestimated intra-operatively. These tumors had undergone NTR but were recategorized as radiographic STR based on the immediate post-operative MRI. The mean volume of these tumors was 8.93 cm^3 (median 7.30 cm^3) compared to a mean volume of 5.27 cm^3 (median 2.89 cm^3) in tumors that were considered as radiographic NTRs and GTRs. This difference, however, did not reach statistical significance ($p = 0.27$).

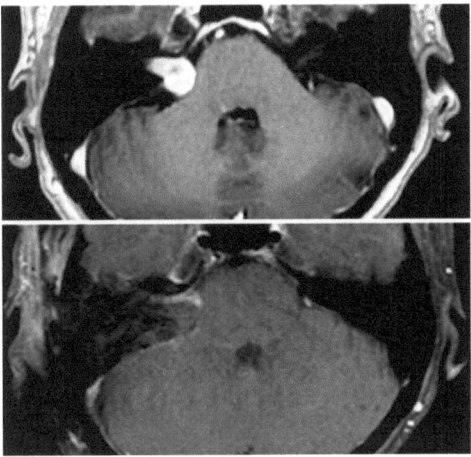

Figure 1. Pre-operative MRI (**top** panel) shows right sided vestibular schwannoma that was resected (**bottom** panel) using a translabyrinthine approach. While this was assessed as a near-total resection, post-operative volumetric analysis classified the residual as subtotal resection (7.9% of original tumor volume).

3.1.3. Follow-Up MRI Evaluation of EOR

All patients had follow-up imaging. Follow-up post-operative MRI (ranging 3 to 22 months) was available for eighteen patients with residual tumors (sixteen NTRs and two STRs). Lack of a residual tumor was confirmed via follow-up MRIs obtained around 3 and/or 12 months post-operatively on all patients in whom the intra-operative assessment was consistent with gross-total resection. As seen in Table 2, the resection assessment changed in six cases in between the immediate and delayed MRIs. In two cases, while a residual was seen on the immediate MRI, the delayed MRI was assessed as radiographic GTR. In two cases, while no residuals were seen on the immediate MRI, the delayed MRIs revealed residual tumors (both radiographic NTR; Figure 2). In the other two cases the assessment changed from radiographic STR to NTR.

Table 2. Comparison of the residual volume ratios between immediate and delayed post-operative MRI.

	Age/Sex	Intra-Operative Assessment	Residual Volume Ratio		Change in Radiographic Assessment
			Immediate MRI	Delayed MRI	
1	29 F	NTR	R-NTR	R-NTR	No
2	55 F	NTR	R-STR	R-GTR	Yes
3	35 F	NTR	R-NTR	R-NTR	No
4	53 F	NTR	R-NTR	R-GTR	Yes
5	62 F	NTR	R-NTR	R-NTR	No
6	58 F	NTR	R-GTR	R-NTR	Yes
7	61 F	NTR	R-STR	R-STR	No
8	57 F	NTR	R-GTR	R-GTR	No
9	50 M	NTR	R-GTR	R-GTR	No
10	65 M	NTR	R-GTR	R-NTR	Yes
11	40 F	NTR	R-NTR	R-NTR	No

Table 2. Cont.

	Age/Sex	Intra-Operative Assessment	Residual Volume Ratio		Change in Radiographic Assessment
			Immediate MRI	Delayed MRI	
12	68 F	NTR	R-STR	R-STR	No
13	52 F	NTR	R-STR	R-NTR	Yes
14	25 F	NTR	R-STR	R-NTR	Yes
15	54 F	NTR	R-GTR	R-GTR	No
16	54 F	NTR	R-GTR	R-GTR	No
17	71 M	STR	R-STR	R-STR	No
18	54 M	STR	R-GTR	R-GTR	No

R-GTR: Radiographic GTR.

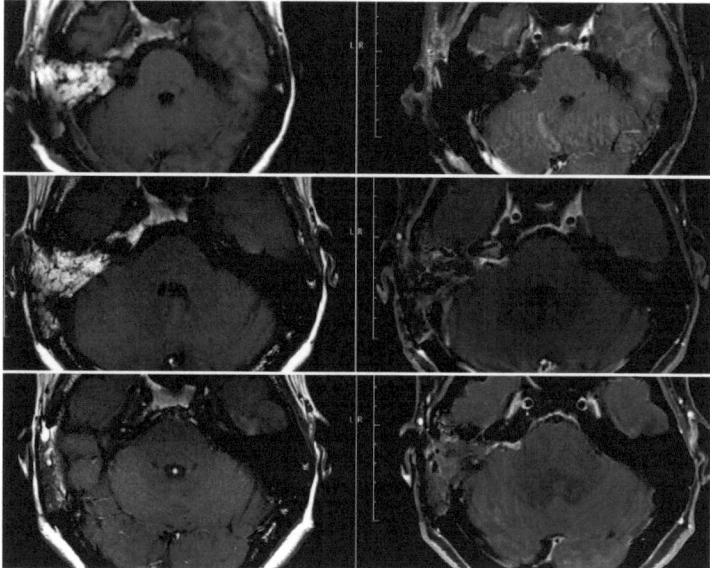

Figure 2. Post-operative MRIs at day 1 (**top**), 3 months (**middle**), and 15 months (**bottom**) after NTR of a right sided vestibular schwannoma. The intra-operative residual estimate was 1 mm. The immediate MRI was a radiographic GTR, but the delayed MRIs were radiographic NTR with stable appearance of the area of enhancement.

4. Discussion

The present study revealed a disparity between the intra-operative assessment of tumor residual size and post-operative radiographic assessments in some cases. When the surgeon was confident in removing the entire tumor, post-operative MRI confirmed GTR. However, when a residual was left behind, the degree of resection was recategorized in 76% of the cases after the post-operative MRI was reviewed. These findings are consistent with a previous study that evaluated residual tumors on post-operative MRIs in fifty vestibular schwannomas including fifteen NTRs and eight STRs. About 73% of the NTRs were actually noted to be radiographic STR, while all STRs were also radiographic STR [6]. By comparison, the percentage of NTRs being recategorized as radiographic STRs in the present study was lower (nine cases, 41%). In these nine cases where the residual tumor was underestimated, the pre-operative tumor volume was, on average, smaller. Although no statistical significance was reached due to the relatively small sample size, this difference can be clinically significant and suggests that in smaller tumors intra-operative estimation of the residual volume relative to the original tumor may be more difficult.

Surgeons' intra-operative assessment is mainly subjective and limited by the location of the residual tumor and extent of the surgical field. The definitions of NTR and STR can also vary between institutions. In our practice, a resection is considered near-total if (a) only a thin, linear layer of the tumor capsule is left on the facial nerve (or other structures), and (b) this residual tumor is estimated to be less than 5% of the original tumor volume. While the 5% volume ratio as the threshold to differentiate between NTR and STR has been used in the literature [6,8], other definitions have also been described. One method considers a resection near-total if the residual tumor is less than 25 mm^2 and 2 mm thick along the facial nerve or brain stem [9,10]. Another method considers residuals less than $5 \times 5 \times 2$ mm as NTR [11]. As seen in these examples, the definitions for NTR are variable and no consensus exists yet.

Our data show that an immediate post-operative MRI can be helpful in establishing the shape and size of the residual and provides a better estimate of the degree of resection than the surgeon's estimation. In the literature, there is no consensus regarding the timing of the first MRI after vestibular schwannoma resection. A 2005 survey of the American Neurotology Society (ANS) and North American Skull Base Society members revealed that 2.3% of neurotologists and 23.4% of neurosurgeons obtained an MRI on post-operative day one, whereas 21.6% of neurotologists and 61.7% of neurosurgeons obtained the first MRI within a year [12]. A more recent survey of the ANS members revealed similarly variable practices in MRI surveillance. Of the survey responders, the first post-operative MRI was obtained by 18.6% during the immediate post-operative inpatient stay, 23.3% at 3 months, 16.3% at 6 months, and the rest at one year or longer. The completeness of resection was found to affect 73.8% of the responders' decision about the timing of the first MRI. Among these surgeons, 25.8% indicated that they would obtain the first imaging study earlier than their usual one-year MRI if the excision was incomplete [13].

While the timing and interval of the first post-operative MRI varies between surgeons and institutions, an early MRI during the post-operative inpatient stay could provide additional information to the surgeon. This immediate MRI is obtained on day one after the surgery at our institution. On the MRIs obtained months after the surgery, it may be difficult to differentiate scar tissue from a growing residual tumor [11,14]. An MRI obtained on post-operative day one does not include these nonspecific enhancements. The patient in Figure 2 (#6 in Table 2) had an extremely small residual about 1 mm and the immediate MRI confirmed the lack of a large residual tumor. While the later MRIs showed a larger area of enhancement than anticipated, comparison with the immediate post-operative MRI resulted in more confidence in the degree of resection and differentiation from later non-specific enhancements due to dural inflammation and/or connective tissue formation. As seen in Figure 2, the noted area of enhancement did not change in size from 3 to 15 months post-operatively. Although some studies have shown that these nonspecific enhancements can disappear with time, they may persist in other cases and continue to enhance after 5 years or longer [15,16]. This persistent enhancement can in turn result in a need for prolonged MRI surveillance. The recent survey of the ANS members revealed that a higher percentage of surgeons would follow linear enhancements for longer than 5 years and 14.3% would never stop ordering surveillance MRIs [13]. In this context, an early post-operative MRI could allow surgeons to evaluate the degree of resection and the presence of a residual tumor more accurately, and prior to any scar tissue formation. We believe that most of the changes between POD#1 and three months are attributable to enhancement seen with scarring. Hence, we anticipate that the three-month MRI may actually overestimate the extent of the residual tumor. In addition, the thickness of the obtained images can potentially result in missing small or thin residuals and a radiographic GTR should not obviate the need for continued surveillance in cases with a known residual. Furthermore, the current study was limited by its sample size and future studies will need to follow a larger cohort and compare the long-term appearances of residual tumors to those in the immediate post-operative MRIs.

5. Conclusions

Preservation of the facial nerve integrity may necessitate leaving a small residual vestibular schwannoma that is then followed by serial MRIs. Intra-operative assessment of the residual size may be inaccurate given its subjective nature. In our series, post-operative MRI changed the assessment of the degree of resection in 76% of the cases where a residual tumor was left behind. While there is no consensus on the timing of the first post-operative MRI among institutions, an early post-operative MRI establishes a baseline for the residual tumor prior to scar formation and could provide a critical point of comparison for long-term surveillance.

Author Contributions: Conceptualization, M.E.M. and G.P.L.; methodology, H.M. and G.P.L.; software, H.M.; resources, W.H.S.III; writing—original draft preparation, H.M.; writing—review and editing, H.M. and G.P.L.; supervision, G.P.L., M.E.M. and W.H.S.III. All authors have read and agreed to the published version of the manuscript.

Funding: This research received no external funding.

Institutional Review Board Statement: The study was conducted according to the guidelines of the Declaration of Helsinki and was approved by the Institutional Review Board (or Ethics Committee) of St. Vincent's Hospital (IRB# SV-018-21).

Informed Consent Statement: Patient consent was waived due to retrospective nature of the study in accordance with institutional IRB policies.

Data Availability Statement: The data presented in this study are available on request from the corresponding author. The data are not publicly available due to concern for patient privacy.

Conflicts of Interest: The authors declare no conflict of interest.

References

1. Ahmed, O.H.; Mahboubi, H.; Lahham, S.; Pham, C.; Djalilian, H.R. Trends in demographics, charges, and outcomes of patients undergoing excision of sporadic vestibular schwannoma. *Otolaryngol. Head Neck Surg.* **2014**, *150*, 266–274. [CrossRef] [PubMed]
2. Carlson, M.L.; Habermann, E.B.; Wagie, A.E.; Driscoll, C.L.; Van Gompel, J.J.; Jacob, J.T.; Link, M.J. The Changing Landscape of Vestibular Schwannoma Management in the United States—A Shift Toward Conservatism. *Otolaryngol. Head Neck Surg.* **2015**, *153*, 440–446. [CrossRef] [PubMed]
3. Goshtasbi, K.; Abouzari, M.; Moshtaghi, O.; Sahyouni, R.; Sajjadi, A.; Lin, H.W.; Djalilian, H.R. The changing landscape of vestibular schwannoma diagnosis and management: A cross-sectional study. *Laryngoscope* **2020**, *130*, 482–486. [CrossRef] [PubMed]
4. Pandrangi, V.C.; Han, A.Y.; Alonso, J.E.; Peng, K.A.; St John, M.A. An Update on Epidemiology and Management Trends of Vestibular Schwannomas. *Otol. Neurotol.* **2020**, *41*, 411–417. [CrossRef] [PubMed]
5. Gurgel, R.K.; Dogru, S.; Amdur, R.L.; Monfared, A. Facial nerve outcomes after surgery for large vestibular schwannomas: Do surgical approach and extent of resection matter? *Neurosurg. Focus.* **2012**, *33*, E16. [CrossRef] [PubMed]
6. Godefroy, W.P.; van der Mey, A.G.; de Bruine, F.T.; Hoekstra, E.R.; Malessy, M.J. Surgery for large vestibular schwannoma: Residual tumor and outcome. *Otol. Neurotol.* **2009**, *30*, 629–634. [CrossRef] [PubMed]
7. Sorensen, A.G.; Patel, S.; Harmath, C.; Bridges, S.; Synnott, J.; Sievers, A.; Yoon, Y.-H.; Lee, E.J.; Yang, M.C.; Lewis, R.F.; et al. Comparison of diameter and perimeter methods for tumor volume calculation. *J. Clin. Oncol.* **2001**, *19*, 551–557. [CrossRef] [PubMed]
8. Kemink, J.L.; Langman, A.W.; Niparko, J.K.; Graham, M.D. Operative management of acoustic neuromas: The priority of neurologic function over complete resection. *Otolaryngol. Head Neck Surg.* **1991**, *104*, 96–99. [CrossRef] [PubMed]
9. Bloch, D.C.; Oghalai, J.S.; Jackler, R.K.; Osofsky, M.; Pitts, L.H. The fate of the tumor remnant after less-than-complete acoustic neuroma resection. *Otolaryngol. Head Neck Surg.* **2004**, *130*, 104–112. [CrossRef] [PubMed]
10. Strickland, B.A.; Ravina, K.; Rennert, R.C.; Jackanich, A.; Aaron, K.; Bakhsheshian, J.; Russin, J.J.; Friedman, R.A.; Giannotta, S.L. Intentional Subtotal Resection of Vestibular Schwannoma: A Reexamination. *J. Neurol. Surg. B Skull Base* **2020**, *81*, 136–141. [CrossRef] [PubMed]
11. Carlson, M.L.; Van Abel, K.M.; Driscoll, C.L.; Neff, B.A.; Beatty, C.W.; Lane, J.I.; Castner, M.L.; Lohse, C.M.; Link, M.J. Magnetic resonance imaging surveillance following vestibular schwannoma resection. *Laryngoscope* **2012**, *122*, 378–388. [CrossRef] [PubMed]

12. Lee, W.J.; Isaacson, J.E. Postoperative imaging and follow-up of vestibular schwannomas. *Otol. Neurotol.* **2005**, *26*, 102–104. [CrossRef] [PubMed]
13. Bukoski, R.S.; Appelbaum, E.N.; Coelho, D.H. Postoperative MRI Surveillance of Vestibular Schwannomas: Is There a Standard of Care? *Otol. Neurotol.* **2020**, *41*, 265–270. [CrossRef] [PubMed]
14. Miller, M.E.; Lin, H.; Mastrodimos, B.; Cueva, R.A. Long-term MRI surveillance after microsurgery for vestibular schwannoma. *Laryngoscope* **2017**, *127*, 2132–2138. [CrossRef] [PubMed]
15. Weissman, J.L.; Hirsch, B.E.; Fukui, M.B.; Rudy, T.E. The evolving MR appearance of structures in the internal auditory canal after removal of an acoustic neuroma. *AJNR Am. J. Neuroradiol.* **1997**, *18*, 313–323. [PubMed]
16. Bennett, M.L.; Jackson, C.G.; Kaufmann, R.; Warren, F. Postoperative imaging of vestibular schwannomas. *Otolaryngol. Head Neck Surg.* **2008**, *138*, 667–671. [CrossRef] [PubMed]

Disclaimer/Publisher's Note: The statements, opinions and data contained in all publications are solely those of the individual author(s) and contributor(s) and not of MDPI and/or the editor(s). MDPI and/or the editor(s) disclaim responsibility for any injury to people or property resulting from any ideas, methods, instructions or products referred to in the content.

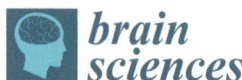
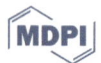

Case Report

Two-Stage Surgical Management for Acutely Presented Large Vestibular Schwannomas: Report of Two Cases

Abdullah Keles , Burak Ozaydin, Ufuk Erginoglu and Mustafa K. Baskaya *

Department of Neurological Surgery, University of Wisconsin—Madison School of Medicine and Public Health, Madison, WI 53792, USA; abdullah.keles@wisc.edu (A.K.); burakozaydin@icloud.com (B.O.); erginoglu@wisc.edu (U.E.)
* Correspondence: baskaya@neurosurgery.wisc.edu; Tel.: +1-(608)-262-7303; Fax: +1-(608)-263-1728

Abstract: The surgical management of vestibular schwannomas should be based on their presentation, neuro-imaging findings, surgeons' expertise, and logistics. Multi-stage surgery can be beneficial for large-sized lesions with acute presentations. Herein, we highlighted the indications for two cases managed initially through the retrosigmoid and, subsequently, translabyrinthine approaches. The first case presented with acute balance and gait issues and a long history of hearing loss and blurred vision. Neuroimaging findings revealed a cerebellopontine angle lesion, resembling a vestibular schwannoma, with significant brainstem compression and hydrocephalus. Due to the rapidly deteriorating clinical status and large-sized tumor, we first proceeded with urgent decompression via a retrosigmoid approach, followed by gross total resection via a translabyrinthine approach two weeks later. The second case presented with gradually worsening dizziness and hemifacial numbness accompanied by acute onset severe headaches and hearing loss. Neuroimaging findings showed a large cerebellopontine angle lesion suggestive of a vestibular schwannoma with acute intratumoral hemorrhage. Given the acute clinical deterioration and large size of the tumor, we performed urgent decompression with a retrosigmoid approach followed by gross total resection through a translabyrinthine approach a week later. Post-surgery, both patients showed excellent recovery. When managing acutely presented large-sized vestibular schwannomas, immediate surgical decompression is vital to avoid permanent neurological deficits.

Keywords: facial nerve; nervus intermedius; retrosigmoid approach; staged surgery; translabyrinthine approach; vestibular schwannoma

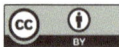

Citation: Keles, A.; Ozaydin, B.; Erginoglu, U.; Baskaya, M.K. Two-Stage Surgical Management for Acutely Presented Large Vestibular Schwannomas: Report of Two Cases. *Brain Sci.* **2023**, *13*, 1548. https://doi.org/10.3390/brainsci13111548

Academic Editor: Miguel Lopez-Gonzalez

Received: 26 September 2023
Revised: 30 October 2023
Accepted: 2 November 2023
Published: 4 November 2023

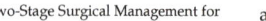

Copyright: © 2023 by the authors. Licensee MDPI, Basel, Switzerland. This article is an open access article distributed under the terms and conditions of the Creative Commons Attribution (CC BY) license (https://creativecommons.org/licenses/by/4.0/).

1. Introduction

Vestibular schwannomas (VSs) account for 90–95% of tumors found in the cerebellopontine angle (CPA). Depending on their size and location, these tumors present with a range of symptoms. These can be as mild as mild headaches, tinnitus, vertigo, disequilibrium, and mild unilateral hearing loss, whereas large VSs might present with severe symptoms of other cranial nerves (mainly trigeminal, facial, and lower cranial nerves), intentional tremor, gait ataxia, and hydrocephalus. Furthermore, sizeable tumors can occasionally bleed internally, resulting in sudden onset hearing loss, new or exacerbated symptoms of cranial nerves, CPA syndrome, and even sudden alterations in mental status [1].

The treatment of VSs should be individualized for every patient. Depending on the patient's specifics, observation, surgery, radiosurgery, or a combination of these can be chosen. Elderly asymptomatic patients with tumors confined to the internal auditory canal (IAC) are best suited for observation. Regardless of tumor size, surgery aiming for complete tumor removal offers a cure while preserving the facial nerve functionality. For those who have residual tumors or with small- to medium-size tumors who cannot tolerate surgery, radiosurgery is a viable option.

For the surgical management of VSs, three main approaches can be utilized: the retrosigmoid, the translabyrinthine, and the middle fossa approach, or sometimes combinations or variations of these [1–5]. Besides these most widely used approaches, there are other combinations and variations that could be utilized in some selected cases, but with limited indications [6–9]. Factors such as the size and extension of the tumor and the patient's hearing status play crucial roles in the choice of surgical approach.

Regardless of the selected surgical approach, surgical treatment of large VSs (>3 cm) presents significant challenges. Surgical treatment of large VSs is often associated with higher morbidity, increased complications, and less favorable facial nerve outcomes compared to smaller VSs [10–12]. For the surgical treatment of large VSs, two-stage surgery was introduced to enhance the outcomes, and several two-stage surgical series have been published [10–16].

In this report, we present two large VS cases in which both initially underwent emergency surgery using the retrosigmoid approach, followed by an elective secondary procedure for gross total removal through the translabyrinthine approach. However, the rationale for the staging varied between the two cases. We highlight these cases to illustrate the criteria for employing multi-stage surgeries to manage large VSs.

2. Results

2.1. Case 1

A 52-year-old man presented with a progressive decline in his left ear hearing and blurry vision over the past 18 months. In addition, he recently began to experience balance and gait problems which had notably worsened in the past few weeks. Following an episode of dizziness that resulted in a fall and subsequent emergency room admission, a CT scan of the head revealed a large lesion in the left CPA. His initial audiogram showed sensorineural hearing loss in the left ear, accompanied by a total lack of word recognition.

The patient immediately had a cranial MRI that displayed a sizeable (4 cm × 3.5 cm × 3.3 cm) left CPA lesion, consistent with a vestibular schwannoma (Figure 1). The lesion caused marked compression on the brainstem and fourth ventricle, resulting in hydrocephalus.

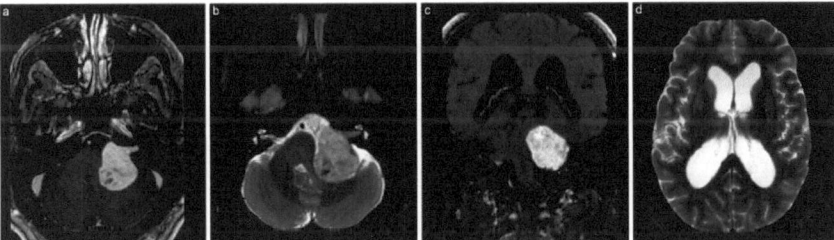

Figure 1. Case 1, preoperative neuroimaging. (**a**) Axial T1-weighted postcontrast, (**b**) axial T2-weighted, (**c**) coronal T1-weighted postcontrast, and (**d**) axial T2-weighted MRI scans show a large CPA lesion suggesting a vestibular schwannoma along with hydrocephalus.

Considering the large size of the tumor, the significant compression it caused on the brainstem and fourth ventricle, the accompanying hydrocephalus, and the rapidly deteriorating balance and gait problems, we decided to urgently commence with initial decompression through a retrosigmoid approach. We had also planned for an elective second stage to achieve gross total resection using a translabyrinthine approach (Supplementary Video).

Before the initial surgery, a ventriculostomy catheter was inserted in the left frontal region.

With the patient positioned supine, we slightly rotated the head to the right and used neuronavigation to mark the locations of the sigmoid and transverse sinuses. We then made a postauricular C-shape skin incision and lifted a myocutaneous flap. Subsequently, a retrosigmoid craniotomy was carried out using a single burr hole, located just below the junction of the sigmoid and transverse sinus.

The dura was opened in a C-shaped fashion, followed by the draining of cerebrospinal fluid from the lateral cerebellomedullary cistern to relax the cerebellum. As the arachnoid dissection progressed, the tumor came into view. Once we confirmed the facial nerve-free tumor regions with a facial nerve stimulator, the tumor capsule was incised. Central tumor debulking commenced with the use of an ultrasonic aspirator and piecemeal resection using microsurgical techniques. As we proceeded with alternating debulking and dissection, cranial nerves IX and X, the basilar artery, and the origin of the anterior inferior cerebellar artery (AICA) were visualized and carefully detached from the tumor. After sufficient tumor debulking, the pressure on the neurovascular structures was relieved, hemostasis was achieved, and the wound was closed in standard fashion.

The patient woke up with House–Brackmann grade I facial nerve function. The histopathological diagnosis was confirmed as a WHO grade I schwannoma. An early postoperative MRI revealed partial resection of the tumor and decompression of the brainstem and surrounding structures, along with regressed hydrocephalus (Figure 2).

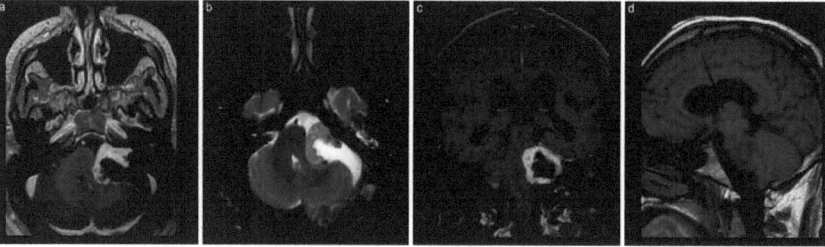

Figure 2. Case 1 post-stage 1 neuroimaging findings. (**a**) Axial T1-weighted postcontrast, (**b**) axial T2-weighted, (**c**) coronal T1-weighted postcontrast, and (**d**) sagittal T1-weighted MRI scans show partial resection with decompression of the brainstem and surrounding structures along with regressed hydrocephalus.

Two weeks afterward, we initiated the second stage of the surgery, the translabyrinthine approach, to achieve gross total resection. The patient was positioned supine, and the previous wound was reopened. Bony exposure, labyrinthectomy, and 270-degree IAC drilling were performed. Afterward, the IAC dura was incised and the intracanalicular part of the tumor was exposed. By employing facial nerve stimulation, the intracanalicular part of the facial nerve was mapped out and carefully detached from the tumor. We then proceeded with presigmoid dural opening, which revealed the tumor and prior resection cavity. At the upper boundary of the tumor, the trigeminal nerve was identified and detached from the tumor. At the lower boundary of the tumor, the vestibulocochlear nerve and the lower cranial nerves were discerned and separated from the tumor. We then delineated the tumor–brainstem border, and the facial nerve root exit zone was detected and confirmed with a nerve simulator. Further piecemeal tumor resection allowed us to find the brainstem origin of the vestibulocochlear nerve in the pontomedullary sulcus.

Once the facial nerve was entirely separated from the tumor, the rest of the tumor was removed en bloc, and hemostasis was achieved. Following that, we removed the incus and packed the eustachian tube with previously harvested stripes of temporalis fascia to avoid postoperative cerebrospinal fluid (CSF) leak. The post-resection cavity was then packed using abdominal fat grafts that had been previously harvested.

As part of our standard neuromonitoring protocol, we continuously monitor and record the compound muscle action potential (CMAP) of the orbicularis oculi and orbicularis oris muscles. In addition, throughout surgery, we use a facial nerve stimulator with a minimum stimulation threshold (MST) of 0.05–0.1 mA for the identification and verification of the facial nerve, for assessing the proximity to the nerve, for monitoring the nerve integrity, and for predicting the postoperative facial nerve outcome. In the majority of the VS cases, the facial nerve could be detached from the tumor by employing gentle traction-counter traction, along with microvascular sharp dissection techniques.

The patient woke up with House–Brackmann grade 2 facial nerve function without any new neurological deficits. The patient's postoperative recovery was uneventful and he eventually had normal facial nerve function at the 3-month follow-up. A postoperative MRI confirmed a gross total resection (Figure 3).

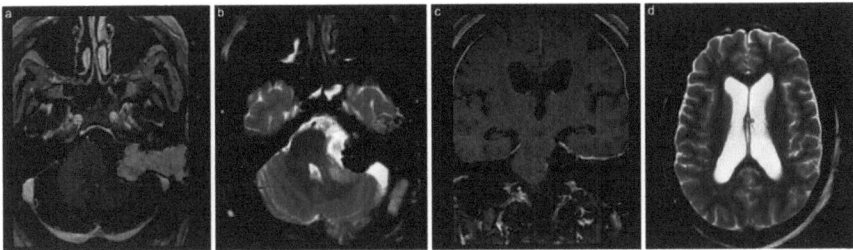

Figure 3. Case 1 post-stage 2 neuroimaging findings. (**a**) Axial T1-weighted postcontrast, (**b**) axial T2 fat suppressed, (**c**) coronal T1-weighted, and (**d**) axial T2-weighted MRI scans show gross total resection with decompression of the brainstem and surrounding structures along with decreased hydrocephalus.

2.2. Case 2

The second case is a 48-year-old man who had presented with dizziness and numbness on the left side of his face for the past six weeks. These symptoms had been escalating, and were accompanied by a severe, newly developed headache. An MRI scan revealed a large cystic left cerebellopontine angle lesion (4.1 cm × 2.5 cm × 2.8 cm), suggestive of a VS, along with signs of recent hemorrhage within the lesion (Figure 4). An initial audiogram revealed moderate to severe sensorineural hearing loss, with no serviceable hearing on the left side.

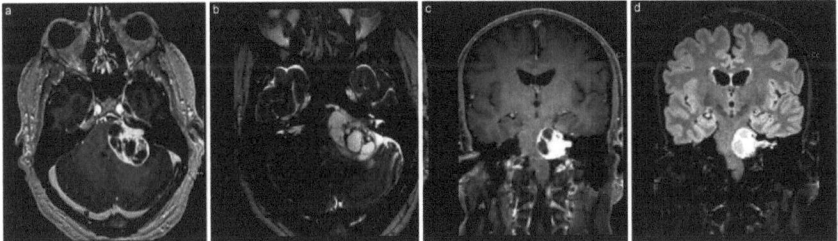

Figure 4. Case 2 preoperative neuroimaging. (**a**) Axial T1-weighted postcontrast, (**b**) axial T2-weighted, (**c**) coronal T1-weighted postcontrast, and (**d**) coronal T2 FLAIR MRI scans show a large cystic CPA lesion, suggesting a vestibular schwannoma along with recent intratumoral hemorrhage.

Given the recent intratumoral hemorrhage and significant tumor size, which resulted in acute increased compression of the surrounding neurovascular structures, we decided to proceed with a two-stage approach. Initially, we performed emergency decompression via the retrosigmoid approach, followed by an elective translabyrinthine approach for a gross total resection (Supplementary Video). Once the patient was positioned supine and the head was slightly rotated, a standard C-shape skin incision, myofascial flap elevation, and craniotomy for a retrosigmoid approach were performed. The tense posterior fossa dura was cautiously incised. The cerebellum was notably swollen because of the heightened pressure in the posterior fossa caused by the tumor and recent intratumoral hemorrhage. We then navigated the lateral cerebellomedullary cistern and drained the CSF to relax the posterior fossa, which facilitated the exposure of the tumor.

Once we verified the area was clear of the facial nerve using nerve stimulation, we incised the tumor capsule. We then accessed the hemorrhagic cavity and removed its content. After sufficient tumor debulking, hemostasis was achieved, and the surgical wound was closed in layers.

The patient woke up with House–Brackmann grade I facial nerve function. Histopathological analysis identified it as a WHO grade I schwannoma. An early postoperative MRI displayed a decompressed brainstem and extent of resection (Figure 5).

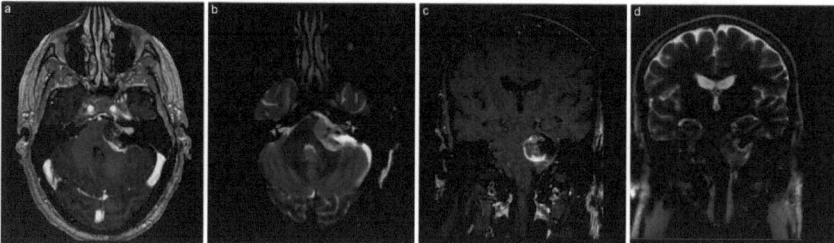

Figure 5. Case 2 post-stage 1 neuroimaging findings. (**a**) Axial T1-weighted postcontrast, (**b**) axial T2-weighted, (**c**) coronal T1-weighted postcontrast, and (**d**) coronal T2-weighted MRI scans show partial resection with decompression of the brainstem and surrounding structures, with evacuation of the cystic and hemorrhagic portion of the lesion.

A week afterward, we initiated the second planned stage to achieve gross total removal through a translabyrinthine approach. The second stage began with the placement of a lumbar drain and obtaining a fat graft from the abdomen. As detailed in the previous case, opening of the previous wound, bony exposure, labyrinthectomy, 270-degree IAC drilling, and intracanalicular tumor removal were performed. We then proceeded with an incision of the presigmoid dura. Once the presigmoid dura opened, the tumor came into view. Then, extending the arachnoid dissection around the tumor, we exposed and released the trigeminal nerve in the upper part of the tumor.

Upon confirming the facial nerve-free zone, the tumor capsule was incised, and piecemeal removal was commenced. Notably, the remaining tumor was less vascular than in the initial stage. On the lateral part of the surgical field, cranial nerves VII and VIII became visible. The facial nerve was identified with nerve stimulation and the vestibulocochlear nerve was cut. As we proceeded with the tumor removal, the nervus intermedius came into view. Every attempt should be made to preserve the nervus intermedius when it is encountered during surgery.

We then turned our attention to the IAC portion of the tumor. We traced the facial nerve in the IAC and meticulously detached it from the tumor, employing sharp and semi-sharp microsurgical dissection techniques. Subsequently, all the remaining arachnoid adhesions were cleared, and the rest of the tumor was removed en bloc. At the final stage of surgery, the facial nerve was stimulated at 0.05 milliampere in the brainstem zone as well as along its entire length. We then proceeded with wound closure.

Postoperative examinations revealed House–Brackmann grade 1 facial nerve function and an early postoperative MRI confirmed the gross total resection of the tumor (Figure 6). The patient remained tumor-free with normal facial nerve function at the 1-year follow-up.

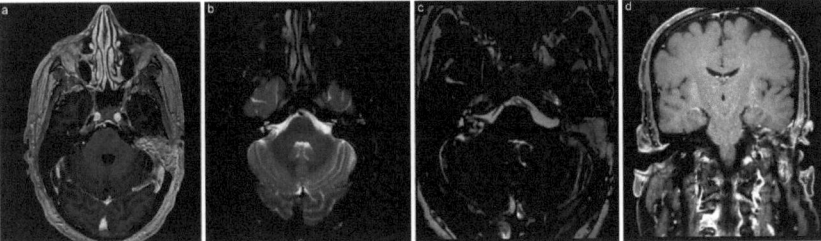

Figure 6. Case 2 post-stage 2 neuroimaging findings. (a) Axial T1-weighted postcontrast, (b) axial T2-weighted, (c) axial FIESTA, and (d) coronal T1-weighted postcontrast MRI scans show gross total resection with decompression of the brainstem and surrounding structures.

3. Discussion

The first successful complete removal of a VS was carried out by Balance in 1894 and reported in 1907 [14,17]. Later, in 1913, pioneer neurosurgeons, Horsley of London, v. Eiselsberg of Vienna and Krause of Berlin presented their VS surgical outcomes at the International Congress of Medicine in London. They reported mortality rates of 67%, 77% and 84%, respectively. Given the challenging nature of the cases, surgical interventions were commonly performed in two stages, notably by v. Eiselsberg and Horsley [14].

In 1917, Cushing introduced his revolutionary technique of partial removal through the intracapsular enucleation method, which remarkably reduced the mortality rates first to 35%, and later further to 11% [18]. In 1925, Dandy shared his expertise on 23 VSs, which he had performed since 1915. He incorporated the finger technique to achieve gross complete removal after the intracapsular enucleation [14]. With the advent of the microsurgery era, new microsurgical approaches were introduced by House (translabyrinthine approach), Kurze and Doyle (subtemporal transpetrosal approach), and Rand and Kurze (suboccipital transmeatal approach) [19–21]. Since the early days of microsurgery, numerous case series have been published in the literature [4,22–32].

The introduction of intraoperative electromyography for monitoring the facial nerve, along with new techniques, has not entirely resolved the complexities of preserving facial nerve functionality, especially in cases with large tumors. Even with a success rate of 86–92% in preserving the anatomical continuity of the facial nerve, there are instances where patients experience facial nerve dysfunctions after surgery, even when their nerves are anatomically preserved [10,28,33–36]. Tumors larger than 3 cm often have less favorable outcomes, while those 2 cm or less have better outcomes [10,25,33]. Samii et al. reported a 100% gross total removal rate, with a 44% rate of good facial nerve outcome in cases larger than 3.9 cm in size [28]. In addition, a recent study by Gazia and colleagues revealed an association between tumor size, MST, CMAP, and facial function in the short and long term, which aids in improving predictions of facial performance [37].

When dealing with large and complex VSs, it is essential to consider staged surgeries preoperatively. Besides the tumor size, various other factors can complicate the surgical approaches to VSs. These include variations in vascular and bony anatomy (thrombosed or missing sigmoid sinus, elevated jugular bulb, anteriorly positioned sigmoid sinus, and a contracted or small mastoid bone), existence of cystic components, and brainstem compression, along with hydrocephalus, intratumoral hemorrhage, prior treatments (either surgical or stereotactic radiation), the tumor's vascularity, and the patient's pre-existing comorbidities [1,12,13].

In the literature, studies have shown that for selective large VSs, staged surgeries improve facial nerve outcomes, reduce morbidity, and have a higher likelihood of achieving gross total removal [10–13,15,16]. One potential rationale for achieving better outcomes with staged surgeries might be that the most delicate dissections can be performed separately, minimizing the impact of surgeon fatigue. Often, detaching the tumor from the facial nerve in the IAC and brainstem, the most important part of the surgery, takes place towards the end of the surgery. Although multi-stage surgery may not be scheduled in advance, it should be considered intraoperatively if a surgeon experiences fatigue during the most crucial parts of the surgery. This might be the safest and most efficient solution for the selected cases.

In prior published series, two-stage surgeries were predominantly performed for the treatment of large vestibular schwannomas. Given that these patients exhibited severe hearing loss preoperatively, hearing preservation was not the primary goal in these surgeries. In these same series, a lower or no additional incidence of morbidity and mortality was associated with staged surgery for the resection of large vestibular schwannomas [10,12,15]. Abe et al. reported a postoperative increase in hearing loss for both of their presented cases where the tumors originated from vestibular nerves [13].

Tinnitus is one of the most common initial symptoms of VSs along with hearing loss, occurring in 60–80% of VS patients [1]. In some of those patients, tinnitus could worsen and significantly influence a patient's quality of life [38–41]. In the published two-stage surgeries for vestibular schwannomas series, no postoperative tinnitus was reported, as seen in our cases.

During the surgical resection of large tumors, it is not always possible to determine the origin of the tumor. As illustrated in our video, sometimes even the identification of the vestibular nerve branches and cochlear nerve is not feasible. Therefore, during our surgeries, we cut the vestibulocochlear nerve to achieve gross total resection. In cases where the cochlear nerve can be preserved, cochlear implantation should be considered in the same sittings [42–45].

Indications and Timing Interval for the Staged Surgeries

As of now, there remains a lack of consensus on the indications and the timing between the two stages in the management of VSs [10,15].

Raslan et al. made staging decisions intraoperatively based on facial nerve anatomical condition and stimulation, tumor adherence, as well as the conditions of the brainstem and cerebellum. They determined the time interval based on facial nerve outcome after the first stage. For those with a House–Brackmann grade I and II, the second stage was scheduled between two and four weeks after the first stage, while the remainder waited for six months, aiming to maximize their recovery in the interim [15]. In contrast, Comey et al. chose to perform second stage surgery once postoperative imaging studies verified the residual tumor's decompression away from the pons. Their time interval between the stages ranged widely from 0.5 to 32 weeks, averaging 4.5 weeks [10]. On the other hand, Abe et al. recommended determining the timing of the second stage based on verifying decreases in vascularity for cases with hypervascularity [13].

Ideally, the second stage surgery should be conducted prior to the formation of arachnoid adhesions or tumor revascularization [31]. To prevent such adhesions, a thin gelatin sponge layer can be used during the initial surgery's closure [46]. In our experience, the second stage should not be delayed more than 2–3 weeks at maximum to avoid arachnoid adhesion. As documented in various studies, the remaining tumor often exhibits decreased vascularity and less adherence, which allows for a relatively easier dissection in the second stage surgery [10,13,14]. This was observed in our second case as well.

In theory, multi-stage surgeries could bring additional operative risks related to multiple anesthesia administration, potential surgical site infections, and issues with wound recovery. However, in both the published series and our series, there were no evident complications due to the aforementioned reasons.

Lastly, rapidly gathering neuro-otology and neurosurgery teams might not be viable in some emergency cases. In such scenarios, a multi-stage approach must be strongly considered to minimize the risk of permanent neurological deficits and ensure the best patient care.

In summary, the literature suggests that a two-stage surgical approach for large VSs offers numerous advantages. In selected cases, this enhances facial nerve outcomes, reduces patient morbidity, and increases the likelihood of complete tumor removal. With a two-stage approach, surgeons can tackle intricate dissections with more focus, thereby minimizing mistakes from extended operations. Moreover, in urgent scenarios, like those we have experienced where rapid setup and team assembly were challenging, the two-stage approach ensures that patients receive the best care without compromising the intricacy of the procedures or the necessary preparations.

4. Conclusions

In summary, even in cases with large VSs, a single-stage gross total removal is feasible if the tumor has well-defined arachnoid borders and appropriate consistency. Immediate surgical decompression should be performed for selected large and acutely presented VSs to achieve gross total removal with little or no additional morbidity.

Supplementary Materials: The following supporting information can be downloaded at: https://www.mdpi.com/article/10.3390/brainsci13111548/s1, Video S1: Two-stage Surgical Management for Acutely Presented Large Vestibular Schwannomas: Report of Two Cases with Operative Video Demonstrations.

Author Contributions: M.K.B.; completed surgical procedures, conceptualization, review and editing. U.E.; review and editing. B.O.; writing—original draft preparation, review and editing. A.K.; writing—original draft preparation, review and editing. All authors have read and agreed to the published version of the manuscript.

Funding: This research received no external funding.

Institutional Review Board Statement: Ethical approval is not required for retrospective case report studies without identifiable information in accordance with the University of Wisconsin—Madison Institutional Review Board guidelines.

Informed Consent Statement: Patient consent is not required for retrospective case report studies without identifiable information in accordance with University of Wisconsin—Madison Institutional Review Board guidelines.

Data Availability Statement: Not Applicable.

Acknowledgments: We thank Steven L. Goodman, Distinguished Editor, for his contributions to the editing of this work.

Conflicts of Interest: The authors declare no conflict of interest.

References

1. Baskaya, M.K.; Pyle, G.M.; Roche, J.P. *Vestibular Schwannoma Surgery: A Video Guide*; Springer: Berlin/Heidelberg, Germany, 2019.
2. Chamoun, R.; MacDonald, J.; Shelton, C.; Couldwell, W.T. Surgical approaches for resection of vestibular schwannomas: Translabyrinthine, retrosigmoid, and middle fossa approaches. *Neurosurg. Focus* **2012**, *33*, E9. [CrossRef] [PubMed]
3. Nickele, C.M.; Akture, E.; Gubbels, S.P.; Baskaya, M.K. A stepwise illustration of the translabyrinthine approach to a large cystic vestibular schwannoma. *Neurosurg. Focus* **2012**, *33*, 5. [CrossRef] [PubMed]
4. Ocak, P.E.; Dogan, I.; Ocak, U.; Dinc, C.; Baskaya, M.K. Facial nerve outcome and extent of resection in cystic versus solid vestibular schwannomas in radiosurgery era. *Neurosurg. Focus* **2018**, *44*, 8. [CrossRef]
5. Sayyahmelli, S.; Roche, J.; Baskaya, M.K. Microsurgical Gross Total Resection of a Large Residual/Recurrent Vestibular Schwannoma via Translabyrinthine Approach. *J. Neurol. Surg. Part B* **2018**, *79*, S387–S388. [CrossRef]
6. Marchioni, D.; Carney, M.; Rubini, A.; Nogueira, J.F.; Masotto, B.; Alicandri-Ciufelli, M.; Presutti, L. The Fully Endoscopic Acoustic Neuroma Surgery. *Otolaryngol. Clin. N. Am.* **2016**, *49*, 1227–1236. [CrossRef]
7. Molinari, G.; Calvaruso, F.; Presutti, L.; Marchioni, D.; Alicandri-Ciufelli, M.; Friso, F.; Fernandez, I.J.; Francoli, P.; Di Maro, F. Vestibular schwannoma removal through expanded transcanal transpromontorial approach: A multicentric experience. *Eur. Arch. Oto-Rhino-Laryn.* **2023**, *280*, 2165–2172. [CrossRef]
8. Bi, Y.K.; Ni, Y.J.; Gao, D.D.; Zhu, Q.W.; Zhou, Q.Y.; Tang, J.J.; Liu, J.; Shi, F.; Li, H.C.; Yin, J.; et al. Endoscope-Assisted Retrosigmoid Approach for Vestibular Schwannomas With Intracanalicular Extensions: Facial Nerve Outcomes. *Front. Oncol.* **2022**, *11*, 774462. [CrossRef]
9. Presutti, L.; Magnaguagno, F.; Pavesi, G.; Cunsolo, E.; Pinna, G.; Alicandri-Ciufelli, M.; Marchioni, D.; Prontera, A.; Gioacchini, F.M. Combined endoscopic-microscopic approach for vestibular schwannoma removal: Outcomes in a cohort of 81 patients. *Acta Otorhinolaryngol. Ital.* **2014**, *34*, 427–433.

10. Comey, C.H.; Jannetta, P.J.; Sheptak, P.E.; Jho, H.D.; Burkhart, L.E. Staged Removal of Acoustic Tumors—Techniques and Lessons Learned from a Series of 83 Patients. *Neurosurgery* **1995**, *37*, 915–920. [CrossRef]
11. Kim, E.; Nam, S.-I. Staging in vestibular schwannoma surgery: A modified technique. *J. Korean Neurosurg. Soc.* **2008**, *43*, 57–60. [CrossRef]
12. Patni, A.H.; Kartush, J.M. Staged resection of large acoustic neuromas. *Otolaryngol. Head Neck Surg.* **2005**, *132*, 11–19. [CrossRef]
13. Abe, T.; Izumiyama, H.; Imaizumi, Y.; Kobayashi, S.; Shimazu, M.; Sasaki, K.; Matsumoto, K.; Kushima, M. Staged resection of large hypervascular vestibular schwannomas in young adults. *Skull Base-Interdiscip. Appr.* **2001**, *11*, 199–206. [CrossRef]
14. Dandy, W.E. An operation for the total removal of cerebellopontine (acoustic) tumors. *Surg Gynecol Obs.* **1925**, *41*, 129–148.
15. Raslan, A.M.; Liu, J.K.; McMenomey, S.O.; Delashaw, J.B., Jr. Staged resection of large vestibular schwannomas. *J. Neurosurg.* **2012**, *116*, 1126–1133. [CrossRef] [PubMed]
16. Sheptak, P.E.; Jannetta, P.J. The two-stage excision of huge acoustic neurinomas. *J. Neurosurg.* **1979**, *51*, 37–41. [CrossRef] [PubMed]
17. Ballance, C.A. *Some Points in the Surgery of the Brain and Its Membranes*; Macmillan: London, UK, 1907.
18. Cushing, H. *Tumors of the Nervous Acusticus and the Syndrome of the Cerebellopontile Angle*; WB Saunders: Philadelphia, PA, USA, 1917.
19. House, W.F. Surgical exposure of the internal auditory canal and its contents through the middle, cranial fossa. *Laryngoscope* **1961**, *71*, 1363–1385. [PubMed]
20. Kurze, T.; Doyle, J.B. Extradural Intracranial (Middle Fossa) Approach to Internal Auditory Canal. *J. Neurosurg.* **1962**, *19*, 1033–1037. [CrossRef]
21. Rand, R.; Kurze, T. Micro-neurosurgical resection of acoustic tumors by a transmeatal posterior fossa approach. *Bull. Los Angeles Neurol. Soc.* **1965**, *30*, 17–20.
22. Arts, H.A.; Telian, S.A.; El-Kashlan, H.; Thompson, B.G. Hearing preservation and facial nerve outcomes in vestibular schwannoma surgery: Results using the middle cranial fossa approach. *Otol. Neurotol.* **2006**, *27*, 234–241. [CrossRef]
23. Brackmann, D.E.; Cullen, R.D.; Fisher, L.M. Facial nerve function after translabyrinthine vestibular schwannoma surgery. *Otolaryngol. Head Neck Surg.* **2007**, *136*, 773–777. [CrossRef]
24. Irving, R.M.; Jackler, R.K.; Pitts, L.H. Hearing preservation in patients undergoing vestibular schwannoma surgery: Comparison of middle fossa and retrosigmoid approaches. *J. Neurosurg.* **1998**, *88*, 840–845. [CrossRef]
25. Lanman, T.H.; Brackmann, D.E.; Hitselberger, W.E.; Subin, B. Report of 190 consecutive cases of large acoustic tumors (vestibular schwannoma) removed via the translabyrinthine approach. *J. Neurosurg.* **1999**, *90*, 617–623. [CrossRef]
26. Noudel, R.; Gomis, P.; Duntze, J.; Marnet, D.; Bazin, A.; Roche, P.H. Hearing preservation and facial nerve function after microsurgery for intracanalicular vestibular schwannomas: Comparison of middle fossa and restrosigmoid approaches. *Acta Neurochir.* **2009**, *151*, 935–945. [CrossRef]
27. Samii, M.; Gerganov, V.; Samii, A. Improved preservation of hearing and facial nerve function in vestibular schwannoma surgery via the retrosigmoid approach in a series of 200 patients. *J. Neurosurg.* **2006**, *105*, 527–535. [CrossRef]
28. Samii, M.; Gerganov, V.M.; Samii, A. Functional outcome after complete surgical removal of giant vestibular schwannomas Clinical article. *J. Neurosurg.* **2010**, *112*, 860–867. [CrossRef] [PubMed]
29. Yamakami, I.; Uchino, Y.; Kobayashi, E.; Yamaura, A.; Oka, N. Removal of large acoustic neurinomas (vestibular schwannomas) by the retrosigmoid approach with no mortality and minimal morbidity. *J. Neurol. Neurosurg. Psychiatry* **2004**, *75*, 453–458. [CrossRef] [PubMed]
30. Yasargil, M. *Microneurosurgery, Volume IVB: Microneurosurgery of CNS Tumors*; Georg Thieme Verlag: Stuttgart, Germany, 1996.
31. Yaşargil, M.; Smith, R.; Gasser, J. Microsurgical Approach to Acoustic Neurinomas. *Adv. Technol. Stand. Neurosurg.* **1977**, *4*, 93–129.
32. Yaşargil, M.G. *Microsurgery Applied to Neurosurgery*; Georg Thieme: Stuttgart, Germany, 1969.
33. Kaylie, D.M.; Gilbert, E.; Horgan, M.A.; Delashaw, J.B.; McMenomey, S.O. Acoustic neuroma surgery outcomes. *Otol. Neurotol.* **2001**, *22*, 686–689. [CrossRef]
34. Godefroy, W.P.; van der Mey, A.G.L.; de Bruine, F.T.; Hoekstra, E.R.; Malessy, M.J.A. Surgery for Large Vestibular Schwannoma: Residual Tumor and Outcome. *Otol. Neurotol.* **2009**, *30*, 629–634. [CrossRef]
35. Silva, J.; Cerejo, A.; Duarte, F.; Silveira, F.; Vaz, R. Surgical Removal of Giant Acoustic Neuromas. *World Neurosurg.* **2012**, *77*, 731–735. [CrossRef]
36. Sughrue, M.E.; Yang, I.; Rutkowski, M.J.; Aranda, D.; Parsa, A.T. Preservation of facial nerve function after resection of vestibular schwannoma. *Br. J. Neurosurg.* **2010**, *24*, 666–671. [CrossRef] [PubMed]
37. Gazia, F.; Callejo, A.; Perez-Grau, M.; Lareo, S.; Prades, J.; Roca-Ribas, F.; Amilibia, E. Pre- and intra-operative prognostic factors of facial nerve function in cerebellopontine angle surgery. *Eur. Arch. Oto-Rhino-Laryn.* **2022**, *280*, 1055–1062. [CrossRef] [PubMed]
38. Andersson, G.; Kinnefors, A.; Ekvall, L.; RaskAndersen, H. Tinnitus and translabyrinthine acoustic neuroma surgery. *Audiol. Neuro-Otol.* **1997**, *2*, 403–409. [CrossRef] [PubMed]
39. Fahy, C.; Nikolopoulos, T.P.; O'Donoghue, G.M. Acoustic neuroma surgery and tinnitus. *Eur. Arch. Oto-Rhino-Laryn.* **2002**, *259*, 299–301. [CrossRef]
40. Kojima, T.; Oishi, N.; Nishiyama, T.; Ogawa, K. Severity of Tinnitus Distress Negatively Impacts Quality of Life in Patients With Vestibular Schwannoma and Mimics Primary Tinnitus. *Front. Neurol.* **2019**, *10*, 389. [CrossRef]

41. West, N.; Bunne, M.; Sass, H.; Caye-Thomasen, P. Cochlear Implantation for Patients with a Vestibular Schwannoma: Effect on Tinnitus Handicap. *J. Int. Adv. Otol.* **2022**, *18*, 382–387. [CrossRef] [PubMed]
42. Conway, R.M.; Tu, N.C.; Sioshansi, P.C.; Porps, S.L.; Schutt, C.A.; Hong, R.S.; Jacob, J.T.; Babu, S.C. Early Outcomes of Simultaneous Translabyrinthine Resection and Cochlear Implantation. *Laryngoscope* **2021**, *131*, E2312–E2317. [CrossRef]
43. Salem, N.; Galal, A.; Piras, G.; Sykopetrites, V.; Di Rubbo, V.; Talaat, M.; Sobhy, O.; Sanna, M. Management of Vestibular Schwannoma with Normal Hearing. *Audiol. Neuro-Otol.* **2023**, *28*, 12–21. [CrossRef]
44. Sorrentino, F.; Tealdo, G.; Cazzador, D.; Favaretto, N.; Brotto, D.; Montino, S.; Caserta, E.; Bovo, R.; Denaro, L.; Baro, V.; et al. Cochlear implant in vestibular schwannomas: Long-term outcomes and critical analysis of indications. *Eur. Arch. Oto-Rhino-Laryn.* **2022**, *279*, 4709–4718. [CrossRef]
45. Wick, C.C.; Butler, M.J.; Yeager, L.H.; Kallogjeri, D.; Durakovic, N.; McJunkin, J.L.; Shew, M.A.; Herzog, J.A.; Buchman, C.A. Cochlear Implant Outcomes Following Vestibular Schwannoma Resection: Systematic Review. *Otol. Neurotol.* **2020**, *41*, 1190–1197. [CrossRef]
46. Gonzalez-Lopez, P.; Harput, M.V.; Türe, H.; Atalay, B.; Türe, U. Efficacy of placing a thin layer of gelatin sponge over the subdural space during dural closure in preventing meningo-cerebral adhesion. *World Neurosurg.* **2015**, *83*, 93–101. [CrossRef] [PubMed]

Disclaimer/Publisher's Note: The statements, opinions and data contained in all publications are solely those of the individual author(s) and contributor(s) and not of MDPI and/or the editor(s). MDPI and/or the editor(s) disclaim responsibility for any injury to people or property resulting from any ideas, methods, instructions or products referred to in the content.

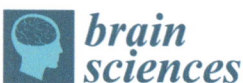 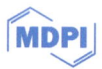

Review

Jugular Foramen Tumors: Surgical Strategies and Representative Cases

Andrea L. Castillo [1,2,*], Ali Tayebi Meybodi [1,2] and James K. Liu [2,3,*]

1. Department of Neurological Surgery, New Jersey Medical School, Newark, NJ 07103, USA; at1085@njms.rutgers.edu
2. Department of Neurosurgery, Cooperman Barnabas Medical Center, RWJ Barnabas Health, Livingston, NJ 07039, USA
3. Skull Base Institute of New Jersey, Neurosurgeons of New Jersey, Livingston, NJ 07039, USA
* Correspondence: alcm91@gmail.com (A.L.C.); jliu@neurosurgerynj.com (J.K.L.)

Abstract: (1) Background: Jugular foramen tumors are complex lesions due to their relationship with critical neurovascular structures within the skull base. It is necessary to have a deep knowledge of the anatomy of the jugular foramen and its surroundings to understand each type of tumor growth pattern and how it is related to the surrounding neurovascular structures. This scope aims to provide a guide with the primary surgical approaches to the jugular foramen and familiarize the neurosurgeons with the anatomy of the region. (2) Methods and (3) Results: A comprehensive description of the surgical approaches to jugular foramen tumors is summarized and representative cases for each tumor type is showcased. (4) Conclusions: Each case should be carefully assessed to find the most suitable approach for the patient, allowing the surgeon to remove the tumor with minimal neurovascular damage. The combined transmastoid retro- and infralabyrinthine transjugular transcondylar transtubercular high cervical approach can be performed in a stepwise fashion for the resection of complex jugular foramen tumors.

Keywords: jugular; tumor; foramen; paraglanglioma; combined

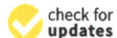

Citation: Castillo, A.L.; Meybodi, A.T.; Liu, J.K. Jugular Foramen Tumors: Surgical Strategies and Representative Cases. *Brain Sci.* **2024**, *14*, 182. https://doi.org/10.3390/brainsci14020182

Academic Editor: Miguel Lopez-Gonzalez

Received: 10 December 2023
Revised: 7 February 2024
Accepted: 15 February 2024
Published: 17 February 2024

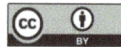

Copyright: © 2024 by the authors. Licensee MDPI, Basel, Switzerland. This article is an open access article distributed under the terms and conditions of the Creative Commons Attribution (CC BY) license (https:// creativecommons.org/licenses/by/ 4.0/).

1. Introduction

Tumors found in the jugular foramen are complex to approach due to the intricate surrounding neurovascular anatomy of the craniocervical junction [1]. Paragangliomas are the most frequently found tumors in the jugular foramen, with schwannomas following closely behind. Other less common tumors found in this area include meningiomas, chordomas, chondrosarcomas, and plasmacytomas. Metastases and malignant tumors that originate in nearby anatomical structures like the nasopharynx, parotid, and temporal bone can also spread to the jugular foramen during later stages [1]. Lastly, endolymphatic sac tumors can potentially extend to the jugular foramen and originate from the posterior medial region of the petrous bone [1,2].

The jugular foramen is a hiatus between the temporal and occipital bones [3]. The petrous portion of the temporal bone forms its anterolateral margin, and the occipital bone's condylar part forms its posteromedial margin [4]. The jugular foramen is at the crossroads of the caudal cranial nerves and the sigmoid and inferior petrosal sinuses with the otic capsule and lower brainstem in close proximity. The internal carotid artery is related to it anteromedially. These anatomic relationships pose a genuine challenge from a surgical perspective [3,5–7].

It is crucial to have a deep knowledge of the anatomy of the jugular foramen and its surroundings to comprehend each tumor growth pattern and its relation to the neurovascular structures surrounding them. These essential tools will allow the neurosurgeon to develop the appropriate surgical techniques to remove these tumors safely and effectively.

This work aims to provide a guide with the primary surgical approaches to the jugular foramen and familiarize neurosurgeons with the anatomy of the region. Although there are a variety of surgical approaches, it is paramount to individualize each case and tailor the approach for the patient to provide the appropriate necessary exposure to remove the most amount of tumor with the least amount of neurovascular morbidity.

2. Materials and Methods

A comprehensive description of the surgical approaches for jugular foramen tumors is summarized and detailed. Representative cases for different types of tumors were selected based on the senior author's experience to describe the combined transmastoid retro- and infralabyrinthine high cervical approach used in large jugular foramen tumors. Operative pearls, proper selection approach, and avoidance of complications are also discussed.

3. Results

The jugular foramen can be approached through several pathways depending on the tumor's configuration. Each case must be carefully assessed before selecting the adequate approach. Frequently, subtle nuances distinguish each approach from others, adding complexity for proper understanding. To simplify this, we can divide the approaches based on anterolateral and posterolateral perspectives [8]. The anterolateral approaches include the dissection of the structures located in front and lateral to the sigmoid sinus and jugular foramen, and the posterolateral approaches are accessed via the dissection of structures behind and lateral to the sigmoid sinus and jugular foramen [8]. Every approach has its advantages and disadvantages, and their specific indications for each type of tumor are shown in Table 1. Also, a combined approach can be used, maximizing the advantages from both anterolateral and posterolateral corridors [9].

Table 1. Surgical approaches classification for jugular foramen tumors.

Anterolateral	Posterolateral	Combined
Postauricular transtemporal approach	Retrosigmoid approach	Combined transmastoid retro- and infralabyrinthine transjugular transcondylar trans tubercular high cervical approach
Preauricular Subtemporal infratemporal approach	Far-Lateral approach -Transcondylar approach -Supracondylar approach -Paracondylar approach	

3.1. Posterolateral Approaches

3.1.1. Retrosigmoid Approach

This approach is the workhorse for posterior fossa lesions. It is the most common and well-known approach for jugular foramen tumors in neurosurgery. It is indicated predominantly for intradural tumors with little or no extension to the extradural compartment [10]. A C-shaped retroauricular skin incision is created, posterior and parallel to the outline of the pinna, followed by a lateral suboccipital craniotomy exposing the dura inferior and posterior to the transverse and sigmoid sinuses [3]. The dura is also opened in a C or U shape manner. The cerebellum is gently displaced medially away from the posterior petrous surface of the temporal bone to expose the lateral aspect of the brainstem and intracranial segments of the cranial nerves exiting through the internal acoustic meatus and jugular foramen [3,8] Figure 1A.

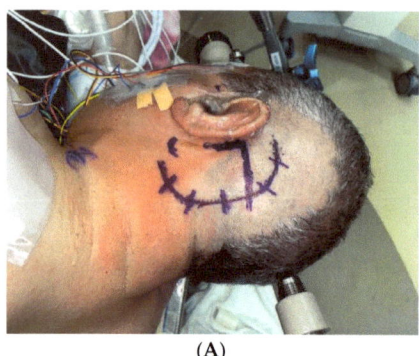 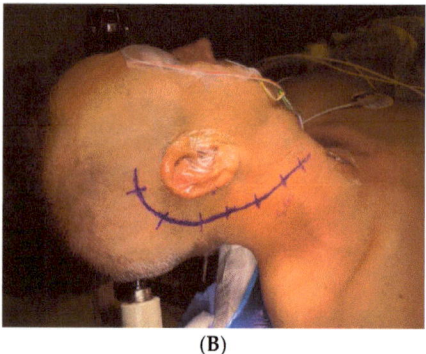

Figure 1. (**A**). Retrosigmoid C-shaped retroauricular skin incision posterior and parallel to the outline of the pinna (**B**). Combined approach right-sided C-shaped retro-auricular incision. The incision is started approximately 2 to 3 cm posterior to the upper border of the ear. It continues posteroinferiorly into the neck over the anterior border of the sternocleidomastoid muscle and under the mandibular angle.

Even though it is a straightforward approach, this is unsuitable for large tumors that go out the jugular foramen's extracranial compartment [11]. A suprajugular extension of the retrosigmoid approach was described by Matsushima et al. in 2014. The area inferior to the internal acoustic meatus, medial to the endolymphatic depression, and the surrounding superior half of the glossopharyngeal dural fold is drilled to access the suprajugular aspect of the jugular foramen. This approach is suitable for tumors extending into the jugular foramen's upper part and above the jugular bulb [12].

3.1.2. Far-Lateral Approach

The far-lateral approach is a more inferior extension of the retrosigmoid approach and involves extending further laterally from the lateral suboccipital approach [13,14]. It provides a better access to the foramen magnum and craniocervical junction, extending the corridor inferior and lateral to the lower cranial nerves [15]. Its primary indication is tumors that extend to the foramen magnum anteriorly or laterally to the lower brainstem at the craniocervical junction [13,14]. The jugular foramen is exposed posteriorly [3]. The skin can be incised using a retro auricular C-shaped incision, or by a classic hockey stick incision beginning from the mastoid tip; the line runs posteriorly to the inion and finally ends inferiorly to the spinous process of C2. The muscles attached to the occipital bone are detached en bloc and reflected inferiorly. A retrosigmoid suboccipital craniotomy that unroofs the foramen magnum and C1 hemilaminectomy is performed. It has three variations depending on which area is desired for access: the jugular foramen, the lower clivus, and the premedullary area [8,15,16]. Some lesions located along the anterolateral margin of the foramen magnum might only need a basic far-lateral approach without drilling the condyle (retrocondylar). Nevertheless, the far-lateral approach can provide a route through which the transcondylar, supracondylar, and paracondylar extensions can be completed with a further increase in the working space along the anterior border of the foramen magnum, jugular tubercle area, and posterior margin of the jugular foramen, respectively [15–18].

The degree of drilling the occipital condyle will depend on the access area needed.

The transcondylar approach is performed by drilling the posterior condyle, which gradually expands the working space to the anterior brainstem and petroclival area [19,20]. The percentage of condyle to be removed can vary from only the posterior one third with no instability of the craniovertebral junction to as far as the posterior half, which will require fixation of the craniovertebral junction due to instability of the atlanto-occipital joint [21,22]. The complete trans-condylar approach during which the posterior two thirds of the condyle is removed will have the hypoglossal canal as the anterior limit and can provide a dramatic increase in petroclival exposure, especially if the jugular tuberculum is also removed [13,20]. This approach is generally used to reach the premedullary area [13,23].

The supracondylar extension is the approach used to reach the jugular tubercle. It involves drilling the occipital bone above and behind the occipital condyle by completely preserving the occipital condyle and including the drilling of the condylar fossa. The condylar fossa contains the posterior condylar canal below, and drilling it results in a defect in the posterior part of the jugular tubercle [8,13,16].

Lesions affecting the posterior section of the jugular foramen may be approached using the paracondylar extension. These can include paragangliomas of the jugular foramen and dumbbell schwannomas of the lower cranial nerves. The approach is tailored towards the jugular process of the occipital bone, which is located lateral to the occipital condyle and is the site of attachment of the rectus capitis lateralis muscle. It involves the skeletonization and opening of the hypoglossal canal, partial drilling of the lateral portion of the occipital condyle, and the mastoid tip [8,13,16,17].

The preservation of the occipital condyle and the C-1 lateral mass, as well as the attachments of the alar and transverse ligaments to the anterior one third of the occipital condyle and the anterior one third of the C-1 lateral mass, are among the key variables that are responsible for maintaining the stability of the occipitocervical junction [15,17]. An occipital-cervical fusion operation is required when the integrity of these structures has been impaired, whether through a complete trans-condylar approach, a transplacental approach, or tumor destruction of these areas. Fusion is usually performed as a second-stage operation and when there is no sign of cerebrospinal fluid leakage [15,17,20].

3.2. Anterolateral Approaches

3.2.1. Postauricular Transtemporal Approach

This approach can provide excellent exposure to the jugular foramen and lateral skull base. It is accessed from a lateral approach through the mastoid and the neck (mastoid-neck approach) [8]. A post-auricular C-shaped skin incision provides exposure for a mastoidectomy and neck dissection. The external auditory canal can be either preserved or transected with blind sac closure, depending on the anterior extension of the tumor [3]. The mastoidectomy primarily involves the infralabyrinthine region with exposure of the sigmoid sinus, jugular bulb, and mastoid segment of the facial nerve. Hearing does not have to be sacrificed, and it can be preserved by maintaining the footplate of the stapes. Nevertheless, to fully expose the lateral half of the jugular foramen, the mastoid portion of the facial nerve is mobilized anteriorly (which can cause facial nerve palsy), the styloid process must be resected, and detachment of the rectus capitis lateralis muscle from the jugular process of the occipital bone is performed [8,24,25]. The middle and posterior cranial fossa dura in front (Trautman's triangle) and behind the sigmoid sinus are exposed [26].

3.2.2. Preauricular Subtemporal Infratemporal Approach

This approach exposes the jugular foramen anteriorly, and it may be suitable for selected tumors that extend along the petrous portion of the internal carotid artery, through the eustachian tube, or the cancellous portion of the petrous apex [3]. A preauricular skin incision is performed extending across the zygomatic process of the temporal bone into the cervical region. A fronto-temporal craniotomy with or without the superior and lateral orbital rim removal is performed. The middle cranial fossa floor is removed from lateral to medial until the carotid canal is reached. Both the eustachian tube and tensor tympani muscle are removed. Removal of the styloid process allows anterior mobilization of the internal carotid artery and access to the clival region. The drilling of Kawase's triangle allows resection of the petrous apex and provides a corridor to the posterior fossa [8,25,27].

In 1978, Fisch described three types of tumor classification and infratemporal fossa approaches to the lateral skull base. Type A tumors are jugulotympanic paragangliomas. Type B tumors are jugular paragangliomas with no destruction of the bone, and type C tumors are jugular paragangliomas with the destruction of the infralabyrinthine compartment of the temporal bone. The Type A approach allows access to the temporal bone in its infralabyrinthine component and is suitable for jugular foramen tumors. The external auditory canal is transected at the bone-cartilage junction [28,29]. However, this approach is often combined with a lateral approach to access tumors with more anterior extension (Type B or C Fisch's classification of paraganglioma tumors), requiring two-staged surgeries with a bigger chance of auditory loss and facial nerve damage [29].

3.3. Combined Approach

Combined Transmastoid Retro- and Infralabyrinthine Transjugular Transcondylar Transtubercular Transcervical Approach

From an anterolateral perspective, we can use a combined approach to reach total exposure of the jugular foramen in a single-stage surgery. This approach allows radical resection of tumors around the jugular foramen, the lower clivus, and the high cervical region. It combines the transmastoid, retro- and infra-labyrinthine transcondylar transtubercular and transcervical approaches. Multidirectional angles of attack and working corridors can be performed, including suprajugular, transjugular, and infrajugular exposures, maximizing the advantages of the abovementioned approaches. Both intracranial and extracranial tumors can be removed in a one-stage procedure. Blind sac closure of the external ear canal can be performed selectively as indicated (tumor extension into middle ear), and permanent facial nerve re-routing and mandibular translocation are generally unnecessary, minimizing postoperative complications. Nevertheless, these maneuvers can be performed selectively based on the indicated pathology. Furthermore, access to the lower clivus is facilitated by anterior translocation of the vertical portion of the internal carotid artery and inferior translocation of the lower cranial nerves, if needed [9,30].

This complex approach to entirely expose the jugular foramen can be simplified stepwise: 1. Postauricular C-shaped infratemporal incision; 2. Retrolabyrinthine mastoidectomy; 3. High cervical exposure; 4. Skeletonization and anterior translocation of the facial nerve; 5. Lateral suboccipital craniotomy and transcondylar transtubercular exposure; 6. Exposure of the internal jugular vein, jugular bulb, and sigmoid sinus; 7. Intradural exposure (for tumors with intracranial extension) [9,30] Figure 1B-3.

The patient is positioned supine with the head turned contralaterally. A retroauricular curvilinear C-shaped skin incision 2 to 3 cm posterior to the upper border of the ear is performed (Figure 1B). It continues posteroinferiorly into the neck crossing the anterior boundary of the sternocleidomastoid muscle and reaching underneath the mandibular angle. Prior to mastoidectomy, the entire body and tip of the mastoid, the spine of Henle, the posterior end of the root of the zygoma, the supramastoid crest, and the asterion must be exposed [9,30].

From that point, we skeletonize the semicircular canals, fallopian canal, sigmoid sinus, and jugular bulb (Figure 2A). The extracranial sections of the lower cranial nerves, the internal carotid artery, and the internal jugular vein are identified using a high cervical exposure (Figure 2B). After dividing the subcutaneous tissue and platysma muscle, the posterior angle of the mandible and the anterior boundary of the sternocleidomastoid muscle are identified by blunt dissection. Later, the facial nerve in the fallopian canal is totally skeletonized with a diamond burr from the genu to the stylomastoid foramen. The fallopian bridge technique involves leaving the facial nerve invested in its protective bone shell to avoid facial nerve damage. The mastoid tip is then removed with a high-speed drill to decompress the facial nerve from the stylomastoid foramen [9,30].

Exposure of the deeply seated suboccipital triangle provides a crucial anatomical landmark for this portion of the approach. It is important to open it by separating the superior and inferior oblique muscle insertions from the transverse process of C1 and reflecting them medially. The dorsal ramus of the C1 nerve root and the V3 horizontal portion of the vertebral artery can be found in this triangle. A lateral suboccipital craniectomy is then performed. Extradural reduction in the occipital condyle and jugular tubercle are the critical maneuvers of this step (Figure 3A,B). Removal of the posterior and medial one third of the occipital condyle is generally enough to increase the surgical corridor to the ventral foramen magnum [9,30].

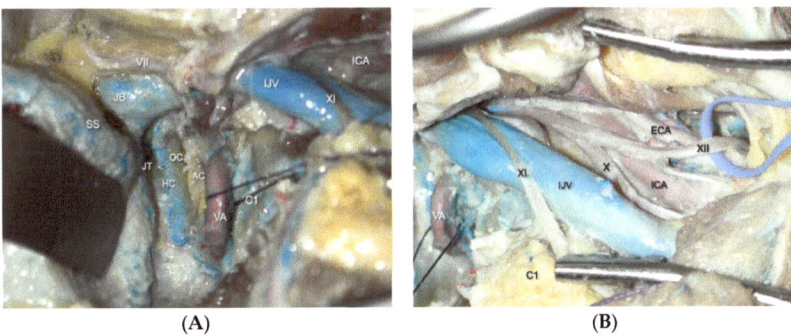

Figure 2. (**A**) Lateral view of the combined transmastoid retro- and infralabyrinthine transjugular transcondylar transtubercular high cervical approach, reflecting the posterior fossa dura. The JB passing through the jugular foramen. The IJV descends along the ICA with the lower cranial nerves. The vertebral artery ascends through the transverse process of C1 and usually passes behind the atlantal condyle. (**B**) Extracranial transcervical perspective of the glossopharyngeal, vagus, accessory, and hypoglossal nerves. The IX and XII nerve pass anteriorly along the lateral surface of the ICA. The XI nerve descends posteriorly across the lateral surface of the IJV. The vagus descends inferiorly within the carotid sheath. *AC.*, atlantal Condyle. *C1.*, atlas. *ECA.*, external carotid artery. *HC.*, hypoglossal canal. *ICA.*, internal carotid artery. *IJV.*, internal jugular vein. *JB.*, jugular bulb. *JT.*, jugular tubercule *OC.*, occipital condyle. *PFD.*, posterior fossa dura. *SS.*, sigmoid sinus. *VA.*, vertebral artery. *VII.*, facial nerve. *XI.*, accessory nerve. *IX.*, glossopharyngeal nerve. *X.*, vagus nerve. *XII.*, hypoglossal nerve.

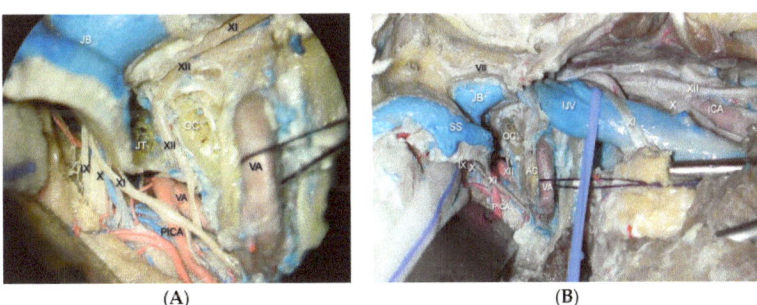

Figure 3. (**A**). Intradural and extradural views of the lower cranial nerves passing through the jugular foramen. The glossopharyngeal, vagus, and accessory nerves arise from the medulla in the postolivary sulcus and pierce the dural roof of the jugular foramen to pass through it. The IX nerve enters the jugular foramen through the glossopharyngeal meatus, and the X and XI nerves through the vagus meatus. The PICA arises from the posterior or lateral surfaces of the VA. The XII exits through the hypoglossal canal above the OC. (**B**) Final view of the combined approach with high cervical exposure. From the intradural perspective, the lower cranial nerves leaving the medulla and enter the jugular foramen. Hypoglossal nerve exits through the hypoglossal canal. Vertebral artery below the OC. Sigmoid sinus empties into the jugular foramen after coursing down the sigmoid sulcus, crossing the occipitomastoid suture at the site of the jugular bulb. From the jugular bulb, the flow is directed downward into the IJV. *AC.*, atlantal condyle *ICA.*, internal carotid artery., *IJV.*, internal jugular vein. *JB.*, jugular bulb. *JT.*, jugular tubercule. *OC.*, occipital condyle., *PICA.*, postero-inferior cerebellar artery. *SS.*, sigmoid sinus. *VA.*, vertebral artery. *VII.*, facial nerve. *IX.*, glossopharyngeal nerve. *X.*, vagus nerve. *XI.*, accessory nerve. *XII.*, hypoglossal nerve.

The tumor mass is generally palpable within the venous structures after entire exposure of the sigmoid sinus, jugular bulb, and internal jugular vein. We can then coagulate all of the tumor's arterial feeders and ligate the internal jugular vein slightly inferior to the tumor bulk. A suture ligature is used to occlude the sigmoid sinus immediately above the tumor. Alternatively, an endoluminal occlusion using gelfoam packing can also be used to avoid any durotomies (for entirely extradural tumors). This involves incising the lateral wall of the sigmoid sinus and inserting gelfoam pledgets proximally into the sigmoid sinus. Care is taken to avoid occluding the transverse sigmoid junction where the vein of Labbe enters. Control of back bleeding from the inferior petrosal sinus is controlled by injecting a flowable hemostatic matrix (Surgiflo, Ethicon, Inc., Bridgewater, NJ, USA) distally towards the jugular bulb. The lateral wall of the internal jugular vein is incised and the intraluminal tumor within the IJV, jugular bulb and sigmoid sinus is removed. If needed, for intradural pathology, the posterior fossa dura including the retrosigmoid, transsigmoid, and/or presigmoid dural incision, can be made to access the intradural portion of the tumor [9,30].

3.4. Representative Cases

The selection for the approach for jugular foramen tumors must be tailored case by case, considering the tumor's configuration, the patient's neurological status, and the neurosurgeon's experience. Here, we present four cases in which the combined approach can be used to treat large complex jugular foramen tumors.

Case 1:

A 69-year-old female patient presented to our institution with progressive headaches, dysphagia, dysphonia, hearing loss, and severe gait ataxia from a left jugular foramen paraganglioma invading the jugular bulb and internal jugular vein with intradural compression of the brainstem (Figure 4A,B). After preoperative tumor embolization, the tumor was resected via a combined transmastoid infralabyrinthine transjugular transcervical approach. The internal jugular vein was ligated, and the sigmoid sinus was occluded endoluminally. The jugular bulb and vein were opened to remove the intraluminal invasion by the tumor. The intradural tumor was then removed to decompress the brainstem. Postoperatively, the patient remained at her neurological baseline with no new cranial nerve deficits. Severe gait ataxia improved. Postoperative MRI showed gross total resection of the tumor (Figure 4C,D).

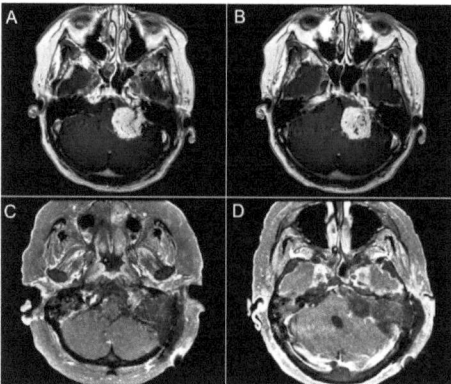

Figure 4. Pre-op and Post-op MRI demonstrating a left jugular paraganglioma (glomus jugulare). (**A,B**) The images show a large jugular paraganglioma that invaded into the cervical IJV and had significant extension intradurally into the cerebellopontine angle with compression of the brainstem. (**C,D**) The images show gross total resection of the tumor by the combined transmastoid retro- and infralabyrinthine transjugular transcondylar transtubercular high cervical approach.

Case 2:

A 24-year-old female patient presented with progressive headaches, dysphagia, and right-sided weakness from a left jugular foramen meningioma invading the jugular bulb and internal jugular vein with compression of the brainstem (Figure 5A,B). The tumor was resected via a combined transmastoid infralabyrinthine transjugular transcervical approach. In this case, blind sac closure was unnecessary since the tumor had no extension into the middle ear. The retrosigmoid corridor was opened to remove the intradural portion of the tumor. Then, the internal jugular vein was ligated, and the sigmoid sinus was occluded endoluminally (Figure 6A–D). The jugular bulb and vein were opened to remove the intraluminal invasion by the tumor. Postoperatively, the patient was neurologically intact with no cranial nerve deficits. Postoperative MRI showed gross total resection of the tumor (Figure 5C,D).

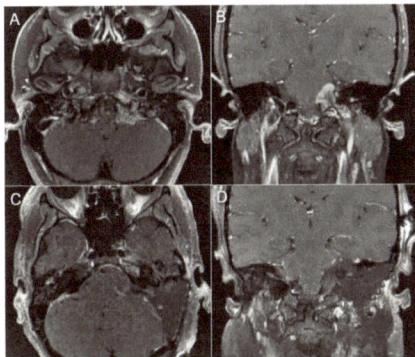

Figure 5. Pre-operative and post-operative MRI views of a left jugular foramen meningioma invading the internal jugular vein. (**A,B**) The images show T1 gadolinium- enhanced images of a homogenous mass in the jugular foramen with intradural extension. (**C,D**) The images show gross total resection of the tumor by the combined transmastoid retro- and infralabyrinthine transjugular transcondylar trans tubercular high cervical approach.

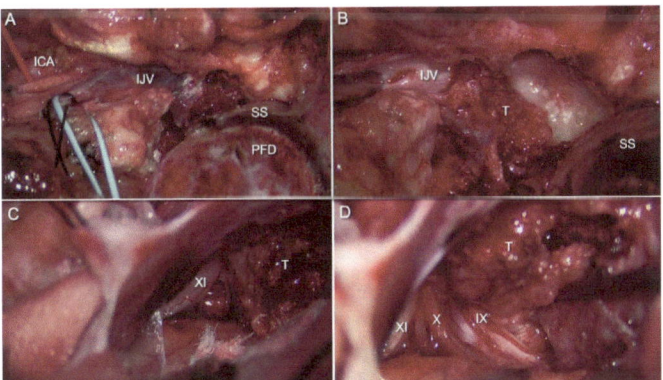

Figure 6. (**A**) Left-sided exposure of jugular foramen via extended anterolateral infralabyrinthine transjugular approach for resection of jugular foramen meningioma. (**B**) After tying off the IJV and endoluminal occlusion of the sigmoid sinus, the lateral wall of the sigmoid sinus, jugular bulb and internal jugular vein are excised to expose the intraluminal tumor in the jugular bulb. (**C,D**) Retrosigmoid exposure of the intradural portion of the tumor at the jugular fossa. The tumor is carefully dissected from the lower cranial nerves. ICA., internal carotid artery. IJV., internal jugular vein. PFD., posterior fossa dura. SS., sigmoid sinus. T., tumor.

Case 3:

A 51-year-old male presented with progressive dysphagia and significant weight loss with 9th through 12th cranial nerve palsies. MRI demonstrated a giant craniocervical junction chordoma with jugular foramen invasion, extension into the right parapharyngeal space and intradural cervicomedullary junction, and near-complete erosion of the right occipital condyle (Figure 7A–C). The tumor was resected via a right combined infralabyrinthine transjugular transclival transcervical approach. The internal jugular vein was ligated, and the sigmoid sinus was occluded endoluminally with gelfoam. The jugular bulb was opened to reveal intrabulbar chordoma. A gross total tumor resection in all the invaded spaces was achieved, and the pre-clival dura was resected (Figure 7D,F). Multi-layered reconstruction with an alloderm graft and fat graft was performed. A second-stage occipital cervical fusion was performed because of the craniocervical instability caused by tumor invasion into the right occipital condyle. Postoperatively, the patient remained at his preoperative neurological baseline without any new neurological deficits.

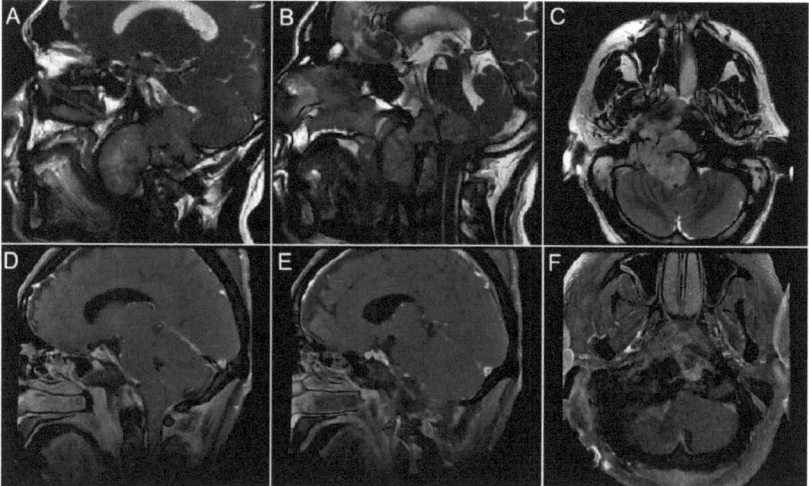

Figure 7. Pre-op and Post-op MRI views of an extensive cranio-cervical chordoma invading the jugular foramen, cerebello-medullary cistern and parapharyngeal space. (**A–C**) The images show a T2 MRI signal with a large lobulated mass centered on the right parapharyngeal space with intradural and extradural extension. The tumor is compressing the anterior pons and the airway deviated to the left side. (**D–F**) The images show a gross total resection of the tumor using the combined transmastoid retro- and infralabyrinthine transjugular transcondylar transtubercular high cervical approach.

Case 4:

A 34-year-old female presented with left-sided hearing loss, left vocal cord paralysis, and severe gait ataxia from a left dumbbell jugular foramen schwannoma involving the cerebellopontine angle (Figure 8A,B). A gross total resection was achieved via a combined infralabyrinthine, trans-sigmoid transjugular approach (Figure 8C,D). Postoperatively, the patient improved gait function and incurred no new cranial nerve deficits.

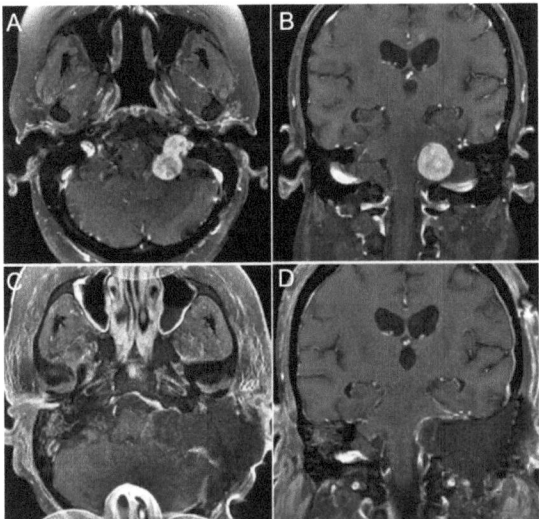

Figure 8. Pre-op and post-op MRI views of a jugular foramen schwannoma. (**A,B**) The images show a gadolinium enhanced T1 weighted MR images with a well- circumscribed dumbbell shaped Schwannoma invading the jugular foramen. (**C,D**) The images show gross total resection of the tumor using a combined transmastoid retro- and infralabyrinthine transjugular transcondylar transtubercular high cervical approach.

4. Discussion

The approach selection for jugular foramen tumors can vary significantly according to the lesion's type, size, and configuration. Also, experience and extensive knowledge of the region's anatomy are critical for achieving optimal clinical results. We aim to have a philosophy of maximal safe resection, avoiding neurovascular injury, and optimal preservation of functioning cranial nerves. A more aggressive approach can be considered in cases with pre-existing irreversible cranial nerve palsies [31].

The posterolateral approaches, especially the retrosigmoid approach, are indicated for tumors predominantly intradural with little or no extension to the extradural compartment. The anterolateral approaches can provide an excellent pathway when the tumor is extending to the infratemporal ICA or when the middle fossa approach is needed for tumors extending to the petrous apex.

The combined transmastoid retro- and infralabyrinthine transjugular transcondylar transtubercular transcervical approach described above with a high cervical C-shaped retroauricular incision allows a single-staged radical resection of large complex jugular foramen tumors. This approach has the advantage of delivering a total exposure of the jugular foramen through various attack angles. Without transection of the external ear canal, permanent facial nerve re-routing, or mandibular translocation, the infratemporal carotid artery can be exposed [9].

The permanent transposition of the facial nerve is a regular step during most of the trans-labyrinthine approaches [24]. After opening the stylomastoid foramen, the bone in the pre-facial area needs to be drilled. This drilling should be performed in the area that corresponds to the base of the styloid process. When this portion is drilled, it results in the detachment of the process. This detachment and the further permanent re-routing of the facial nerve provide exposure to the carotid canal, which contains the vertical C7 segment of the ICA [24,28,29]. Nevertheless, other authors have advocated performing an anterior, slightly vertical translocation of the facial nerve instead of permanent rerouting with less chance of facial nerve palsy when there is no need to expose the infratemporal segment

(C7) of the carotid artery [9,31]. Translocating the facial nerve can often lead to temporary facial nerve palsy, so this technique, as well as permanent rerouting of the nerve, must be used with caution. It is important to keep the periosteum, which surrounds the facial nerve and contains the blood supply to the nerve, intact to ensure optimal preservation of the facial nerve [9].

Surgery of jugular foramen tumors often requires vascular control of the jugular venous system by ligating the internal jugular vein and sigmoid sinus to allow intrabulbar access. Occlusion of the sigmoid sinus traditionally involves pre- and retrosigmoid durotomies to allow the application of vascular clips or suture ligatures, with the risk of postoperative cerebrospinal fluid (CSF) leakage and pseudomeningoceles. An endoluminal sigmoid sinus occlusion with the gelfoam technique that is entirely extradural can avoid any durotomies that can result in postoperative CSF leaks. It can be performed by placing pieces of gel foam endoluminally into the proximal sigmoid sinus after the jugular vein is tied off. Care must be taken to avoid occlusion of the venous outflow of the vein of Labbe at the transverse-sigmoid junction to avoid temporal lobe venous infarction.

CSF leakage rate in jugular foramen tumors after surgery may vary according to the tumor size, type, configuration, intradural or extradural localization, and extension. There are several variables that must be taken into consideration when comparing one approach to another regarding CSF occurrence. There is little information in the literature because most of the case series presented have several approach selections, and none of them are designed to compare CSF outcomes from one approach to another. Nevertheless, some authors have reported low rates of CSF leaks, from 0% [10] in the retrosigmoid approach to higher rates of 4.5% [32,33], 5.3% [34], and 10% [35,36] in the translabyrinthine approach for other types of tumors. More studies should be conducted to give a more accurate CSF leak rate for each approach and each type of jugular foramen tumor.

Nevertheless, there are general pearls and tricks that the surgeon must follow in other to decrease the chances of CSF leakage. The first step involved is to perform a watertight dural repair using the dural sling technique with autologous fascia lata [37]. This involves suturing a piece of autologous fascial lata graft to the borders of the dural defect with interrupted 4-0 Nurolon (Ethicon) sutures producing a dural sling. Next, Tachosil (fibrin sealant on a collagen carrier) is placed on the edges, creating an additional layer of protection and further reinforcing the repair. After the repair has been reinforced, a fat graft is placed on top of the fascial sling and fills the mastoidectomy defect. Creating a facial sling prevents the fat from being in direct contact and compression with the intradural structures such as the brainstem and cranial nerves, and reduces the chances of fat necrosis, subarachnoid fat embolism and lipoid meningitis [38–40]. Then, a Medpor titanium plate may be used to reconstruct the bony defect and also buttresses the fat graft against the dural closure to further prevent a csf leak. It is important to seal off the entrance of the mastoid antrum into the middle ear with a bone wax plate and also to wax off any air cells as these may sometimes provide alternate accessory pathways to the middle ear. We usually reinforce this with another layer of calcium phosphate bone substitute (Hydroset, Stryker). The remaining dead space in the mastoid cavity is filled with fat graft and buttressed with a Medpor Titan plate. Additionally, lumbar drainage is performed for 3–5 days postoperatively at 5–10 cc per hour to help reduce the risk of pseudomeningocele formation and CSF leakage [37].

Endoscopic assistance can also be performed to assess the degree of tumor resection and improve visualization of the lower cranial nerves after removing the tumor. The need to perform a tracheostomy and/or gastrostomy is tailored on a case by case basis and will depend mostly on postoperative assessment with video laryngoscopy and modified barium swallow. Patients with dysphonia, either pre-existing preoperatively or newly developed postoperatively, may require vocal cord injections to improve voice function. Additional maneuvers with botox injection or esophageal balloon dilatation can be considered based on the assessment by our laryngology team.

A multidisciplinary team comprising neurosurgeons, otolaryngologists (including neuro-otologist, laryngologist, head and neck surgeon), radiation oncologist, and neurinterventionalist is critical for management of complex jugular foramen tumors. We encourage all neurosurgeons to first have extensive anatomical knowledge of the jugular foramen through cadaveric dissections or 3D simulations before attempting to perform these types of approaches.

5. Conclusions

Surgery for jugular foramen tumors can be complex and laborious. Each case should be thoroughly evaluated to determine the best strategy for the patient, allowing the surgeon to achieve maximal safe removal of the tumor while avoiding neurological complications. Our workhorse is the combined transmastoid retro- and infralabyrinthine transjugular transcondylar transtubercular high cervical approach which can be used to resect difficult jugular foramen tumors such as paragangliomas, schwannomas, meningiomas, and chordomas. Total exposure of the jugular foramen can be achieved, and multidirectional approaches can be performed, including suprajugular, infrajugular, and transjugular corridors. A multidisciplinary team and extensive understanding of the surgical anatomy are essential to offer the patient with the greatest chance of optimal postoperative outcomes.

Author Contributions: Conceptualization: A.L.C., A.T.M. and J.K.L. Methodology: A.L.C. and A.T.M.; software: A.L.C. and A.T.M.; validation A.L.C., A.T.M. and J.K.L.; formal analysis, A.L.C., A.T.M. and J.K.L.; investigation, A.L.C. and A.T.M.; resources, A.L.C. and A.T.M.; data curation, A.L.C. and A.T.M. writing—original draft preparation, A.L.C., A.T.M. and J.K.L.; writing—review and editing, A.L.C., A.T.M. and J.K.L.; visualization, A.L.C., A.T.M. and J.K.L.; supervision, J.K.L.; project administration, J.K.L. All authors have read and agreed to the published version of the manuscript.

Funding: This research received no external funding.

Institutional Review Board Statement: Not applicable.

Informed Consent Statement: Written informed consent has been obtained from the patients to publish this paper.

Data Availability Statement: No new data were created or analyzed in this study. Data sharing is not applicable to this article.

Conflicts of Interest: The authors declare no conflicts of interest.

References

1. Ramina, R.; Maniglia, J.J.; Fernandes, Y.B.; Paschoal, J.R.; Pfeilsticker, L.N.; Neto, M.C.; Borges, G. Jugular foramen tumors: Diagnosis and treatment. *Neurosurg. Focus* **2004**, *17*, E5. [CrossRef] [PubMed]
2. Weber, A.L.; McKenna, M.J. Radiologic evaluation of the jugular foramen. Anatomy, vascular variants, anomalies, and tumors. *Neuroimaging Clin. N. Am.* **1994**, *4*, 579–598. [PubMed]
3. Rhoton, A.L. Jugular Foramen. In *Rhoton Cranial Anatomy and Surgical Approaches*, Oxford University Press: Oxford, UK, 2019.
4. Inserra, M.M.; Pfister, M.; Jackler, R.K. Anatomy involved in the jugular foramen approach for jugulotympanic paraganglioma resection. *Neurosurg. Focus* **2004**, *12*, E6. [CrossRef] [PubMed]
5. Shapiro, R. Compartmentation of the jugular foramen. *J. Neurosurg.* **1972**, *36*, 340–343. [CrossRef] [PubMed]
6. Tekdemir, I.; Tuccar, E.; Aslan, A.; Elhan, A.; Deda, H.; Ciftci, E.; Akyar, S. The Jugular Foramen A Comparative RadioAnatomic Study. *Surg. Neurol.* **1998**, *50*, 557–562. [CrossRef] [PubMed]
7. Ayeni, S.A.; Ohata, K.; Tanaka, K.; Hakuba, A. The microsurgical anatomy of the jugular foramen. *J. Neurosurg.* **1995**, *83*, 903–909. [CrossRef]
8. McGrew, B.; Matusz, P.; De Caro, R.; Loukas, M.; Tubbs, R.; Griessenauer, C. Surgical Approaches to the Jugular Foramen: A Comprehensive Review. *J. Neurol. Surg. Part B Skull Base* **2016**, *77*, 260–264. [CrossRef]
9. Liu, J.K.; Sameshima, T.; Gottfried, O.N.; Couldwell, W.T.; Fukushima, T. The combined Transmastoid Retro- and Infralabyrinthine Transjugular Transcaondylar Transtubercular High Cervical approach for resection of Glomus jugulare Tumors. *Neurosurgery* **2006**, *59* (Suppl. 1), ONS115–ONS125. [CrossRef]
10. Matsushima, K.; Kohno, M.; Nakajima, N.; Izawa, H.; Ichimasu, N.; Tanaka, Y.; Sora, S. Retrosigmoid Intradural Suprajugular Approach to Jugular Foramen Tumors with Intraforaminal Extension: Surgical Series of 19 Cases. *World Neurosurg.* **2019**, *125*, e984–e991. [CrossRef] [PubMed]

11. Jackson, G.G.; Kaylie, D.M.; Coppit, G.; Gardner, E.K. Glomus Jugulare Tumors with intracranial extension. *Neurosurg. Focus* **2004**, *17*, E7. [CrossRef] [PubMed]
12. Matsushima, K.; Michihiro, K.; Komune, N.; Miki, K.; Matsushima, T.; Rhoton, A.L. Suprajugular extension of the retrosigmoid approach: Microsurgical anatomy. *J. Neurosurg.* **2014**, *121*, 397–407. [CrossRef]
13. Luzzi, S.; Lucifero, A.G.; Bruno, N.; Baldoncini, M.; Campero, A.; Galio, R. Far Lateral Approach. *Acta Biomed.* **2021**, *92*, e2021352. [CrossRef]
14. Chaddad-Neto, F.; Doria-Netto, H.L.; Campos-Filho, J.M.; Reghin-Neto, M.; Rothon, A.L., Jr.; de Oliveria, E. The Far-lateral craniotomy: Tips ans Tricks. *Arq. Neuropsiquiatr.* **2014**, *72*, 699–705. [CrossRef]
15. Rhoton, A.L., Jr. The Far-Lateral Approach and Its Transcondylar, Supracondular, and Paracondylar Extensions. *Neurosurgery* **2000**, *47*, S195–S209. [CrossRef]
16. Wen, H.T.; Albert LRothon, A.L.; Katsuta, T.; de Oliveira, E. Microsurgical anatomy of the transcondylar, supracondylar, and paracondylar extensions of the far-lateral approach. *J. Neurosurg.* **1997**, *87*, 555–585. [CrossRef]
17. Salas, E.; Sekhar, L.N.; Ziyal, I.M.; Caputy, A.J.; Wright, D.C. Variations of the extreme-lateral craniocervical approach: Anatomical study and clinical analysis of 69 patients. *J. Neurosurg. Spine* **1999**, *90*, 206–219. [CrossRef]
18. Sen, C.N.; Sekhar, L.N. Surgical Management of Anteriorly Placed Lesions at the Craniocervical Junction-an Alternative Approach. *Acta Neurochir.* **1991**, *108*, 70–77. [CrossRef]
19. Sato, A.; Hirai, S.; Obata, Y.; Maehara, T.; Aoyagi, M. Muscular-Stage Dissection during Far Lateral Approach and Its Transcondylar Extension. *J. Neurol. Surg. Part B Skull Base* **2018**, *79* (Suppl. 4), S356–S361. [CrossRef]
20. Spektor, S.; Anderson, G.J.; McMenomey, S.O.; Horgan, M.A.; Kellogg, J.X.; Delashaw, J.B. Quantitative description of the far-lateral transcondylar transtubercular approach to the foramen magnum and clivus. *J. Neurosurg.* **2000**, *92*, 824–831. [CrossRef] [PubMed]
21. Babu, R.P.; Sekhar, L.N.; Wright, D.C. Extreme lateral transcondylar approach: Technical improvements and lessons learned. *J. Neurosurg.* **1994**, *81*, 49–59. [CrossRef] [PubMed]
22. Açikbaş, S.C.; Tuncer, R.; Demirez, I.; Rahat, Ö.; Kazan, S.; Sindel, M.; Saveren, M. The effect of condylectomy on extreme lateral transcondylar approach to the anterior foramen magnum. *Acta Neurochir.* **1997**, *139*, 546–550. [CrossRef] [PubMed]
23. Hosoda, K.; Fujita, S.; Kawaguchi, T.; Yamada, H. A transcondylar approach to the arteriovenous malformation at the ventral cervicomedullary junction: Report of three cases. *Neurosurgery* **1994**, *34*, 748–752. [CrossRef] [PubMed]
24. Fukushima, T.; Nonaka, Y. *Fukushima Manual of Skull Base Dissection*, 3rd ed.; AF-Neuro Video: Raleigh, NC, USA, 2010.
25. Sanna, M.; Saleh, E.; Khrais, T.; Mancini, F.; Piazza, P.; Russo, A.; Taibah, A. *Atlas of Microsurgery of the Lateral Skull Base*, 2nd ed.; Thieme: New York, NY, USA, 2008.
26. Shane Tubbs, R.; Griessenauer, C.; Loukas, M.; Shaheryar FAnsari, S.F.; Fritsch, M.H.; Cohen-Gadol, A. Trautmann's Triangle Anatomy With Application to Posterior Transpetrosal and Other Related Skull Base Procedures. *Clin. Anat.* **2014**, *27*, 994–998. [CrossRef] [PubMed]
27. Al-Mefty, O.; Fox, J.L.; Rifai, A.; Smith, R.R. A Combined Infratemporal and Posterior Fossa Approach for the Removal of Giant Glomus Tumors and Chondrosarcomas. *Surg. Neurol.* **1987**, *28*, 423–431. [CrossRef] [PubMed]
28. Fisch, U. Infratemporal fossa approach to tumours of the temporal bone and base of the skull. *J. Laryngol. Otol.* **1978**, *92*, 949–967. [CrossRef] [PubMed]
29. Fisch, U.; Pillsbury, H.C. Infratemporal Fossa Approach to Lesions in the Temporal Bone and Base of the Skull. *Arch. Otolaryngol.* **1979**, *105*, 99–107. [CrossRef] [PubMed]
30. Liu, J.K.; Zhao, K.; Baredes, S.; Jyung, R.W. Extended Anterolateral Infralabyrinthine Transjugular Approach for Microsurgical Resection of Giant Glomus Vagale Tumor: Operative Video and Technical Nuances. *J. Neurol. Surg. Part B Skull Base* **2021**, *82* (Suppl. 1), S59–S60. [CrossRef]
31. Al-Mefty, O.; Teixeira, A. Complex tumors of the glomus jugulare: Criteria, treatment, and outcome. *J. Neurosurg.* **2002**, *97*, 1356–1366. [CrossRef]
32. Sanna, M.; Bacciu, A.; Falcioni, M.; Taibah, A. Surgical management of jugular foramen schwannomas with hearing and facial nerve function preservation: A series of 23 cases and review of the literature. *Laryngoscope* **2006**, *116*, 2191–2204. [CrossRef]
33. Jackson, G.G.; McGrew, B.M.; Forest, J.A.; Netterville, J.L.; Hampf, C.F.; Glasscock, M.E. Lateral Skull Base Surgery for Glomus Tumors: Long-Term Control. *Otol. Neurotol.* **2001**, *22*, 377–382. [CrossRef]
34. Makiese, O.; Chibbaro, S.; Marsella, M.; Tran Ba Huy, P.; George, B. Jugular Foramen Paragangliomas: Manegement, outcome and avoidance of complications in a series of 75 cases. *Neurosurg. Rev.* **2012**, *35*, 185–194. [CrossRef]
35. Goodard, J.C.; Oliver, E.R.; Lambert, P.L. Prevention of cerebroespinal fluid leak after translabyrinthine resection of vesticular schwannoma. *Otol. Neurotol.* **2010**, *31*, 473–477. [CrossRef] [PubMed]
36. Selesnick, S.H.; Liu, J.C.; Jen, A.; Newman, J. The Incidence of cerebrospinal fluid leak after vestibular schwannoma surgery. *Otol. Neurotol.* **2004**, *25*, 387–393. [CrossRef] [PubMed]
37. Liu, J.K.; Patel, S.K.; Podolski, A.J.; Jyung, R.W. Fascial sling technique for dural reconstruction after translabyrinthine resection of acoustic neuroma: Technical note. *Neurosurg. Focus* **2016**, *33*, E17. [CrossRef] [PubMed]
38. Ray, J.; D'Souza, A.R.; Chavda, S.V.; Irving, R.M. Dissemination of fat in CSF: A common finding following translabyrinthine acoustic neuroma surgery. *Clin. Otolaryngol.* **2005**, *30*, 405–408. [CrossRef]

39. Ricaurte, J.C.; Murali, R.; Mandell, W. Uncomplicated Postoperative lipoid Meningitis secondary to autologous fat graft necrosis. *Clin. Infect. Dis.* **2000**, *30*, 613–615. [CrossRef]
40. Taha, A.N.; Almefty, R.; Pravdenkova, S.; Al-Mefty, O. Sequelae of autologous fat graft used for reconstruction in skull base surgery. *World Neurosurg.* **2011**, *75*, 692–695. [CrossRef]

Disclaimer/Publisher's Note: The statements, opinions and data contained in all publications are solely those of the individual author(s) and contributor(s) and not of MDPI and/or the editor(s). MDPI and/or the editor(s) disclaim responsibility for any injury to people or property resulting from any ideas, methods, instructions or products referred to in the content.

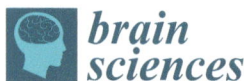

Article

Multi-Disciplinary Approach to Skull Base Paragangliomas

Steven D. Curry [1,2], Armine Kocharyan [1,2] and Gregory P. Lekovic [1,3,*]

1. House Clinic, Los Angeles, CA 90017, USA
2. Department of Head and Neck Surgery, University of California Los Angeles Medical Center, Los Angeles, CA 90095, USA
3. Department of Neurosurgery, University of California Los Angeles Medical Center, Los Angeles, CA 90095, USA
* Correspondence: glekovic@mednet.ucla.edu

Abstract: The treatment of skull base paragangliomas has moved towards the use of cranial nerve preservation strategies, using radiation therapy and subtotal resection in instances when aiming for gross total resection would be expected to cause increased morbidity compared to the natural history of the tumor itself. The goal of this study was to analyze the role of surgery in patients with skull base paragangliomas treated with CyberKnife stereotactic radiosurgery (SRS) for definitive tumor control. A retrospective review identified 22 patients (median age 65.5 years, 50% female) treated with SRS from 2010–2022. Fourteen patients (63.6%) underwent microsurgical resection. Gross total resection was performed in four patients for tympanic paraganglioma ($n = 2$), contralateral paraganglioma ($n = 1$), and intracranial tumor with multiple cranial neuropathies ($n = 1$). Partial/subtotal resection was performed for the treatment of pulsatile tinnitus and conductive hearing loss ($n = 6$), chronic otitis and otorrhea ($n = 2$), intracranial extension ($n = 1$), or episodic vertigo due to perilymphatic fistula ($n = 1$). Eighteen patients had clinical and imaging follow-up for a mean (SD) of 4.5 (3.4) years after SRS, with all patients having clinical and radiological tumor control and no mortalities. Surgery remains an important component in the multidisciplinary treatment of skull base paraganglioma when considering other outcomes besides local tumor control.

Keywords: paraganglioma; glomus tumor; skull base surgery; stereotactic radiosurgery; CyberKnife; microsurgery

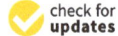

Citation: Curry, S.D.; Kocharyan, A.; Lekovic, G.P. Multi-Disciplinary Approach to Skull Base Paragangliomas. *Brain Sci.* **2023**, *13*, 1533. https://doi.org/10.3390/brainsci13111533

Academic Editor: Miguel Lopez-Gonzalez

Received: 26 September 2023
Revised: 25 October 2023
Accepted: 28 October 2023
Published: 31 October 2023

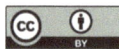

Copyright: © 2023 by the authors. Licensee MDPI, Basel, Switzerland. This article is an open access article distributed under the terms and conditions of the Creative Commons Attribution (CC BY) license (https://creativecommons.org/licenses/by/4.0/).

1. Introduction

Paragangliomas are rare tumors overall but are the most common tumors of the jugular foramen and middle ear; hence, they are of importance to skull base surgeons [1,2]. Paragangliomas are slow-growing, benign-acting, neuroendocrine neoplasms that develop from the embryonic neural crest. In the vicinity of the skull base, these tumors can develop from cells in the adventitia of the jugular bulb (jugular paraganglioma, glomus jugulare), middle ear (tympanic paraganglioma, glomus tympanicum), or along one of the three ganglia of the vagus nerve (vagal paraganglioma) [3,4]. Patients with temporal bone paragangliomas (jugular or tympanic paraganglioma) commonly present with hearing loss and pulsatile tinnitus [5–9]. Less commonly, patients with jugular paragangliomas can present with symptoms of facial or lower cranial neuropathy that can manifest as dysphonia, dysphagia, shoulder weakness, or tongue hemiparesis [10]. Vagal paragangliomas can be found incidentally on imaging, but they may also present initially with lower cranial nerve deficits [11].

The management of head and neck paragangliomas has traditionally involved surgical excision with a goal of gross total resection. Tympanic paragangliomas (Fisch class A and B) can be managed surgically to achieve tumor control while improving symptoms of hearing loss and pulsatile tinnitus [12–14]. The surgical management of larger (Fisch class C and D) jugulotympanic paragangliomas (JTP) is challenging due to the complex anatomy, including the great vessels, cranial nerves, and proximity to intracranial structures. Similarly, the excision of vagal paragangliomas has resulted in high rates of vagus nerve injury leading to persistent dysphagia and dysphonia [15–18].

Advances in neuroimaging, refinements in radiation therapy, and an interest in less invasive treatment paradigms for these usually benign-acting lesions have led to a movement away from radical removal to achieve gross total resection of skull base paragangliomas towards more conservative approaches focused on functional preservation [19–21]. This has led to the use of individualized treatment using one or more modalities during the course of treatment including surgery, radiation therapy, or observation with serial imaging ("wait-and-scan approach") as part of a multidisciplinary team approach. These modalities can be combined or used sequentially based on contingencies and patient-specific factors including tumor size, growth, and location; cranial nerve function (ipsilateral and contralateral); patient age; and patient preferences. Understanding the utility of these options can aid in the treatment planning of complex cases. Subtotal surgical resection has been used in symptomatic patients, either alone or together with radiotherapy, to manage large JTPs while maintaining the functionality of the lower cranial nerves [22–24]. Stereotactic radiosurgery (SRS) has been shown to be effective when used to arrest tumor growth but often does not lead to the improvement of symptoms such as pulsatile tinnitus and hearing loss; hence, there is a need to consider surgical management options in order to achieve the dual goals of tumor control and symptom reduction [25].

Numerous prior studies have examined outcomes including tumor control and cranial nerve function among patients with head and neck paragangliomas treated with either surgery or radiation therapy to contrast the relative merits of these treatment modalities [21,26–28]. The goal of this study was to examine treatment management strategies in patients who underwent CyberKnife SRS to determine the role of surgery in the contemporary multidisciplinary treatment of complex skull base paragangliomas.

2. Materials and Methods

A retrospective chart review was performed for patients at a tertiary care neurotology clinic who were treated for paragangliomas by the senior author (G.P.L.). The inclusion criteria were patients with tympanic, jugular, vagal paraganglioma, or a combination of these who underwent CyberKnife for definitive management of their tumor from 2010–2022. Patient charts were reviewed, and demographic and clinical data were collected, including sex, age, diagnosis, prior treatment, clinical history and presentation, radiation therapy (treatment modality, dose, and dates treated), pre-operative embolization, surgical management (indication for treatment, operation performed, date treated, extent of resection, surgical pathology), pertinent imaging records, and length of follow-up after treatment. Tumor extent was stratified using the Fisch classification of paragangliomas. Data on outcome measures were collected including, post-surgery and -radiotherapy new or worsening cranial neuropathy or other treatment-related complications, length of follow-up with tumor control, and mortality.

All patients were treated with CyberKnife radiosurgical ablation using a prescription dose of 27 Gy in three fractions. Prior to treatment, an Aquaplast mask was fabricated to immobilize the patient, and thin-section magnetic resonance imaging (MRI) with multiplanar, multisequence reconstructions in the axial, coronal, and sagittal planes performed prior to and following the administration of intravenous contrast and computed tomography (CT) images using a high resolution multidetector CT scanner with post-processed reformations was obtained to delineate the target tumor volume and critical anatomic structures for treatment planning using the CyberKnife Multiplan software (Accuray Incorporated, Sunnyvale, CA, USA).

Patients were followed after treatment with contrast-enhanced MRI and clinical examination. Tumor control was defined as unchanged (<2 mm growth in any dimension) or decreased tumor volume determined by the greatest linear measurements in the craniocaudal, axial, and transverse dimensions on MRI studies and no new or worsening cranial neuropathies identified on clinical examination.

Descriptive statistics were calculated to summarize the patient series. Continuous variables were reported as mean and standard deviation if normally distributed, or median and interquartile range (IQR) if skewed as determined by the Shapiro–Wilk test. Associations between continuous variables were assessed using independent samples t-tests. Statistical analysis was performed in R version 4.3.1 (R Foundation for Statistical Computing, Vienna, Austria). A threshold of $p < 0.05$ was considered significant for all statistical tests.

3. Results

3.1. Patient Demographics and Clinical Characteristics

There were 22 patients who met inclusion criteria and were retrospectively analyzed. The mean (SD) age was 61.2 (16.8) years (range 15 to 83 years), and 50% were female (Table 1).

Table 1. Patient demographic and clinical characteristics.

Variable	Value
Age, mean (SD)	61.2 (16.8) years
Female (%)	11 (50%)
Tumor classification	
Jugulotympanic paraganglioma	19
Fisch class A	0
Fisch class B	3
Fisch class C	15
Fisch class D	1
Vagal paraganglioma	3

Abbreviations: SD, standard deviation.

Nineteen patients were treated for jugulotympanic paragangliomas, including Fisch class B tympanic paragangliomas ($n = 3$), and Fisch class C ($n = 15$) and class D ($n = 1$) jugular paragangliomas. Three patients were treated for vagal paragangliomas. No tumors were found to be functional/secreting.

3.2. Surgical Management

Fourteen patients (63.6%) underwent microsurgical resection. Tympanomastoidectomy with or without an extended facial recess approach was used in half ($n = 7$) of the cases, including all class B tumors ($n = 3$) for both tumor and symptom control, and three class C tumors in cases in which the goal of surgery was relief of otologic symptoms. An infratemporal fossa approach with modifications including with or without closure of the external ear canal, and with or without facial nerve rerouting, was used for the remaining jugular and all cases of vagal paragangliomas. In terms of extent of resection, gross total resection was obtained in four patients for tympanic paraganglioma ($n = 2$), contralateral paraganglioma ($n = 1$), or intracranial tumor with multiple cranial neuropathies ($n = 1$). Figure 1 shows pre- and post-operative imaging results from a patient with a class D tumor with brainstem compression.

Subtotal resection was performed for treatment of pulsatile tinnitus and conductive hearing loss ($n = 6$), chronic otitis and otorrhea ($n = 2$), intracranial extension ($n = 1$), or episodic vertigo due to perilymphatic fistula ($n = 1$). Figure 2 shows imaging results from a patient with a class C tumor who underwent subtotal resection for debilitating pulsatile tinnitus.

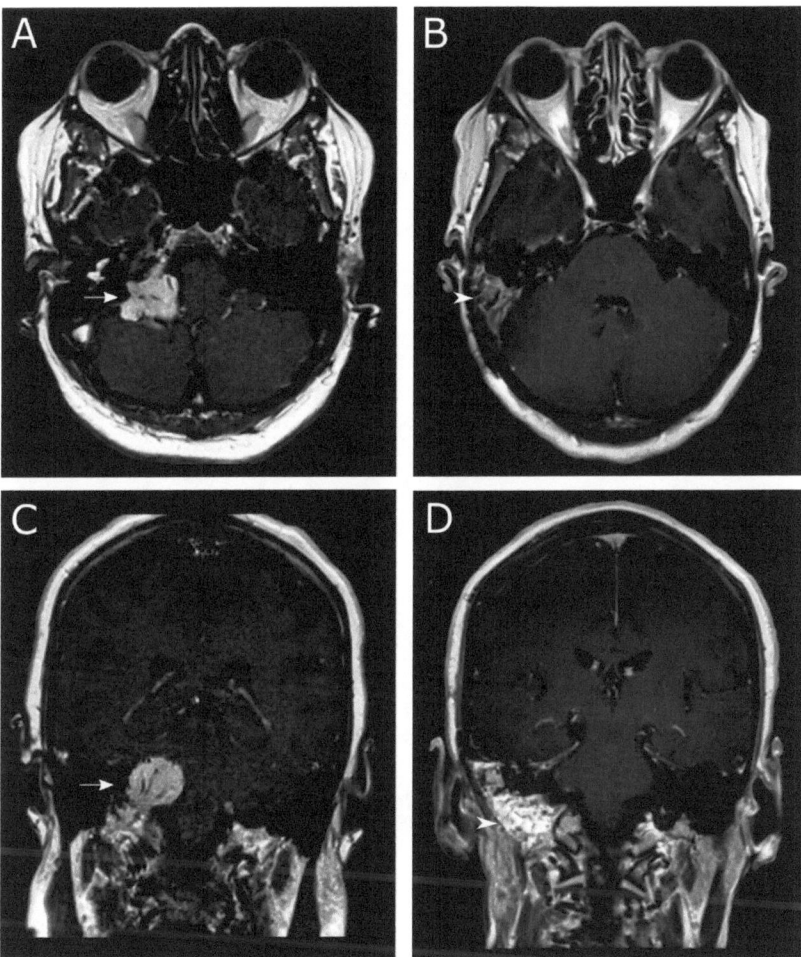

Figure 1. T1-weighted contrast-enhanced MRI of a patient with a Fisch class D jugular paraganglioma who underwent an infratemporal fossa approach for gross total resection of the tumor. The axial pre-surgery image in (**A**) shows brainstem compression from a contrast-enhancing tumor. Part (**B**) shows an axial image slightly more cranial compared to the image in (**A**) showing a fat graft that was used to reconstruct the surgical defect. The coronal pre-surgery image in (**C**) shows contrast-enhancing tumor extending from the jugular bulb to the cerebellopontine angle. The post-surgery image in (**D**) shows the removal of intracranial tumor, with a fat graft visible. Arrows in (**A**,**C**) indicate tumor. Arrowheads in (**B**,**D**) indicate fat graft.

Five patients underwent revision surgery for tumor growth or recurrence ($n = 4$) or persistent conductive hearing loss ($n = 1$) following prior infratemporal fossa ($n = 2$) or tympanomastoidectomy ($n = 3$) approaches. This included tumors classified as Fisch class B ($n = 2$), class C ($n = 2$), or class D ($n = 1$) prior to the patients' first paraganglioma resection. Revision surgical approaches used included tympanomastoidectomy ($n = 3$), infratemporal fossa ($n = 1$), and far lateral ($n = 1$) approaches.

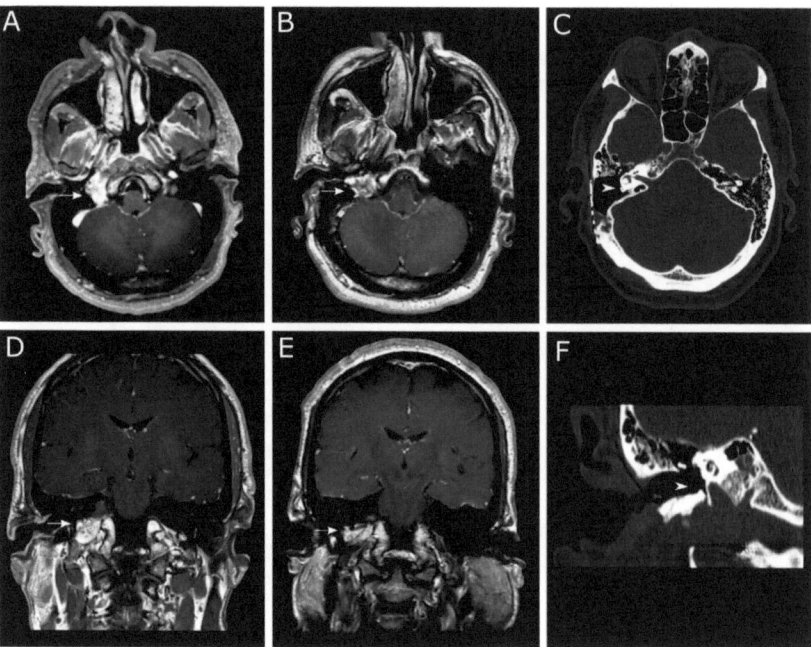

Figure 2. MRI and CT imaging of a patient with a Fisch class C jugular paraganglioma who underwent a modified infratemporal fossa approach for subtotal tumor resection for relief of pulsatile tinnitus and conductive hearing loss. Axial T1-weighted contrast-enhanced MRI presurgical (**A**) and postsurgical (**B**) imaging shows persistent tumor in the area of the jugular bulb. Axial CT bone window (**C**) postsurgical imaging shows no persistent tumor adjacent to the cochlea. Coronal T1-weighted contrast-enhanced MRI presurgical (**D**) and postsurgical (**E**) images show an interval decreased in tumor. Coronal CT bone window (**F**) postsurgical imaging shows no persistent tumor in the mesotympanum or hypotympanum. Arrows in (**A**,**B**,**D**,**E**) indicate tumor. Arrowheads in (**C**,**F**) show the absence of tumor in the middle ear.

3.3. Outcomes

Six patients (43% of patients treated surgically) had new or worsening cranial neuropathies after surgery. Facial nerve palsy occurred in three patients; all improved to House–Brackmann grade 1 or 2. Other cranial neuropathies included worsened dysphonia ($n = 3$) and worsened dysphagia ($n = 2$). No patients required a tracheostomy or gastrostomy.

Patients were treated with SRS a median of 1.4 years (IQR 0.4 to 3.1 years) after initial surgical treatment. The extent of surgical resection (gross total versus subtotal resection) was not associated with a statistically significant difference in time between initial surgery and SRS ($p = 0.41$). Four patients were reported to have new or worsened cranial neuropathies after SRS including dysphagia ($n = 2$), dysphonia ($n = 1$), vertigo ($n = 1$), facial numbness ($n = 1$), and facial spasm ($n = 1$). Eighteen patients had clinical and radiological follow-up for a mean (SD) of 4.5 (3.4) years after SRS, with all patients having clinical and radiological tumor control. There were no mortalities.

4. Discussion

Over half (63.6%) of the patients in this series of 22 patients with skull base paragangliomas who were treated with CyberKnife stereotactic radiation for tumor control of skull base paragangliomas underwent surgery. Patients treated with subtotal surgical resection comprised 10 (45.5%) of the series and the majority (10 out of 14, 71.4%) of patients who were treated surgically. Overall, rates of new or worsening cranial neuropathies treatment using approaches directed towards preserving function were much lower compared to the published literature on patients who were treated using surgical approaches focused on gross total resection, thus showing that a management approach ordered towards functional preservation in advanced skull base paragangliomas is practical [15,27,29–31].

Despite the typically indolent growth of these tumors, mass effect and local invasion can produce symptoms and warrant management. Operative management of skull base paragangliomas serves a role for alleviating otologic symptoms of conductive hearing loss and pulsatile tinnitus, as well as controlling the effects of secreting tumors, though functional tumors are uncommon among paragangliomas of the head and neck. Surgery may also be indicated in patients with intracranial extension causing brainstem compression or obstructive hydrocephalus [24,32–35]. The World Health Organization Classification of Head and Neck Tumors now classifies paraganglioma as a tumor of indeterminate biology, rather than benign or malignant, with a spectrum of malignant potential [36]. Known or suspected cases of metastasis may result in additional surgical indications. In the present series, otologic symptoms including pulsatile tinnitus, conductive hearing loss, and external ear canal extension comprised the symptomatic indications for surgery. Other surgical indications in this series included intracranial extension and tympanic paraganglioma treated with an intent to cure. There were no instances of secreting tumors or suspected metastases.

The treatment of skull base paragangliomas is challenging due to the complex anatomy, infiltrative growth though air cell tracts and along foramina and vascular pathways, and the risk of damage to cranial nerves and blood vessels with treatment [25]. The surgical management of jugular foramen tumors can result in high rates of new or worsening cranial nerve deficits, especially to cranial nerves IX to XII as they pass through the jugular foramen and the hypoglossal canal, though lower rates of cranial nerve dysfunction have been reported for surgical management of paragangliomas compared to schwannomas or meningiomas of the jugular foramen [31,37]. The majority of skull base paragangliomas are slow-growing, non-secreting, benign-appearing tumors; thus, it is important that interventions minimize added morbidity and deliver better long-term outcomes than patients would have with the natural course of the disease. These considerations have led to an interest in alternatives to methods such as the infratemporal fossa type A approach, with facial nerve transposition and jugular vein resection, as described by Fisch in 1978 for jugulotympanic paragangliomas [38,39].

Treatment that is more conservative compared to complete surgical extirpation and that encompasses multiple goals, including tumor control, symptom reduction, the relief of brainstem compression if present, and the prevention of late complications while maintaining cranial nerve function, can be individualized based on tumor and patient factors. For patients with symptomatic or growing tumors, subtotal resection with adjuvant or salvage radiation therapy can result in high rates of tumor control with low rates of new or worsening lower cranial neuropathies [27,29,30]. Microsurgical techniques including preservation of the medial wall of the jugular bulb in surgical resection of jugular paragangliomas allow for protection of the lower cranial nerves that pass through the jugular foramen [40–42].

Special consideration should be given to paragangliomas of the vagus nerve. Operative management of vagal paragangliomas carries an especially high risk of vagus nerve injury compared to surgery for jugular paragangliomas. In a series of vagal paragangliomas, 37 out of 40 patients treated surgically had sacrifice of the ipsilateral vagus nerve, and all 40 patients had permanent ipsilateral vocal fold paralysis [15]. A systematic review of 226 vagal paragangliomas treated surgically found that the vagus nerve was functionally preserved in only 11 (4.9%) patients [26]. In addition to the laryngeal deficits from vagal nerve injury, high vagal paralysis causes ipsilateral soft palate paralysis and subsequent nasal regurgitation and voice changes. Among elderly or debilitated patients especially, multiple cranial neuropathies, as can occur with aggressive surgical resection of these tumors, may prevent rehabilitation to adequate oral diet [43]. Bilateral vagal nerve palsy can lead to the need for permanent tracheostomy and enteral nutrition. In contrast to these reasons for avoiding surgery, vagal paragangliomas have higher rates of metastasis compared to jugulotympanic paragangliomas [44–46]. The management of these tumors should be individualized in light of these considerations.

Radiation therapy, especially SRS with CyberKnife, has emerged as an option for both primary or salvage treatment of skull base paragangliomas [26,28,47]. SRS has excellent rates of tumor control, with decreased morbidity compared to surgery in these cases [21,26]. After a planned subtotal resection for indications including pulsatile tinnitus or conductive hearing loss, SRS can be useful to arrest tumor growth in enlarging tumors, especially in younger patients to reduce the risk of future complications such as cranial neuropathies. In the absence of surgical indications, SRS can be used as a primary therapy to arrest tumor growth. Overall, the incidence of new cranial neuropathy after SRS is low [24,48]. Among patients in our series, two patients had more severe vagal neuropathies (worse dysphagia and/or dysphonia) after SRS, and one patient developed facial numbness and facial spasms after SRS. One important limitation of SRS compared to surgery is that radiation therapy may yield improvement in symptoms in less than half of patients [25].

In the present series, while all patients underwent SRS for definitive control of their paragangliomas (according to the inclusion criteria of this study), most of the patients additionally underwent surgical management for indications including improvement in conductive hearing loss, reducing pulsatile tinnitus, treating otorrhagia and chronic otitis from tumor extension into the external ear canal, and reducing the radiation dose to the cochlea sustained during SRS. Dual-modality treatment (subtotal microsurgical resection with stereotactic radiotherapy) should be considered in patients with bothersome symptoms that are amenable to surgical therapy and who are appropriately counseled regarding the risks and benefits of these treatment modalities.

Angiography with embolization was a commonly used adjunct to surgery. A retrospective study of patients who underwent pre-operative embolization prior to resection of jugular paraganglioma showed a >50% reduction in tumor blush in 86% of patients, with no new or worsening cranial nerve deficits after embolization [49]. Nevertheless, embolization carries risks as the overlapping blood supply between tumors and cranial nerves has been shown to cause facial or lower cranial neuropathies after preoperative embolization with onyx or ethylene vinyl alcohol [50,51]. Cerebrovascular accident can occur due to anastomotic connections between branches of the external carotid artery (e.g., branches of the ascending pharyngeal, deep cervical, ascending cervical, and occipital arteries) and the vertebral artery [52].

Non-operative management should be considered especially in patients who are elderly or who have contralateral lower cranial nerve deficits, poor health or life expectancy, or are unable to tolerate surgery. Observation can be considered in asymptomatic and non-growing tumors to avoid treatment-related morbidities. Reports show that a significant portion of jugular paragangliomas may remain stable in size with observation with serial MRI for years, allowing patients to potentially avoid either surgery or radiation therapy [53–56].

Other considerations in the comprehensive management of skull base paragangliomas include genetic and biochemical testing. The prevalence of germline mutations in head and neck paragangliomas is now recognized to be about 40%, and the results of genetic testing can provide information for risk stratification. This can include stratifying the risk of aggressive tumor behavior and the development of future tumors, whether metastatic, synchronous, or metachronous paragangliomas, or other tumors that can present as part of a syndrome including renal cell carcinoma, papillary thyroid carcinoma, neuroblastoma, or gastrointestinal stroma tumors [57]. Mutations in subunits of succinate dehydrogenase (SDH) are the most common, and tumors with SDHB mutations have the highest risk for metastasis [36,58–60]. Clinical practice and clinical consensus guidelines recommend referral for genetic testing for all patients diagnosed with paragangliomas, and initial biochemical testing with either plasma free metanephrines or urinary fractionated metanephrines is recommended to evaluate for the presence of secreting tumors [57,61,62].

Given the rarity of these tumors, the present study comprises a relatively large number of patients treated with definitive SRS. This series illustrates multiple indications for surgery apart from tumor control, showing that in the multidisciplinary treatment of patients with skull base paragangliomas both surgery and radiation therapy may have value, and the comprehensive treatment of these patients should address both tumor control and symptom amelioration. One of the limitations of this study is that it encompasses a heterogenous group of patients, with a variety of presenting symptoms, tumor locations and sizes, patient ages, and comorbidities. Treatment decisions were determined by shared decision making between surgeons and patients for diverse reasons rather than per a defined protocol. Given these limitations, the ability to quantitatively analyze the outcomes and generalize them to other patient populations may be limited.

5. Conclusions

The management of head and neck paragangliomas has evolved to focus on long term preservation of function, with many tumors being treated more conservatively than they would have been in the past, and radiotherapy is a common treatment modality for achieving tumor control. Among patients with skull base paragangliomas who are treated with CyberKnife SRS for definitive management of their tumors, surgery remains an important component in the multidisciplinary treatment when considering other outcomes beyond local tumor control including the treatment of pulsatile tinnitus, conductive hearing loss, chronic otitis and otorrhea, intracranial extension of tumor, or episodic vertigo due to perilymphatic fistula.

Author Contributions: S.D.C.: Conceptualization, Methodology, Investigation, Formal analysis, Writing—original draft, Writing—review and editing, Visualization. A.K.: Conceptualization, Methodology, Investigation, Writing—review and editing. G.P.L.: Conceptualization, Methodology, Resources, Writing—review and editing, Supervision. All authors have read and agreed to the published version of the manuscript.

Funding: This research received no external funding.

Institutional Review Board Statement: The study was conducted according to the guidelines of the Declaration of Helsinki, and performed in accordance with Institutional Review Board policies under which it was exempt by the Institutional Review Board of PIH Health (9 April 2020).

Informed Consent Statement: Patient consent was waived due to the retrospective design without identifiable information.

Data Availability Statement: Data used for the current original research are available from the corresponding author upon reasonable request.

Conflicts of Interest: The authors declare no conflict of interest.

References

1. Wasserman, P.G.; Savargaonkar, P. Paragangliomas: Classification, Pathology, and Differential Diagnosis. *Otolaryngol. Clin. N. Am.* **2001**, *34*, 845–862. [CrossRef]
2. Ramina, R.; Maniglia, J.J.; Fernandes, Y.B.; Paschoal, J.R.; Pfeilsticker, L.N.; Coelho Neto, M. Tumors of the Jugular Foramen: Diagnosis and Management. *Neurosurgery* **2005**, *57*, 59–68. [CrossRef]
3. Szymańska, A.; Szymański, M.; Czekajska-Chehab, E.; Gołąbek, W.; Szczerbo-Trojanowska, M. Diagnosis and Management of Multiple Paragangliomas of the Head and Neck. *Eur. Arch. Otorhinolaryngol.* **2015**, *272*, 1991–1999. [CrossRef]
4. Graham, N.J.; Smith, J.D.; Else, T.; Basura, G.J. Paragangliomas of the Head and Neck: A Contemporary Review. *Endocr. Oncol.* **2022**, *2*, R153–R162. [CrossRef]
5. Ramos Macías, A.; Bueno Yanes, J.; Bolaños Hernández, P.; Lisner Contreras, I.; Osorio Acosta, A.; Vicente Barrero, M.; Zaballos González, M.L. Temporal paragangliomas. A 12-year experience. *Acta Otorrinolaringol. Esp.* **2011**, *62*, 375–380. [CrossRef]
6. Waldvogel, D.; Mattle, H.P.; Sturzenegger, M.; Schroth, G. Pulsatile Tinnitus—A Review of 84 Patients. *J. Neurol.* **1998**, *245*, 137–142. [CrossRef]

7. Hofmann, E.; Behr, R.; Neumann-Haefelin, T.; Schwager, K. Pulsatile Tinnitus: Imaging and Differential Diagnosis. *Dtsch. Arztebl. Int.* **2013**, *110*, 451–458. [CrossRef]
8. Song, J.-J.; An, G.S.; Choi, I.; De Ridder, D.; Kim, S.Y.; Choi, H.S.; Park, J.H.; Choi, B.Y.; Koo, J.-W.; Lee, K. Objectification and Differential Diagnosis of Vascular Pulsatile Tinnitus by Transcanal Sound Recording and Spectrotemporal Analysis: A Preliminary Study. *Otol. Neurotol.* **2016**, *37*, 613–620. [CrossRef]
9. Thomsen, K.; Elbrond, O.; Andersen, A.P. Glomus Jugulare Tumours. (A Series of 21 Cases). *J. Laryngol. Otol.* **1975**, *89*, 1113–1121. [CrossRef]
10. Kaylie, D.M.; O'Malley, M.; Aulino, J.M.; Jackson, C.G. Neurotologic Surgery for Glomus Tumors. *Otolaryngol. Clin. N. Am.* **2007**, *40*, 625–649. [CrossRef]
11. Offergeld, C.; Brase, C.; Yaremchuk, S.; Mader, I.; Rischke, H.C.; Gläsker, S.; Schmid, K.W.; Wiech, T.; Preuss, S.F.; Suárez, C.; et al. Head and Neck Paragangliomas: Clinical and Molecular Genetic Classification. *Clinics* **2012**, *67* (Suppl. S1), 19–28. [CrossRef]
12. Sanna, M.; Fois, P.; Pasanisi, E.; Russo, A.; Bacciu, A. Middle Ear and Mastoid Glomus Tumors (Glomus Tympanicum): An Algorithm for the Surgical Management. *Auris Nasus Larynx* **2010**, *37*, 661–668. [CrossRef]
13. Carlson, M.L.; Sweeney, A.D.; Pelosi, S.; Wanna, G.B.; Glasscock, M.E.; Haynes, D.S. Glomus Tympanicum: A Review of 115 Cases over 4 Decades. *Otolaryngol. Head Neck Surg.* **2015**, *152*, 136–142. [CrossRef] [PubMed]
14. Prasad, S.C.; Mimoune, H.A.; Khardaly, M.; Piazza, P.; Russo, A.; Sanna, M. Strategies and Long-Term Outcomes in the Surgical Management of Tympanojugular Paragangliomas. *Head Neck* **2016**, *38*, 871–885. [CrossRef] [PubMed]
15. Netterville, J.L.; Jackson, C.G.; Miller, F.R.; Wanamaker, J.R.; Glasscock, M.E. Vagal Paraganglioma: A Review of 46 Patients Treated during a 20-Year Period. *Arch. Otolaryngol. Head Neck Surg.* **1998**, *124*, 1133–1140. [CrossRef] [PubMed]
16. Zanoletti, E.; Mazzoni, A. Vagal Paraganglioma. *Skull Base* **2006**, *16*, 161–167. [CrossRef] [PubMed]
17. Bradshaw, J.W.; Jansen, J.C. Management of Vagal Paraganglioma: Is Operative Resection Really the Best Option? *Surgery* **2005**, *137*, 225–228. [CrossRef]
18. Lozano, F.S.; Gómez, J.L.; Mondillo, M.C.; González-Porras, J.R.; González-Sarmiento, R.; Muñoz, A. Surgery of Vagal Paragangliomas: Six Patients and Review of Literature. *Surg. Oncol.* **2008**, *17*, 281–287. [CrossRef]
19. Foote, R.L.; Pollock, B.E.; Gorman, D.A.; Schomberg, P.J.; Stafford, S.L.; Link, M.J.; Kline, R.W.; Strome, S.E.; Kasperbauer, J.L.; Olsen, K.D. Glomus Jugulare Tumor: Tumor Control and Complications after Stereotactic Radiosurgery. *Head Neck* **2002**, *24*, 332–338; discussion 338–339. [CrossRef]
20. Mazzoni, A.; Zanoletti, E. Observation and Partial Targeted Surgery in the Management of Tympano-Jugular Paraganglioma: A Contribution to the Multioptional Treatment. *Eur. Arch. Otorhinolaryngol.* **2016**, *273*, 635–642. [CrossRef]
21. Campbell, J.C.; Lee, J.W.; Ledbetter, L.; Wick, C.C.; Riska, K.M.; Cunningham, C.D.; Russomando, A.C.; Truong, T.; Hong, H.; Kuchibhatla, M.; et al. Systematic Review and Meta-Analysis for Surgery Versus Stereotactic Radiosurgery for Jugular Paragangliomas. *Otol. Neurotol.* **2023**, *44*, 195. [CrossRef] [PubMed]
22. Willen, S.N.; Einstein, D.B.; Maciunas, R.J.; Megerian, C.A. Treatment of Glomus Jugulare Tumors in Patients with Advanced Age: Planned Limited Surgical Resection Followed by Staged Gamma Knife Radiosurgery: A Preliminary Report. *Otol. Neurotol.* **2005**, *26*, 1229–1234. [CrossRef] [PubMed]
23. Cosetti, M.; Linstrom, C.; Alexiades, G.; Tessema, B.; Parisier, S. Glomus Tumors in Patients of Advanced Age: A Conservative Approach. *Laryngoscope* **2008**, *118*, 270–274. [CrossRef] [PubMed]
24. Wanna, G.B.; Sweeney, A.D.; Carlson, M.L.; Latuska, R.F.; Rivas, A.; Bennett, M.L.; Netterville, J.L.; Haynes, D.S. Subtotal Resection for Management of Large Jugular Paragangliomas with Functional Lower Cranial Nerves. *Otolaryngol. Head Neck Surg.* **2014**, *151*, 991–995. [CrossRef]
25. Miller, J.P.; Semaan, M.T.; Maciunas, R.J.; Einstein, D.B.; Megerian, C.A. Radiosurgery for Glomus Jugulare Tumors. *Otolaryngol. Clin. N. Am.* **2009**, *42*, 689–706. [CrossRef]
26. Suárez, C.; Rodrigo, J.P.; Bödeker, C.C.; Llorente, J.L.; Silver, C.E.; Jansen, J.C.; Takes, R.P.; Strojan, P.; Pellitteri, P.K.; Rinaldo, A.; et al. Jugular and Vagal Paragangliomas: Systematic Study of Management with Surgery and Radiotherapy. *Head Neck* **2013**, *35*, 1195–1204. [CrossRef]
27. Ivan, M.E.; Sughrue, M.E.; Clark, A.J.; Kane, A.J.; Aranda, D.; Barani, I.J.; Parsa, A.T. A Meta-Analysis of Tumor Control Rates and Treatment-Related Morbidity for Patients with Glomus Jugulare Tumors. *J. Neurosurg.* **2011**, *114*, 1299–1305. [CrossRef]
28. Lieberson, R.E.; Adler, J.R.; Soltys, S.G.; Choi, C.; Gibbs, I.C.; Chang, S.D. Stereotactic Radiosurgery as the Primary Treatment for New and Recurrent Paragangliomas: Is Open Surgical Resection Still the Treatment of Choice? *World Neurosurg.* **2012**, *77*, 745–761. [CrossRef] [PubMed]
29. Guss, Z.D.; Batra, S.; Limb, C.J.; Li, G.; Sughrue, M.E.; Redmond, K.; Rigamonti, D.; Parsa, A.T.; Chang, S.; Kleinberg, L.; et al. Radiosurgery of Glomus Jugulare Tumors: A Meta-Analysis. *Int. J. Radiat. Oncol. Biol. Phys.* **2011**, *81*, e497–e502. [CrossRef]
30. Manzoor, N.F.; Yancey, K.L.; Aulino, J.M.; Sherry, A.D.; Khattab, M.H.; Cmelak, A.; Morrel, W.G.; Haynes, D.S.; Bennett, M.L.; O'Malley, M.R.; et al. Contemporary Management of Jugular Paragangliomas with Neural Preservation. *Otolaryngol. Head Neck Surg.* **2021**, *164*, 391–398. [CrossRef]
31. Fayad, J.N.; Keles, B.; Brackmann, D.E. Jugular Foramen Tumors: Clinical Characteristics and Treatment Outcomes. *Otol. Neurotol.* **2010**, *31*, 299–305. [CrossRef] [PubMed]
32. Sanna, M.; Jain, Y.; De Donato, G.; Rohit; Lauda, L.; Taibah, A. Management of Jugular Paragangliomas: The Gruppo Otologico Experience. *Otol. Neurotol.* **2004**, *25*, 797–804. [CrossRef] [PubMed]

33. Fayad, J.N.; Schwartz, M.S.; Brackmann, D.E. Treatment of Recurrent and Residual Glomus Jugulare Tumors. *Skull Base* **2009**, *19*, 92–98. [CrossRef] [PubMed]
34. Carlson, M.L.; Driscoll, C.L.W.; Garcia, J.J.; Janus, J.R.; Link, M.J. Surgical Management of Giant Transdural Glomus Jugulare Tumors with Cerebellar and Brainstem Compression. *J. Neurol. Surg. B Skull Base* **2012**, *73*, 197–207. [CrossRef] [PubMed]
35. Moe, K.S.; Li, D.; Linder, T.E.; Schmid, S.; Fisch, U. An Update on the Surgical Treatment of Temporal Bone Paraganglioma. *Skull Base Surg.* **1999**, *9*, 185–194. [CrossRef] [PubMed]
36. Williams, M.D.; Tischler, A.S. Update from the 4th Edition of the World Health Organization Classification of Head and Neck Tumours: Paragangliomas. *Head Neck Pathol.* **2017**, *11*, 88–95. [CrossRef]
37. Lustig, L.R.; Jackler, R.K. The Variable Relationship between the Lower Cranial Nerves and Jugular Foramen Tumors: Implications for Neural Preservation. *Am. J. Otol.* **1996**, *17*, 658–668. [PubMed]
38. Fisch, U. Infratemporal Fossa Approach to Tumours of the Temporal Bone and Base of the Skull. *J. Laryngol. Otol.* **1978**, *92*, 949–967. [CrossRef]
39. Fisch, U.; Fagan, P.; Valavanis, A. The Infratemporal Fossa Approach for the Lateral Skull Base. *Otolaryngol. Clin. N. Am.* **1984**, *17*, 513–552. [CrossRef]
40. Al-Mefty, O.; Fox, J.L.; Rifai, A.; Smith, R.R. A Combined Infratemporal and Posterior Fossa Approach for the Removal of Giant Glomus Tumors and Chondrosarcomas. *Surg. Neurol.* **1987**, *28*, 423–431. [CrossRef] [PubMed]
41. Al-Mefty, O.; Teixeira, A. Complex Tumors of the Glomus Jugulare: Criteria, Treatment, and Outcome. *J. Neurosurg.* **2002**, *97*, 1356–1366. [CrossRef] [PubMed]
42. de Brito, R.; Cisneros Lesser, J.C.; Lopes, P.T.; Bento, R.F. Preservation of the Facial and Lower Cranial Nerves in Glomus Jugulare Tumor Surgery: Modifying Our Surgical Technique for Improved Outcomes. *Eur. Arch. Otorhinolaryngol.* **2018**, *275*, 1963–1969. [CrossRef] [PubMed]
43. Netterville, J.L.; Civantos, F.J. Rehabilitation of Cranial Nerve Deficits after Neurotologic Skull Base Surgery. *Laryngoscope* **1993**, *103*, 45–54. [CrossRef] [PubMed]
44. Heinrich, M.C.; Harris, A.E.; Bell, W.R. Metastatic Intravagal Paraganglioma. Case Report and Review of the Literature. *Am. J. Med.* **1985**, *78*, 1017–1024. [CrossRef]
45. Browne, J.D.; Fisch, U.; Valavanis, A. Surgical Therapy of Glomus Vagale Tumors. *Skull Base Surg.* **1993**, *3*, 182–192. [CrossRef]
46. González-Orús Álvarez-Morujo, R.; Arístegui Ruiz, M.; Martin Oviedo, C.; Álvarez Palacios, I.; Scola Yurrita, B. Management of Vagal Paragangliomas: Review of 17 Patients. *Eur. Arch. Otorhinolaryngol.* **2015**, *272*, 2403–2414. [CrossRef]
47. Sager, O.; Dincoglan, F.; Beyzadeoglu, M. Stereotactic Radiosurgery of Glomus Jugulare Tumors: Current Concepts, Recent Advances and Future Perspectives. *CNS Oncol.* **2015**, *4*, 105–114. [CrossRef]
48. Elshaikh, M.A.; Mahmoud-Ahmed, A.S.; Kinney, S.E.; Wood, B.G.; Lee, J.H.; Barnett, G.H.; Suh, J.H. Recurrent Head-and-Neck Chemodectomas: A Comparison of Surgical and Radiotherapeutic Results. *Int. J. Radiat. Oncol. Biol. Phys.* **2002**, *52*, 953–956. [CrossRef]
49. Helal, A.; Vakharia, K.; Brinjikji, W.; Carlson, M.L.; Driscoll, C.L.; Van Gompel, J.J.; Link, M.J.; Cloft, H. Preoperative Embolization of Jugular Paraganglioma Tumors Using Particles Is Safe and Effective. *Interv. Neuroradiol.* **2022**, *28*, 145–151. [CrossRef]
50. Gaynor, B.G.; Elhammady, M.S.; Jethanamest, D.; Angeli, S.I.; Aziz-Sultan, M.A. Incidence of Cranial Nerve Palsy after Preoperative Embolization of Glomus Jugulare Tumors Using Onyx. *J. Neurosurg.* **2014**, *120*, 377–381. [CrossRef]
51. Gartrell, B.C.; Hansen, M.R.; Gantz, B.J.; Gluth, M.B.; Mowry, S.E.; Aagaard-Kienitz, B.L.; Baskaya, M.K.; Gubbels, S.P. Facial and Lower Cranial Neuropathies after Preoperative Embolization of Jugular Foramen Lesions with Ethylene Vinyl Alcohol. *Otol. Neurotol.* **2012**, *33*, 1270–1275. [CrossRef] [PubMed]
52. De Marini, P.; Greget, M.; Boatta, E.; Jahn, C.; Enescu, I.; Garnon, J.; Dalili, D.; Cazzato, R.L.; Gangi, A. Safety and Technical Efficacy of Pre-Operative Embolization of Head and Neck Paragangliomas: A 10-Year Mono-Centric Experience and Systematic Review. *Clin. Imaging* **2021**, *80*, 292–299. [CrossRef] [PubMed]
53. van der Mey, A.G.; Frijns, J.H.; Cornelisse, C.J.; Brons, E.N.; van Dulken, H.; Terpstra, H.L.; Schmidt, P.H. Does Intervention Improve the Natural Course of Glomus Tumors? A Series of 108 Patients Seen in a 32-Year Period. *Ann. Otol. Rhinol. Laryngol.* **1992**, *101*, 635–642. [CrossRef] [PubMed]
54. Jansen, J.C.; van den Berg, R.; Kuiper, A.; van der Mey, A.G.; Zwinderman, A.H.; Cornelisse, C.J. Estimation of Growth Rate in Patients with Head and Neck Paragangliomas Influences the Treatment Proposal. *Cancer* **2000**, *88*, 2811–2816. [CrossRef] [PubMed]
55. Prasad, S.C.; Mimoune, H.A.; D'Orazio, F.; Medina, M.; Bacciu, A.; Mariani-Costantini, R.; Piazza, P.; Sanna, M. The Role of Wait-and-Scan and the Efficacy of Radiotherapy in the Treatment of Temporal Bone Paragangliomas. *Otol. Neurotol.* **2014**, *35*, 922–931. [CrossRef] [PubMed]
56. Carlson, M.L.; Sweeney, A.D.; Wanna, G.B.; Netterville, J.L.; Haynes, D.S. Natural History of Glomus Jugulare: A Review of 16 Tumors Managed with Primary Observation. *Otolaryngol. Head Neck Surg.* **2015**, *152*, 98–105. [CrossRef] [PubMed]
57. Lloyd, S.; Obholzer, R.; Tysome, J. BSBS Consensus Group British Skull Base Society Clinical Consensus Document on Management of Head and Neck Paragangliomas. *Otolaryngol. Head Neck Surg.* **2020**, *163*, 400–409. [CrossRef]
58. Favier, J.; Amar, L.; Gimenez-Roqueplo, A.-P. Paraganglioma and Phaeochromocytoma: From Genetics to Personalized Medicine. *Nat. Rev. Endocrinol.* **2015**, *11*, 101–111. [CrossRef]

59. Cass, N.D.; Schopper, M.A.; Lubin, J.A.; Fishbein, L.; Gubbels, S.P. The Changing Paradigm of Head and Neck Paragangliomas: What Every Otolaryngologist Needs to Know. *Ann. Otol. Rhinol. Laryngol.* **2020**, *129*, 1135–1143. [CrossRef]
60. Baysal, B.E.; Willett-Brozick, J.E.; Lawrence, E.C.; Drovdlic, C.M.; Savul, S.A.; McLeod, D.R.; Yee, H.A.; Brackmann, D.E.; Slattery, W.H.; Myers, E.N.; et al. Prevalence of SDHB, SDHC, and SDHD Germline Mutations in Clinic Patients with Head and Neck Paragangliomas. *J. Med. Genet.* **2002**, *39*, 178–183. [CrossRef]
61. Lenders, J.W.M.; Duh, Q.-Y.; Eisenhofer, G.; Gimenez-Roqueplo, A.-P.; Grebe, S.K.G.; Murad, M.H.; Naruse, M.; Pacak, K.; Young, W.F. Endocrine Society Pheochromocytoma and Paraganglioma: An Endocrine Society Clinical Practice Guideline. *J. Clin. Endocrinol. Metab.* **2014**, *99*, 1915–1942. [CrossRef] [PubMed]
62. Taïeb, D.; Wanna, G.B.; Ahmad, M.; Lussey-Lepoutre, C.; Perrier, N.D.; Nölting, S.; Amar, L.; Timmers, H.J.L.M.; Schwam, Z.G.; Estrera, A.L.; et al. Clinical Consensus Guideline on the Management of Phaeochromocytoma and Paraganglioma in Patients Harbouring Germline SDHD Pathogenic Variants. *Lancet Diabetes Endocrinol.* **2023**, *11*, 345–361. [CrossRef] [PubMed]

Disclaimer/Publisher's Note: The statements, opinions and data contained in all publications are solely those of the individual author(s) and contributor(s) and not of MDPI and/or the editor(s). MDPI and/or the editor(s) disclaim responsibility for any injury to people or property resulting from any ideas, methods, instructions or products referred to in the content.

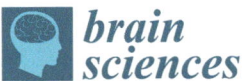

Article

Gruppo Otologico's Experience in Managing the So-Called Inoperable Tympanojugular Paraganglioma

Mario Sanna [1], Mohammed Al-Khateeb [2,*], Melcol Hailu Yilala [3], Mohanad Almashhadani [4] and Giuseppe Fancello [1]

1. Department of Otology and Skull Base Surgery, Gruppo Otologico, 29121 Piacenza, PC, Italy; giuseppe.fancello91@gmail.com (G.F.)
2. Department of ORL-HNS, Rizgary Teaching Hospital, Erbil 44001, Iraq
3. Department of ORL-HNS, School of Medicine, Addis Ababa University, Addis Ababa 9086, Ethiopia; melcol.hailu@aau.edu.et
4. Department of ORL-HNS, Al-Yarmouk Teaching Hospital, Baghdad 10811, Iraq; mohanadhns80@gmail.com
* Correspondence: muh.dlawar@gmail.com

Abstract: Objective: to identify advanced or "so-called inoperable" cases of tympanojugular paragangliomas (PGLs) and analyze how each case is surgically managed and followed afterward. **Study Design**: a retrospective case series study. **Methods**: Out of 262 type C and D TJPs and more than 10 cases of advanced or so-called inoperable cases, files of 6 patients with a diagnosis of advanced tympanojugular PGLs who were referred to an otology and skull-base center between 1996 and 2021 were reviewed to analyze management and surgical outcomes. The criteria for choosing these cases involve having one or more of the following features: (1) a large-sized tumor; (2) a single ipsilateral internal carotid artery (ICA); (3) involvement of the vertebral artery; (4) a considerable involvement of the ICA; (5) an extension to the clivus, foramen magnum, and cavernous sinus; (6) large intradural involvement (IDE); and (7) bilateral or multiple PGLs. **Results**: The age range at presentation was 25–43 years old, with a mean of 40.5 years: two females and four males. The presenting symptoms were glossal atrophy, hearing loss, pulsatile tinnitus, dysphonia, shoulder weakness, and diplopia. The modified Infratemporal Fossa Approach (ITFA) with a transcondylar–transtubercular extension is the principal approach in most cases, with additional approaches being used accordingly. **Conclusions**: The contemporary introduction of carotid artery stenting with the direct and indirect embolization of PGLs has made it possible to operate on many cases, which was otherwise considered impossible to treat surgically. Generally, the key is to stage the removal of the tumor in multiple stages during the management of complex PGLs to decrease surgical morbidities. A crucial aspect is to centralize the treatment of PGLs in referral centers with experienced surgeons who are trained to plan the stages and manage possible surgical complications.

Keywords: tympanojugular paraganglioma; complex tympanojugular PGL; ITFA; carotid artery stenting; preoperative balloon occlusion (PBO); vertebral artery closure

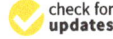

Citation: Sanna, M.; Al-Khateeb, M.; Yilala, M.H.; Almashhadani, M.; Fancello, G. Gruppo Otologico's Experience in Managing the So-Called Inoperable Tympanojugular Paraganglioma. *Brain Sci.* **2024**, *14*, 745. https://doi.org/10.3390/brainsci14080745

Academic Editor: Miguel Lopez-Gonzalez

Received: 6 July 2024
Revised: 19 July 2024
Accepted: 21 July 2024
Published: 25 July 2024

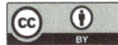

Copyright: © 2024 by the authors. Licensee MDPI, Basel, Switzerland. This article is an open access article distributed under the terms and conditions of the Creative Commons Attribution (CC BY) license (https://creativecommons.org/licenses/by/4.0/).

1. Introduction

Tympanojugular paragangliomas (TJPs) are rare locally aggressive neoplasms of the temporal bone and skull base that arise from the adventitia of the jugular bulb [1]. Because TPJ tumors grow slowly and silently, they often present at later stages, making cases with extensive involvement inoperable in the past.

A TJP presents a challenge to the treating physician because of its high vascularity, locally aggressive nature, and extension and involvement of important neurovascular structures such as the jugular bulb (JB), facial nerve (FN), internal carotid artery (ICA), and lower cranial nerves (LCNs) [1].

Advances in neuroradiology, endovascular interventions, lateral skull-base approaches, neuroanesthesia, and postoperative care make surgical removal a safe and preferred way of treatment [2–5]. Thus, gross total removal remains the mainstay of treatment even in advanced and complex lesions [6].

Some cases, however, are still complex and challenging to treat and require treatment in the hands of highly skilled surgeons in specialized centers. Examples of such cases include large tumors (modified Fisch class C3–4, D, and V); tumors with large intradural extension; tumors involving the cavernous sinus, clivus, and foramen magnum; tumors involving the ICA and vertebral arteries; previously irradiated tumors; recurrent tumors; tumors involving a single carotid artery; bilateral and multiple tumors; and tumors on the side of the dominant or single sigmoid sinus [2,7–12].

A thorough preoperative evaluation and individualized surgical planning are mandatory prerequisites in managing complex and so-called "inoperable" TJPs. A preoperative evaluation of such cases includes a complete otoneurologic clinical examination with an emphasis on the assessment of the function of FN and LCNs, pure-tone audiometry, high-resolution temporal bone CT scans (HRCTs), gadolinium-enhanced magnetic resonance imaging (MRI), and angiography with both arterial and venous phases and four-vessel angiography with cross-compression tests [1,2,5].

In all the cases of complex or so-called "inoperable" TJPs, preoperative embolization is performed 48 h before surgery. Endovascular intervention, such as stenting or permanent balloon occlusion (PBO), however; can be used depending on the presence of indication during the initial MRI and angiography evaluation. Examples of such indications include an encasement of the distal cervical, vertical, and horizontal segments of the ICA between 270 and 360 degrees; evidence of stenosis and irregularity of the arterial lumen; extensive blood supply from branches of ICA; prior irradiation; and past surgery including ICA manipulation [13].

Conversely, extensive involvement of ICA doesn't represent an absolute contraindication to surgery. Therefore, when the tumor invades the ICA and there is adequate collateral blood flow, PBO is carried out. However, we frequently perform intraluminal stenting two to three months prior to surgery in instances with inadequate collateral blood flow [1,13].

Achieving proximal and distal control of the major vessels and maximizing structural exposure while avoiding damage are the objectives of surgical therapy in these instances. Therefore, a surgical strategy that maximizes exposure while minimizing morbidity should be pursued. Since its description by Fisch and Pillsbury in 1979 and its modification by Sanna, the Infratemporal Fossa Approach (ITFA) has come to be recognized as the preferred method for the surgical therapy of TJPs [14,15].

The surgical management and results of several TJP cases that were previously deemed complicated and "inoperable" are presented in this article.

2. Material and Methods

The medical records of patients who have been diagnosed with a TJP at Gruppo Otologico Piacenza-Rome, between 1996 and 2021 were thoroughly examined.

Table 1 shows the updated Fisch classification of TJ PGLs that was used to classify all tumors [16]. The gathered information was examined for age, gender, symptoms at presentation, surgical techniques, tumor size and location as established by radiologic and surgical findings, surgical results, and clinical and radiologic follow-up observations.

A thorough otologic and neurologic examination was performed on each subject. The House–Brackmann (HB) grading system of FN was used to grade the facial function prior to the procedure, right after the procedure, and at each follow-up appointment [17]. In our series, gadolinium-enhanced MRIs and HRCT with bone windows were performed on all patients. In order to investigate the arterial supply, venous circulation, and blood flow of the sigmoid sinus and jugular bulb, arteriovenous magnetic resonance imaging and four-vessel angiography were carried out. A preoperative embolization of the tumor was performed 24 to 48 h before surgery using polyvinyl alcohol. An ICA stent had to be inserted in three patients. Pure-tone audiometry was used to measure hearing levels in each case, and flexible fiber optic naso-pharyngo-laryngoscopy was performed.

Table 1. Modified Fisch classification of TJ PGLs.

Class C	\multicolumn{2}{l}{Tumors extending beyond the tympano-mastoid cavity, destroying the bone of the infra-labyrinthine and apical compartment of the temporal bone and involving the carotid canal}
	C1	Tumors with limited involvement of the vertical portion of the carotid canal
	C2	Tumors invading the vertical portion of the carotid canal
	C3	Tumors with invasions of the horizontal portion of the carotid canal
	C4	Tumors reaching the anterior foramen lacerum
Class D	\multicolumn{2}{l}{Tumors with intracranial extension}
	Di1	Tumors with up to 2 cm of intradural extension
	Di2	Tumors with more than 2 cm of intradural extension
	Di3	Tumors with an inoperable intradural extension
Class V	\multicolumn{2}{l}{Tumors involving the VA}
	Ve	Tumors involving the extradural VA
	Vi	Tumors involving the intradural VA

3. Intraoperative Preparation

The surgical site is shaved following the patient's placement. The patient is placed in a supine position with the head turned to the other side for each approach (Supplementary Materials). Deep vein thrombosis is avoided by using stockings. To enable continuous electromyographic monitoring of the facial nerve, pairs of electrodes are inserted in the orbicularis oculi and orbicularis oris muscles. The surgical area is then prepared with 10 ppm of ether and Citrosil. Furthermore, the abdominal area is cleaned and draped in a similar manner in order to take a piece of fat which is used to obliterate the surgical cavity at the end of the procedure.

4. Postoperative Care

Once the surgery is complete, a tight bandage is applied and left in place for four to five days. There are no drains implanted during intradural operations.

After that, the patients are transferred to the critical care unit, where they will be closely followed for changes in blood pressure, pulse rate, respiratory rate, arterial oxygen saturation, and ECG tracing. Furthermore, the patient's degree of consciousness, pupillary reflexes, and motor responses are assessed every 15 min for the first six hours; then after every half hour for the next 12 to 18 h.

The patients are moved to the ward after 24 h where the vital signs and state of consciousness continue to be monitored. Subsequently, the indwelling urinary catheter is removed and if there is adequate swallowing function the nasogastric tube can be withdrawn, and oral fluids can be initiated. Finally, in order to reduce the risk of pulmonary embolism, early ambulation is advised following the first 24 h.

5. Clinical Cases with Illustrations

5.1. Case 1: (C4Di2)

A 25-year-old male patient with a persistent left TJP was sent to our center following three previous operations performed elsewhere. On admission, he presented with profound hearing loss with LCN palsy. The latest radiological examinations showed a C4Di2 TJ PGL. As there was significant involvement of the ICA, an intra-ICA stent was placed. However, a preoperative angiography showed remarkable residual vascular supply from the ICA, which could not be embolized. One contributing factor was that the stent diameter was inadequate to occlude the vascular supply from the affected ICA. Thus, the decision was made to proceed with PBO after confirming adequate contralateral supply. A first-stage surgery was performed through revision ITFA-A with extradural tumor removal including involved ICA. By using a combination of a translabyrinthine (TLAB) and petro-occipital-trans-sigmoid (POTS) approach, the remnant intradural tumor was removed in the second stage, along with the internal auditory canal (IAC) bone and its contents that the tumor had infiltrated (Figure 1). Three years after the second-stage operation, sural nerve grafting was performed for reconstruction of the FN function with HB-IV in the last follow-up.

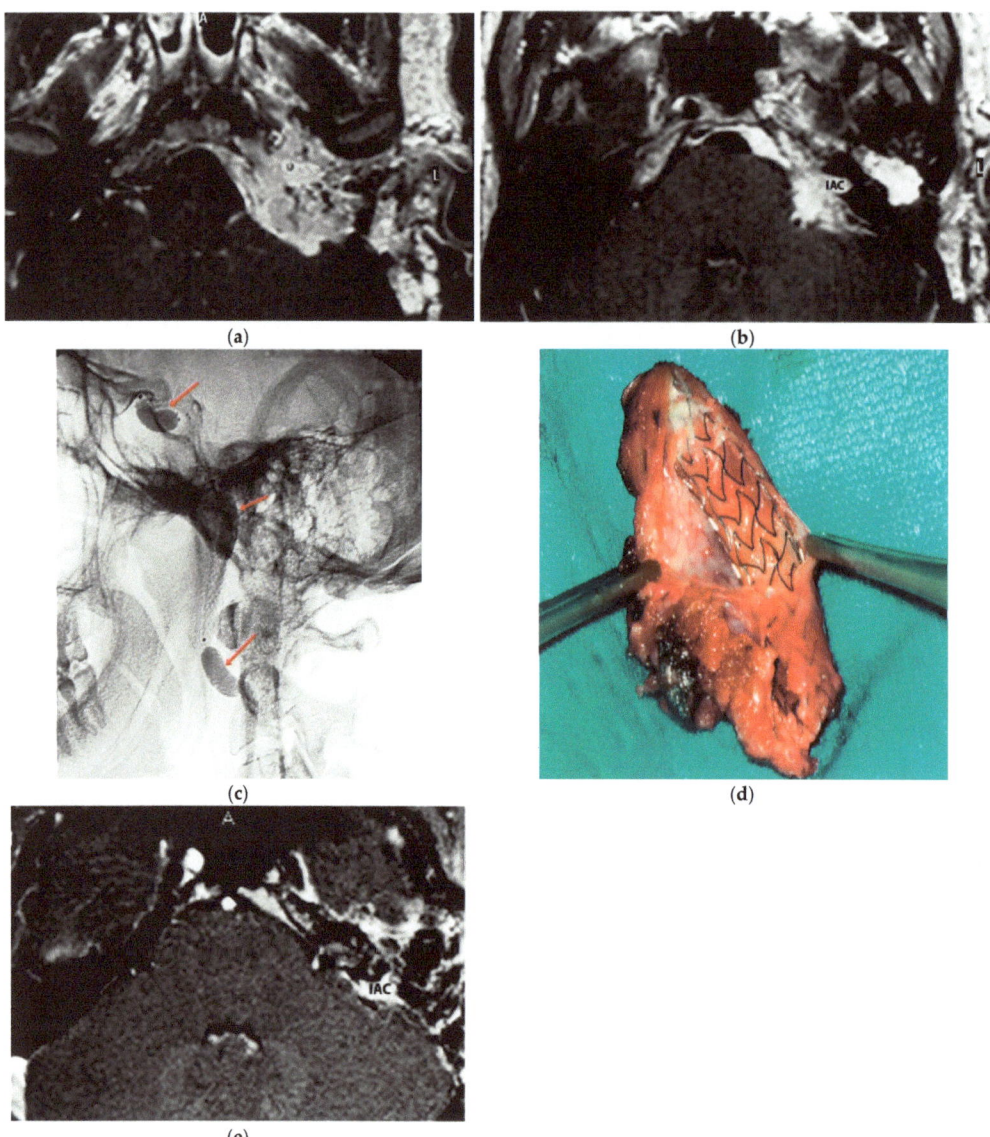

Figure 1. (Case 1) (**a**) Axial-enhanced T1W MRI, with large intradural tumor extension. (**b**) Axial-enhanced T1W MRI, with extensive involvement of posterior fossa dura with intradural and IAC involvement. (**c**) Plain lateral view skull X-ray. Red arrows indicate balloons during permanent occlusion of the IAC. (**d**) Intra-carotid stent was seen after opening the wall of the carotid artery. (**e**) Axial-enhanced T1W MRI revealing dural infiltration and the involvement of IAC.

5.2. *Case 2: (C3Di1 + Stage I VP)*

A 40-year-old male patient [18] was admitted to our center with the diagnosis of right vagal PGL and TJP. The fact that paragangliomas run in his family has been confirmed with genetic tests. The patient underwent surgery at a different facility fifteen years before a left carotid body paraganglioma (CBP), which led to ligation of the left common carotid artery. A clinical examination demonstrated the involvement of right LCN with vocal cord paralysis that was well-compensated.

Two separate masses at the level of the parapharyngeal space and jugular foramen, as well as the involvement of the vertical and horizontal parts of the petrous segment of the ICA, were shown by HRCT and gadolinium-enhanced MRIs (Figure 2). These findings are suggestive of a TJP (class C3Di1) and a VP (stage I). On the other hand, an angiography revealed a left ICA and common carotid artery blockage. The tumor encompassed the distal cervical section and the vertical part of the petrous segment of the right ICA. Therefore, seven weeks before the procedure, the patient had the only right ICA stented. He underwent surgery with an IFTA-A two days after embolization, and total excision was completed successfully and with the preservation of the ICA. After two years of surgery, the right FN function improved from HB-VI in the early postoperative period to HB-III. Contralateral compensation allowed for a good level of tolerance for the paralysis of the right vocal cord. For the first five years, the patient had annual HRCT and MRI scans; after that, they were performed roughly every two years. In October 2021, the last MRI and HRCT with contrast revealed no evidence of tumor recurrence.

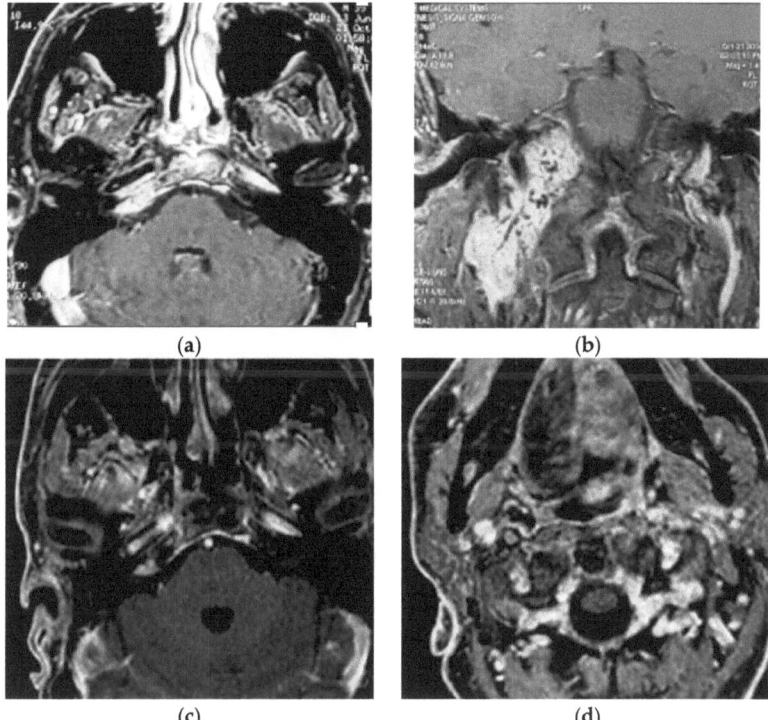

Figure 2. (Case 2) (**a,b**) Enhanced-axial T1W MRI showing C3Di1 + stage I VP. (**c,d**) Postoperative axial and coronal MRI showing no residual tumor.

5.3. Case 3: (C4Di2Vi)

A 32-year-old woman affected by a TJP (class C4Di2Vi) on the right side was brought to the authors' attention (Figure 3). Due to the tumor's invasion of Dorello's canal, the patient suffered from paralysis of the sixth cranial nerve. Because there was no contralateral compensation, the PBO test was unsuccessful.

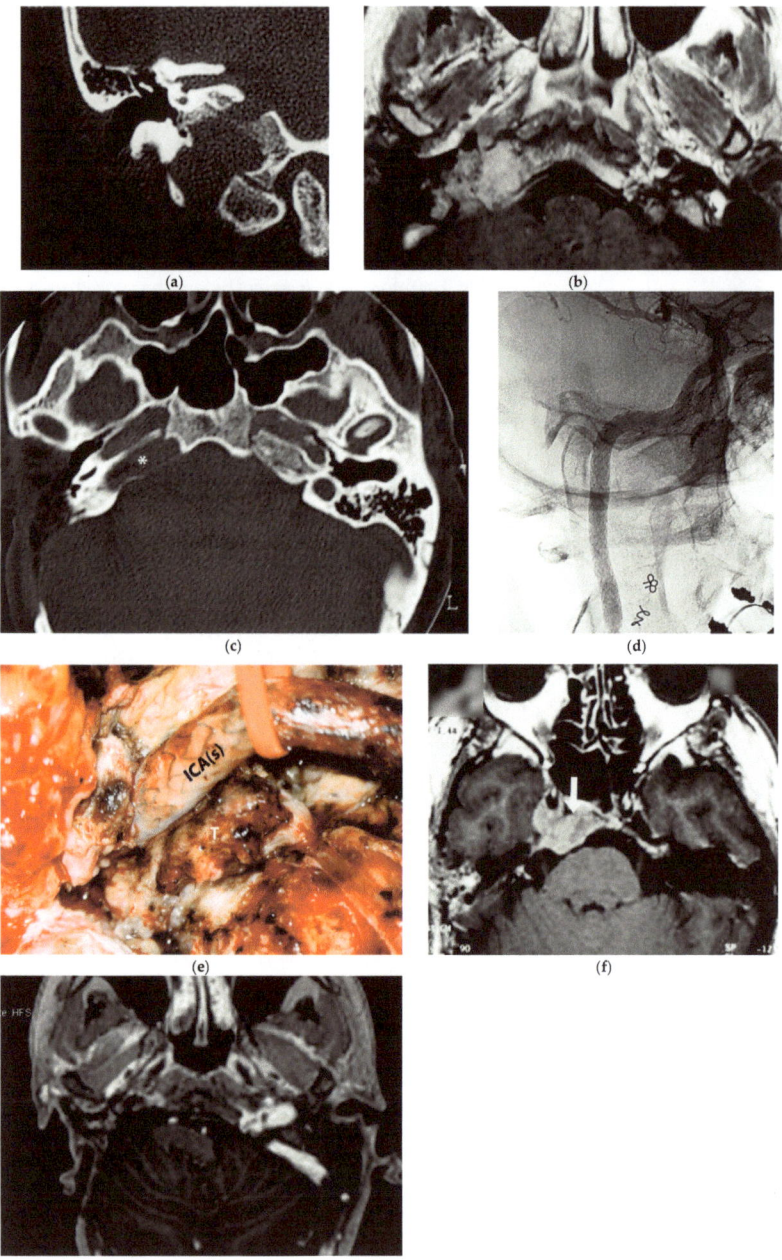

Figure 3. (Case 3) (**a**) CT scan, coronal view, of tumor extending into the craniocervical junction. (**b**) Axial-enhanced T1W MRI showing the tumor extension into the vertical segment of ICA. (**c**) Axial view, CT, after 1st stage showing residual tumor around horizontal ICA and PA. (**d**) X-ray screen shows ICA stenting at the level of foramen lacerum. (**e**) Stented ICA after removal of tumor-invaded adventitia. (**f**) Axial-enhanced T1W MRI showing residual tumor in the cavernous sinus. (**g**) Enhanced T1W MRI after 4th stage [1].

First stage: To minimize the danger of intraoperative arterial rupture, a staged subtotal resection was planned, leaving some tumor remnants at the level of the ICA and at the level of the cavernous sinus to preserve ocular mobility. The first stage was carried out in October 1996 using an IFTA-A following preoperative embolization. During the postoperative phase, the FN function declined to HB-IV. Adjuvant treatment with stereotactic radiation was used for cavernous sinus involvement.

During the second stage, in March 1998, the intradural component of the tumor was excised using a translabyrinthine technique with transapical extension. It seems that the tumor invaded every dura that covers the posterior surface of the petrous bone. A follow-up CT scan revealed that the residual lesion was still present at the ICA level, but there was no tumor growth in the cavernous sinus. All the same, a residual lesion around the ICA grew more noticeable during follow-up surveillance. Since closing the artery was not possible, this was handled conservatively.

Third stage: After the ICA was stented and a fresh embolization was carried out in January 2004, new prospects emerged with the potential to use a stent to fortify the ICA's vascular walls [13]. Subadventitial dissection along the vertical and horizontal segments was necessary for the treatment of the ICA.

Fourth stage: After 8 months from the last operation, the intradural vertebral artery was affected, as determined by an angiography and MRI. As a result, the tumor was completely excised with the involved VA by an extreme lateral approach. HRCT and MRI follow-ups for over 20 years showed no recurrence.

5.4. Case 4: (C3Di2 + Stage II Vagal PGL)

A 53-year-old female patient arrived at our center with the diagnosis of a left-side vagal and TJ PGL. Upon examination of the cranial nerves (CNs), left X and XII CN palsy was found. She has a dead ear on her left side, as determined by the pure-tone audiogram. The radiological examination demonstrated a Fisch stage II vagal PGL and a left-sided modified Fisch class C3Di2 TJ PGL [15]. Severe stenosis and anterior displacement of the cervical ICA were observed by angiography. Well-compensated collateral circulation was found by the preoperative occlusion test. Since there was a genuine risk of an ICA rupture during stent insertion due to severe stenosis, PBO was chosen over stent implantation.

The procedure was delayed for one month in order to give the cerebral vasculature time to adjust to the new hemodynamic conditions. IFTA-A was carried out during the first stage after super-selective embolization and planned subtotal tumor excision. For the second-stage surgery, the bony labyrinth was preserved as a landmark. LCNs with tumor infiltration were sacrificed. A periosteal invasion of the tumor necessitated extensive bone resection from the horizontal segment to the foramen lacerum. The ICA was removed right above the carotid bifurcation to the foramen lacerum. During the first stage, vagal paraganglioma and the extradural portion of the TJP were excised concurrently. After the first-stage surgery, an MRI revealed a remaining intradural component of the tumor. The intradural component of the tumor was entirely excised during the second step of the surgery and was performed using the POTS technique [15]. Following the second round of surgery, the postoperative radiological test revealed the absence of any remaining tumor. The swallowing function was successfully compensated for, and the FN function returned to HB grade III. After four years, there was still no indication of a return.

5.5. Case 5: (C3Di2Vi)

The fifth case was diagnosed with a right TJP (C3Di2Vi) at another center that involved the clivus, the vertebral artery, the foramen magnum, and the occipital condyle and was treated with embolization and radiotherapy. On admission, an MRI showed an enlarging tumor and a clinical examination revealed that there was paralysis of the cranial nerves X, XI, and XII (Figure 4).

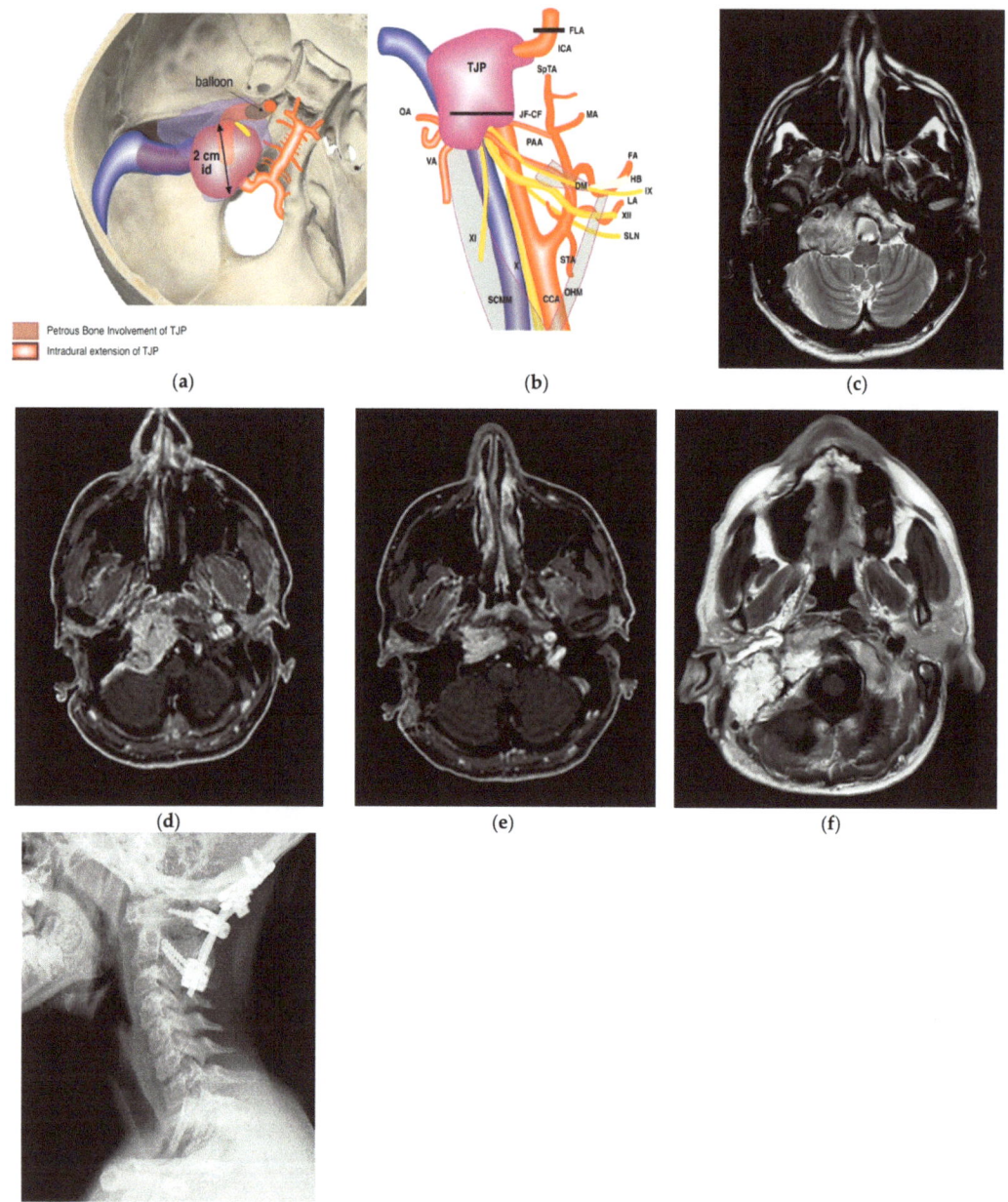

Figure 4. (Case 5) (**a**,**b**) Right tympanojugular paraganglioma (C3Di2Vi) involving the clivus, the vertebral artery, the foramen magnum, and the occipital condyle. (**c**) Axial-enhanced T1-weighted magnetic resonance imaging (MRI) shows a large mass extending to the intradural space up to the foramen magnum. (**d**) Axial-enhanced T1 MRI after first-stage tumor removal. (**e**) Enhanced T1 MRI after second-stage surgery. (**d**,**f**) Axial-enhanced T1 MRI after third-stage tumor removal, which shows total tumor removal with obliteration of the surgical cavity with abdominal fat. (**g**) A sagittal CT scan after total tumor removal during the third stage shows cervical–occipital fixation.

The management plan was to stage the tumor removal to reduce the risk of surgical complications, and the occlusion test revealed good compensation and a preoperative PBO of the ICA and vertebral artery. At the first surgical stage in 2021, the tumor was removed at the jugular foramen, including the ICA, from the carotid bifurcation to the horizontal intra-petrous part through ITFA-A, leaving the tumor at the occipital condyle, clivus, and foramen magnum as well as the intradural part for the second stage. During the second stage, which was carried out in September 2022, the residual tumor from the occipital condyle, clivus, and foramen magnum was removed through revision ITFA-A with transcondylar extension. In February 2023, the third-stage procedure involved the removal of the clival and dural tumors using a trans-cochlear method. Additionally, the clivus was drilled until healthy bone appeared, and concurrent cervical–occipital fixation was carried out (Figure 4g).

5.6. Case 6: (C4Di2Vi)

A 41-year-old man with a right-sided TJP (C4Di2Vi) who had undergone three prior surgeries with partial tumor excision came to our facility. He had HB-IV facial palsy, cranial nerve palsies IX and XII, and a dead ear on the same side at the time of presentation. The management was to stage the tumor resection (Figure 5). During the first stage in 2008, he underwent extradural tumor removal through a modified ITFA-A with transcondylar extension, and the FN and LCNs; IX, X, XI, and XII were sacrificed. During the second stage in 2009, through a modified transcochlear approach (MTCA), he underwent the removal of remnant extradural and intradural tumors. Following the second-stage surgery, coils were used to permanently occlude the tumor-involved vertebral artery (Figure 5j). The third stage was conducted in 2010 through an extreme lateral approach to remove the tumor between the foramen magnum and vertebral artery and drill around the foramen magnum until healthy bone was reached. During the fourth stage in 2011, he underwent a static facial reanimation through a mid-facelift procedure. After receiving gamma knife treatment in 2014 for a sub-centimetric remnant in the cavernous sinus, the tumor remained stable. The most recent follow-up was in 2023.

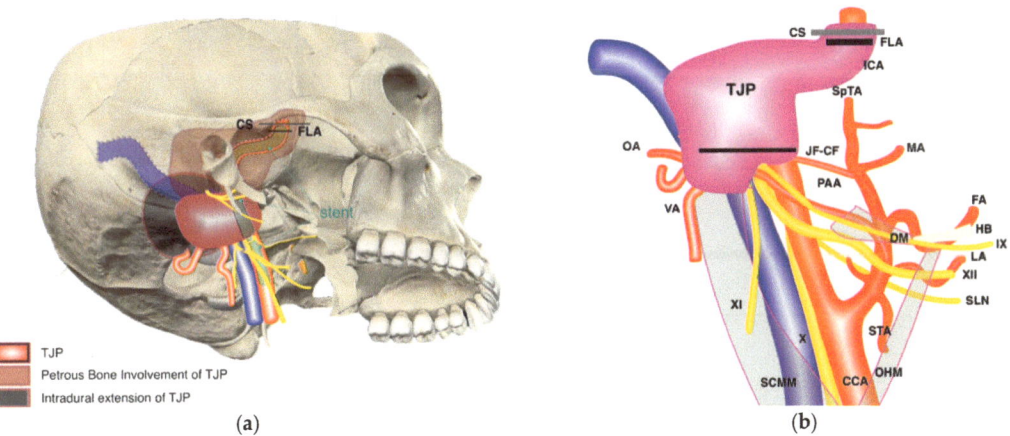

Figure 5. *Cont.*

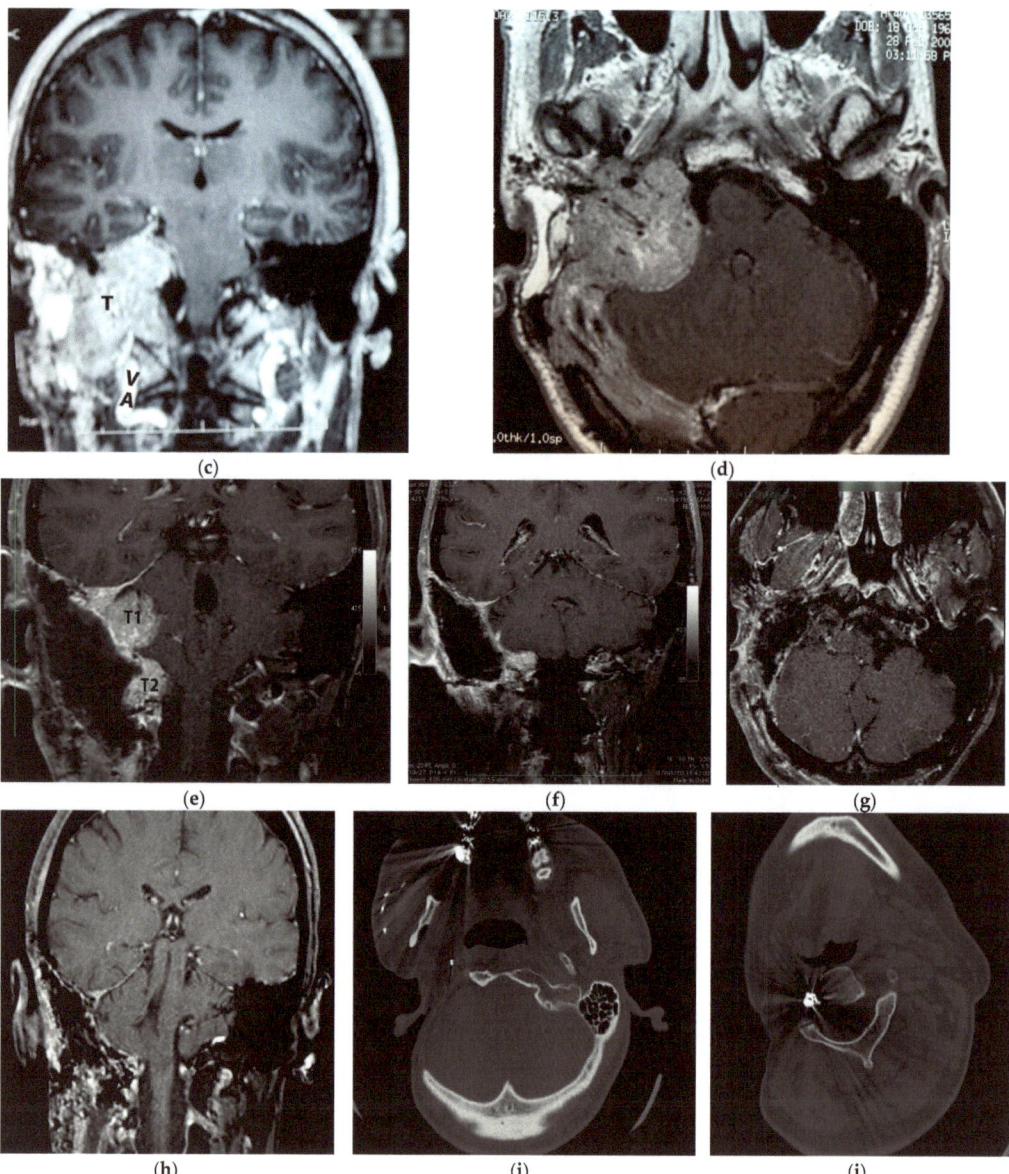

Figure 5. (Case 6) (**a,b**) Right-sided tympanojugular PGL (C4Di2Vi). (**c**) Coronal Gd-enhanced T1-weighted magnetic resonance imaging (MRI) shows a large residual tumor extending to the intradural space involving the vertebral artery. (**d**) Axial Gd-enhanced T1-weighted MRI shows a large residual tumor extending to the intradural space, involving transverse sinus ipsilaterally up to the torcula. (**e**) Coronal Gd-enhanced T1-weighted MRI after first-stage tumor removal. Note the residual tumor: T1 is in the cerebellopontine angle, and T2 is in the foramen magnum. (**f**) Coronal Gd-enhanced T1-weighted MRI after second-stage tumor removal, which shows a small residual tumor at the foramen magnum. (**g,h**) Axial and coronal Gd-enhanced T1-weighted MRI after third-stage tumor removal, which revealed total tumor removal at the level of the foramen magnum. (**i,j**) Axial CT scan after the third stage shows a coil at the internal carotid and vertebral arteries that are used for artery occlusion.

6. Results

Out of the 262 individuals with a pathologically proven TJP treated surgically by the senior author (M.S.), six patients made up the study group. There were four (66.6%) males and two (33.3%) females. At the time of operation, the mean age was 40.5 years old (range: 25–53). There were four (66.6%) tumors on the right side and two (33.3%) on the left. Table 4 includes the pertinent patient demographics, tumor locations, specific surgical techniques performed in each case, and surgical treatment outcomes for the six patients included in the case series. The most common symptoms at the time of presentation were glossal atrophy (GA) (83.3%), hearing loss (66.6%), pulsating tinnitus (66.6%), dysphonia (66.6%), dysphagia (66.6%), shoulder weakness (33.3%), and diplopia (16.6%) (Table 2).

Table 2. Signs and symptoms at presentation at our center.

Symptoms and Signs	No. of Patients (%)
Hearing loss	4 (66.6)
Pulsating tinnitus	4 (66.6)
Vertigo	2 (33.3)
Dysphonia	4 (66.6)
Dysphagia	4 (66.6)
Glossal atrophy	5 (83.3)
Shoulder weakness	3 (50)
Diplopia	1 (16.6)

One patient had paralysis of five cranial nerves (VII, IX, X, XI, and XII); one patient had paralysis of nerves IX, X, XI, and XII; and two other patients presented multiple paralysis of nerves (X, XI, XII, X, and XII). The last patient had palsy of the VI cranial nerve. The FN nerve function; preoperative, immediate postoperative, and during the last follow-up is summarized in (Table 3).

Table 3. Facial nerve function.

	Preoperative, Immediate Postoperative, and Final Facial Nerve Function According to House–Brackmann Scale		
Patient	Preoperative (HB) *	Immediately Postoperative (HB)	At Last Follow-Up (HB)
1	III	VI	IV
2	I	VI	III
3	I	VI	I
4	I	VI	III
5	I	VI	III
6	IV	VI	III (after V–VII anastomosis)

* Status of VII cranial nerve (HB) before surgery at Gruppo Otologico.

All cases showed intradural involvement by the tumor mass (D). Two cases had multiple concomitant paragangliomas (TJ + vagal). All patients were treated with embolization 48 h before surgery. In three cases, it was necessary to place a stent from the carotid bifurcation to the pre-cavernous internal carotid artery at the level of the ICA to proceed with the surgery, and in two cases, the vertebral artery was closed by a coil (Table 4).

Table 4. Patient demographics, PGL classification, type of surgery, and postoperative complications.

Patient	Age at Surgery (y)	Sex	Side	Pre-op. CN Deficits	Class of Tumor	Other Surgeries/ Treatments	Embolization or Stenting	Surgical Approach	New CN Deficits	Tumor Resection	Follow-Up (m)
1	25	M	L	IX, X, XI, and XII	C4Di2	3	Stent of left ICA + PBO	– ITFA-A extended to the parotid gland (extradural portion); – POTS + TLA + sural graft (intradural portion).	-	Total	224
2	40	M	R	IX, X, XI, and XII	C3Di1 + vagal	1 surgery for CB PGL (left side)	Left ICA closed in another surgery and embolization involving stent of right ICA	– ITFA-A	-	Total	95
3	32	F	R	VI	C4Di2Vi	-	Absence of contralateral compensation and embolization involving stent of right-ICA	– ITFA-A (1996) (extradural portion); – POTS (1998) (partial intradural portion); – POTS (2004) recurrence with transcondylar extension (extradural portion); – POTS (2004) (intradural portion);	IX, X, and XII	Total	336
4	53	F	L	X and XII	C3Di2 + vagal	-	Embolization	– ITFA-A (extradural portion); – POTS (intradural portion).	XI	Total	38

Table 4. *Cont.*

Patient Demographics, PGL Classification, Type of Surgery, and Postoperative Complications

Patient	Age at Surgery (y)	Sex	Side	Pre-op. CN Deficits	Class of Tumor	Other Surgeries/ Treatments	Embolization or Stenting	Surgical Approach	New CN Deficits	Tumor Resection	Follow-Up (m)
5	53	M	R	X, XI, and XII	C3Di2Vi	Radiation therapy	Embolization	– ITFA-A transcondylar; – ITFA + TC (intradural portion); – Transcochlear (clivus portion).	IX	Total	35
6	41	M	R	XII	C4Di2Vi	1 surgery in 2002	Embolization	– ITFA-A + TC (extradural portion); – MTCA (intra- and extradural portion); – EL (foramen magnum); – Facial reanimation.	IX, X, and XI	Residual gamma knife (stable)	145

Abbreviation: CB, carotid body tumor; PBO, preoperative balloon occlusion; ITFA-A, Infratemporal Fossa Approach, Type A; TC, transcondylar extension; EL, extreme lateral approach; POTS, petro-occipital trans-sigmoid; TLA, trans-labyrinthine approach; MTCA, modified transcochlear approach.

7. Discussion

Six difficult TJPs make up the current series. Since our center is recognized as one of the world's top referral sites for lateral skull-base conditions, including TJPs, all six cases were referred with advanced tumor stages. Some of them underwent multiple operations at different locations throughout this period.

The mainstay of managing TJPs is total surgical extirpation. However, most of the time, it is not easy to achieve this surgical goal due to the tumor's location in relation to vital neurovascular structures and local infiltrative behaviors [19]. Other options in the management of TJPs include partial excision with adjuvant RTs, stereotactic radiosurgery [20], and active surveillance (wait and scan) once total surgical removal is not possible due to the patient's condition or due to the involvement of critical structures such as the cavernous sinus, AICA, brain parenchyma, and basilar artery [21].

The last few decades have seen a major increase in the use of preoperative direct and intra-arterial embolizations, particularly with polyvinyl alcohol particles, in the treatment of paragangliomas, which is mostly due to developments in high-resolution imaging and super-selective catheterization techniques. The effectiveness of blocking particular tumoral feeders of PGL tumors has significantly increased with the development of super-selective embolization techniques [22,23]. Compared to the surgical resection strategy without embolization, embolizing PGL preoperatively provides a number of advantages. Preoperative embolization has been shown, in numerous studies, to reduce the incidence of bleeding events and blood transfusions after surgery [24–26]. A frequent observation after embolization is a reduction in the tumor size, which raises the possibility of a technically successful excision and could shorten the duration of the procedure [27]. Tumors that were once regarded as inoperable in the old days can now be managed safely. Nevertheless, some TJP cases are too demanding to treat [2,7–12]. Examples of such cases include large tumors; those with a massive intradural extension; tumors involving the cavernous sinus and the ICA or VA and single carotid artery; tumors with the dominant or unilateral sigmoid sinus on the tumor side; previously operated or irradiated tumors; as well as bilateral or multiple tumors [1].

Broadly, the subtype C3 and C4 TJP tumors in Fisch and colleagues' classification are considered large tumors. When TJPs enlarge, they either spread to the petrous apex through an invasion of the carotid canal, or they spread through the medial wall of the jugular bulb into the intradural space, which involves the LCNs [2,28]. As a rule, the classic ITFA can be used for class C1 and certain class C2 tumors, while the class C2–C4 subtype of TJPs—can be managed with the ITFA-A with a transcondylar trans-tubercular extension [1]. However, an additional extension such as the modified transcochlear or extreme lateral transcondylar approach might be required when there is an invasion of the clivus or foramen magnum by the tumor. Furthermore, there is a relationship between the size of the tumor and the probability of maintaining the LCN function. A larger tumor reduces the likelihood of maintaining the LCN function [29,30].

When the intradural extension is large, the frequency of the LCN's involvement and the brainstem compression will be high. It is quite difficult to assess the extent of dural involvement through preoperative radiology or intraoperative findings. If a small area of the dura is invaded, it can be easily removed and managed immediately, whereas, if there is massive dural involvement, it can be managed through staged tumor removal. Widespread intradural recurrence might result from any undetected involvement. Many authors have proposed that single-staged tumor removals are suitable even if there is extensive dural and intradural involvement [3,5,31], but we observed that the risk of cerebrospinal fluid (CSF) leaks is high when resecting a large intradural (Di2) tumor as compared with staged tumor resection, and this is postulated due to several factors: First, the risk of sacrificing LCNs is high when dealing with a large intradural tumor (Di2), which subsequently leads to an increased risk of CSF leaks secondary to increased intracranial pressure from severe aspiration and interactable coughing [28]. Second, larger skull base and dural defects, as well as the direct communication between the intradural and neck space, occur when dealing with Di2 tumors, which in turn leads to a higher incidence of CSF leaks. Thus, for Di2 TJPs, we favor staged tumor removals to prevent postoperative CSF leakage and single-stage removals for tumors with a smaller intradural extension, which is consistent with the practice in other studies [2,15]. Additionally, 5.2% (3.8–33.3) is the average rate of postoperative CSF leaking in a single-stage surgery [5,10,32,33]. In addition, over the years, we have observed that intradural tumor removal is relatively easy during the second stage because the residual tumor has been partly devascularized during the initial stage. A dissection and conservation of the LCN function during the second stage will be more easily achieved, and a preoperative embolization of the feeder vessel during subsequent stages will further help to lower the amount of operative blood loss.

In the second stage, the patient's hearing level and the size and location of the tumor are the main determinant factors for the approach selection. Although the POTS approach [15,34] is the favorable approach among a vast majority of patients, an MTCA or an extreme lateral transcondylar approach may be utilized as well.

The presence of a normal preoperative LCN function does not exclude an intraoperative neural invasion by the tumor [30]. In fact, a tumor extension beyond the dura generally suggests the involvement of the LCN [21]. It has been suggested by some authors to leave the piece of tumor that is attached to LCNs to preserve the function of the LCN, especially in elderly patients [35]. However, in young patients, if total removal is technically reasonable, it is preferred to sacrifice tumor-infiltrated LCNs to avoid recurrence. Most of our patients for whom the LCNs have been sacrificed are well compensated even without postoperative rehabilitation.

If the TJP involves the cavernous sinus, it is recommended to intentionally leave that part of the tumor to avoid sacrificing the cranial nerves III, IV, and VI to maintain ocular mobility. Postoperatively, stereotactic radiotherapy can be given as an adjuvant therapy to control the rate of tumor growth. We have two cases involving the cavernous sinus, and both of them are stable, with no growth of the residual tumor on the cavernous sinus in the most recent follow-up MRI [6].

The modified transcochlear type D or extreme lateral approach is used when there is an involvement of the foramen magnum and lower clivus [10,31]. To avoid leaving the residual tumor, the clivus should be drilled until healthy bone appears because of the infiltrative character of TJPs.

Due to its close anatomical proximity, the ICA is frequently affected by TJPs. The surgical planning and whether the tumor is operable is determined by the degree of the arterial wall involvement by the tumor. When appropriate, the tumor must be dissected from the arterial wall, which can be achieved by either a subperiosteal or subadventitial dissection. A subperiosteal dissection is achieved by finding and dissecting the cleavage plane between the periosteum of the carotid artery canal and the adventitia of the ICA [2]. This method of dissection is appropriate when a tumor involves only the periosteum and is relatively safe and easier in the vertical part of the petrous carotid artery than in the horizontal part of it, as the former has a thicker wall and is more easily accessed. A subadventitial dissection, on the other hand, is a dissection between the adventitia and the muscular layer. This is a delicate step during the surgery and should be carried out with caution, as it may lead to tears in the wall of the ICA. The thickness of the vertical segment of the petrous ICA is around 1.5–2.0 mm, with the adventitia being ~1 mm thick; meanwhile, there is no adventitia in the horizontal segment [17]. Therefore, a subadventitial dissection cannot be carried out at the level of the horizontal part of the petrous ICA.

When the tumor fully encases the artery with extreme narrowing, as evidenced by arteriography, any intervention without sufficient preoperative endovascular control of the ICA may lead to a massive hemorrhage, residual tumor, or stroke [13,35–38]. Whenever there is adequate collateral blood supply, a preoperative balloon occlusion is carried out if the tumor infiltrates the wall of the artery. But if the collateral blood supply is inadequate, we usually reinforce the artery with intraluminal stenting [38], which in turn increases the thickness of and strengthens the arterial wall that allows for generating a dissection plane at the outer surface of the stent to excise the tumor completely without risking an inadvertent carotid rupture. With the advent of these new techniques (endovascular stenting and preoperative balloon occlusion), selected patients who were regarded for a subtotal resection can be safely re-evaluated for a total removal of the tumor.

In order to remove the tumor totally, it is critical to address the ICA preoperatively. Options for those patients with a single carotid artery at the side of the lesion include the following: either wait and scan (especially among elderly patients); an incomplete tumor removal with adjuvant radiotherapy; and total tumor removal (following intraluminal stenting or by utilizing bypass surgery), but the later poses significant risks of cerebral ischemia and strokes. Preoperative intraluminal stenting, however, may be the optimal choice.

So far, at Gruppo Otologico, we have managed two cases with a single ICA on the lesion side with no postoperative complications. One of them is a 55-year-old woman with a previous history of a contralateral ICA occlusion, which had been managed for an intracranial aneurysm, that was found to have a suspected tumor infiltration of the vertical segment of the ICA, as evidenced by angiography. During the observation period, the tumor was noted to have grown, prompting the discussion of a preoperative high-flow carotid artery bypass as a potential management strategy. Ultimately, the surgical team's familiarity and positive experiences with stent insertions in similar cases led them to favor this approach over the bypass procedure, and they proceeded with the stent placement before the tumor resection. Given the patient's advanced age, the substantial extent of the tumor, and the presence of bothersome brainstem compression, the treatment team determined that radiotherapy would not be an appropriate or effective treatment option in this case. The successful placement of the stent enabled the surgical team to subsequently accomplish a complete gross total removal of the tumor. The patients experienced no postoperative complications and were free from disease at 15–20-year follow-ups.

In the case of extradural and/or intradural vertebral artery involvement (Ve/i), we added a new subclass to the Fisch classification of TJPs and removed the De component. This was performed because we observed that, in the case of class D tumors, the tumor had already penetrated the cranial cavity in both the De and Di components and that the general surgical approach for excisions used for both components was nearly the same [16,39].

We discovered that 8 out of the 230 individuals with TJPs had vertebral artery involvement. Six individuals had intradural VA involvement, and one patient had an involvement of the extradural artery. In one patient, both the intradural and extradural VAs were affected at the same time. Out of the eight, seven had surgeries. Through a microdissection, we were able to remove the tumor from the artery in five of the seven patients. A preoperative occlusion was conducted on two patients: one with coils and the other with a balloon. One patient out of the seven underwent surgery to remove a subtotal tumor from the vertebral artery. Tumors surrounding the VA were removed without any significant issues. A gross complete tumor removal without major surgical complications was made possible by the VA's preoperative examination and intervention.

Because a TJP typically results from jugular bulb adventitia, surgical procedures to remove the tumor typically involve closing the sigmoid sinus and ligating the jugular vein. On the other hand, venous congestion, intracranial hypertension, and brain edema may result from a closure of the dominant or sole sigmoid sinus on the lesion side [10]. Therefore, it is crucial to evaluate the brain's venous drainage system prior to the surgery, especially the ipsilateral mastoid emissary vein and condylar vein. The sigmoid sinus should be closed distal to the mastoid emissary vein's exit if their diameters are more than normal. Otherwise, they should be left undisturbed. In cases where the patient lacks adequate collateral venous drainage or where it is not possible to preserve collateral venous drainage, more conservative measures, such as stereotactic radiosurgery, subtotal resection with a preserved sigmoid sinus, or "wait and scan", are advised.

The patient's life is directly and significantly impacted by the management of bilateral paragangliomas. One should never undervalue the significance of neuronal preservation, because bilateral deficiencies in LCNs may occur. The surgeon's primary focus during the initial stage of the surgery should be on removing the tumor while maintaining the LCN's functionality [5,40]. If a larger tumor has an LCN deficit on its side, it should be removed before managing the smaller tumor with radiation therapy or a follow-up. Similarly, a smaller tumor should be removed first if a patient has an LCN deficit on that side, and then the larger tumor on the contralateral side can be monitored. If the tumor grows, it will be managed through a partial removal of the tumor, while maintaining the LCN with adjuvant radiotherapy [1].

However, if both paragangliomas, in the case of bilateral paragangliomas with a normal LCN function, are of the same size, they can be monitored by serial MRIs in addition to the surgery or radiation therapy recommended for tumors that show growth. Surgery is carried out on the side of the larger tumor if the two tumors differ in size to maintain the LCN function. If the function of the LCN is preserved postoperatively, surgery can be considered for the contralateral side as well. On the other hand, if the LCNs are sacrificed, the contralateral tumor needs to be monitored using MRIs regularly and treated with radiation if growth is seen. When dissecting the tumor, it is crucial to protect the jugular bulb's medial wall to maintain the LCN function [5,41].

The cervical section of the vagus nerve should always be recognized and preserved during ITFA-A. Conversely, it is advised to remove both lesions at the same time when vagal paragangliomas and TJPs are present on the same side.

When treating infiltrative skull-base lesions, it is important to remember that persistent or recurring tumors are always a possibility. To ascertain whether radiation, revision surgery, or wait and scan is the best course of action, a thorough radiological appraisal is necessary. It is more difficult to perform revision surgeries because there are no typical tissue planes or surgical landmarks. A history of prior radiation therapy or surgery increases the risk of CSF leaks, injury to LCNs, and damage to the facial nerve [3,10,11,13]. Because irradiated tissue is often hard, removing and dissecting tumors can be challenging [13]. The carotid canal is the most frequent location of recurrence in TJPs, and injuries to the ICA are more likely following prior dissections. Consequently, as was already noted, preoperative treatments of the ICA are quite important.

We performed an anterior FN rerouting with the appropriate extension in all cases during an ITFA. Conservative care of the external auditory canal and FN is not appropriate during revision surgeries. Thirteen individuals in one of our series had received prior therapy; eight of these had undergone different mastoidectomies without rerouting the FN, and following the surgery, a remnant tumor was found under the nerve and surrounding the carotid artery. This was probably caused by either partial excision surrounding the ICA or a lack of facial nerve rerouting.

As a result of the anterior facial nerve rerouting as part of the ITFA-A, the patients experienced a new-onset or worsening facial weakness, which improved within a year (Table 2). One patient experienced a postoperative CSF leak, which was managed with a muscle graft and facia lata to seal the leak. Four patients experienced new-onset LCN palsies (Table 4), which the patients tolerated. None of the six patients had embolization-related complications.

In some instances, complete tumor removal requires a balloon occlusion or intraluminal stenting of the ICA. Due to the infiltrative nature of paragangliomas, wide bone drilling is necessary to prevent residual tumors; preservation of LCNs infiltrated by the tumor should not be attempted, particularly among younger patients.

8. Conclusions

Having one of the biggest series in TJP management has allowed us to draw several conclusions. The cornerstone of this type of surgery is IFTA-A. By rerouting the facial nerve anteriorly, we can lower the likelihood of recurrence and enhance the management of the carotid artery. Planning requires a thorough investigation of the brain's hemodynamics. To prevent jeopardizing the patient's life in situations where there are bilateral tumors, every effort should be taken to maintain the LCN function, if only unilaterally. Complete removal is facilitated by appropriate preoperative endovascular interventions such as PBOT or stenting. Staged removal is advised in cases with a significant intradural component in order to lower the danger of CSF leakage and to make the second stage's intradural tumor removal more manageable and technically straightforward. A preoperative evaluation and intervention, along with the careful management of aggravating variables, can significantly reduce surgical morbidity with a high chance of gross complete removal. Some tumor expansions, such as those enclosing the posterior circulation vasculature, those extending into the cavernous sinus, and those exhibiting a parenchymal brain invasion, are nonetheless incurable without unacceptably high morbidities.

Supplementary Materials: The following supporting information can be downloaded at: https://www.mdpi.com/article/10.3390/brainsci14080745/s1.

Author Contributions: Software, M.A.; resources, M.S.; writing—original draft, M.A.-K. and G.F.; writing—review and editing, M.S. and M.H.Y. All authors have read and agreed to the published version of the manuscript.

Funding: This research received no external funding.

Institutional Review Board Statement: The requirement for informed consent and ethical approval was waived because of the adopted retrospective study design. This study was conducted in accordance with the declaration of Helsinki and Good Clinical Practice guidelines.

Informed Consent Statement: Informed consent was obtained from all subjects involved in this study.

Data Availability Statement: The data presented in this study are available on request from the corresponding author. The data are not publicly available due to the fact that the patient data include preoperative and postoperative follow-up imaging and investigations, which were all archived at Gruppo Otologico.

Conflicts of Interest: The authors declare no conflicts of interest.

References

1. Sanna, M.; Piazza, P.; Shin, S.H.; Flanagan, S.; Mancini, F. *Microsurgery of Skull Base Paraganglioma*; Thieme: Stuttgart, Germany, 2013.
2. Fisch, U.; Fagan, P.; Valavanis, A. The infratemporal fossa approach for the lateral skull base. *Otolaryngol. Clin. North Am.* **1984**, *17*, 513–552. [CrossRef] [PubMed]
3. Green, J.D., Jr.; Brackmann, D.E.; Nguyen, C.D.; Arriaga, M.A.; Telischi, F.F.; De la Cruz, A. Surgical management of previously untreated glomus jugulare tumors. *Laryngoscope* **1994**, *104*, 917–921.
4. Woods, C.I.; Strasnick, B.; Jackson, C.G. Surgery for glomus tumors: The Otology Group experience. *Laryngoscope* **1993**, *103*, 65–70. [CrossRef] [PubMed]
5. Al-Mefty, O.; Teixeira, A. Complex tumors of the glomus jugulare: Criteria, treatment, and outcome. *J. Neurosurg.* **2002**, *97*, 1356–1366. [CrossRef] [PubMed]
6. Sanna, M.; Shin, S.H.; De Donato, G.; Sivalingam, S.; Lauda, L.; Vitullo, F.; Piazza, P. Management of complex tympanojugular paragangliomas including endovascular intervention. *Laryngoscope* **2011**, *121*, 1372–1382. [CrossRef] [PubMed]
7. Brown, J.S. Glomus jugulare tumors revisited: A ten-year statistical follow up of 231 cases. *Laryngoscope* **1985**, *95*, 284–288. [CrossRef]
8. Jackson, C.G.; Glasscock, M.E., III; McKennan, K.X.; Koopmann, C.F., Jr.; Levine, S.C.; Hays, J.W.; Smith, H.P. The surgical treatment of skull-base tumors with intracranial extension. *Otolaryngol. Head Neck Surg.* **1987**, *96*, 175–185. [CrossRef]
9. Spector, G.J.; Sobol, S. Surgery for glomus tumors at the skull base. *Otolaryngol. Head Neck Surg.* **1980**, *88*, 524–530. [CrossRef] [PubMed]
10. Patel, S.J.; Sekhar, L.N.; Cass, S.P.; Hirsch, B.E. Combined approaches for resection of extensive glomus jugulare tumors. A review of 12 cases. *J. Neurosurg.* **1994**, *80*, 1026–1038. [CrossRef]
11. Anand, V.K.; Leonetti, J.P.; Al-Mefty, O. Neurovascular considerations in surgery of glomus tumors with intracranial extensions. *Laryngoscope* **1993**, *103*, 722–728. [CrossRef]
12. Bulsara, K.R.; Al-Mefty, O. Skull base surgery for benign skull base tumors. *J. Neurooncol.* **2004**, *69*, 181–189. [CrossRef] [PubMed]
13. Sanna, M.; Piazza, P.; De Donato, G.; Menozzi, R.; Falcioni, M. Combined endovascular-surgical management of the internal carotid artery in complex tympanojugular paragangliomas. *Skull Base* **2009**, *19*, 26–42. [CrossRef] [PubMed]
14. Fisch, U.; Mattox, D. *Microsurgery of the Skull Base*; Georg Thieme Verlag: Stuttgart, Germany, 1988.

15. Sanna, M.; Saleh, E.; Khrais, T.; Mancini, F.; Piazza, P.; Russo, A. *Atlas of Microsurgery of the Lateral Skull Base*; Georg Thieme Verlag: Stuttgart, Germany, 2008.
16. Sivalingam, S.; Konishi, M.; Shin, S.H.; Lope Ahmed, R.A.; Piazza, P.; Sanna, M. Surgical management of tympanojugular paragangliomas with intradural extension, with a proposed revision of the Fisch classification. *Audiol. Neurotol.* **2012**, *17*, 243–255. [CrossRef] [PubMed]
17. House, J.W.; Brackmann, D.E. Facial nerve grading system. *Otolaryngol. Head Neck Surg.* **1985**, *93*, 146–147. [CrossRef] [PubMed]
18. Piras, G.; Grinblat, G.; Lauda, L.; Caruso, A.; Mardighian, D.; Sanna, M. Long term outcomes of stenting of a single internal carotid artery in complex head and neck paragangliomas. *Clin. Med.* **2023**, *9*, 1–5. [CrossRef]
19. Jackson, C.G.; Haynes, D.S.; Walker, P.A.; Glasscock, M.E., III; Storper, I.S.; Josey, A.F. Hearing conservation in surgery for glomus jugulare tumors. *Am. J. Otol.* **1996**, *17*, 425–437. [PubMed]
20. Dharnipragada, R.; Butterfield, J.T.; Dhawan, S.; Adams, M.E.; Venteicher, A.S. Modern management of complex tympanojugular paragangliomas: Systematic review and meta-analysis. *World Neurosurg.* **2023**, *170*, 149–156. [CrossRef]
21. Fancello, G.; Fancello, V.; Ehsani, D.; Porpiglia, V.; Piras, G.; Caruso, A.; Sanna, M. Tumor progression in tympanojugular paragangliomas: The role of radiotherapy and wait and scan. *Eur. Arch. Oto-Rhino-Laryngol.* **2024**, *281*, 2779–2789. [CrossRef] [PubMed]
22. Ishak, C.; Danda, V. Jugular foramen paragangliomas: Preoperative transcatheter particle embolization. *J. Cerebrovasc. Endovasc. Neurosurg.* **2020**, *22*, 273–281. [CrossRef] [PubMed]
23. Saringer, W.; Kitz, K.; Czerny, C.; Kornfehl, J.; Gstöttner, W.; Matula, C.; Knosp, E. Paragangliomas of the temporal bone: Results of different treatment modalities in 53 patients. *Acta Neurochir.* **2002**, *144*, 1255–1264. [CrossRef]
24. Boedeker, C.C. Paragangliomas and paragangliomas syndromes. *GMS Curr. Top. Otorhinolaryngol-Head. Neck Surg.* **2011**, *10*, 1–26.
25. Karaman, E.; Isildak, H.; Yilmaz, M.; Edizer, D.T.; Ibrahimov, M.; Cansiz, H.; Nazim, K.; Ozgun, E. Management of paragangliomas in otolaryngology practice: Review of a 7-year experience. *J. Craniofac. Surg.* **2009**, *20*, 1294–1297. [CrossRef] [PubMed]
26. Makiese, O.; Chibbaro, S.; Marsella, M.; Tran Ba Huy, P.; George, B. Jugular foramen paragangliomas: Management, outcome and avoidance of complications in a series of 75 cases. *Neurosurg. Rev.* **2012**, *35*, 185–194; discussion 194. [CrossRef] [PubMed]
27. Liscak, R.; Urgosik, D.; Chytka, T.; Simonova, G.; Novotny, J., Jr.; Vymazal, J.; Guseynova, K.; Vladyka, V. Leksell Gamma Knife radiosurgery of the jugulotympanic glomus tumor: Long-term results. *J. Neurosurg.* **2014**, *121*, 198–202. [CrossRef] [PubMed]
28. Farrior, J.B. Infratemporal approach to skull base for glomus tumors: Anatomic considerations. *Ann. Otol. Rhinol. Laryngol.* **1984**, *93 Pt 1*, 616–622. [CrossRef] [PubMed]
29. Fisch, U. Infratemporal fossa approach for glomus tumors of the temporal bone. *Ann. Otol. Rhinol. Laryngol.* **1982**, *91 Pt 1*, 474–479. [CrossRef] [PubMed]
30. Makek, M.; Franklin, D.J.; Zhao, J.C.; Fisch, U. Neural infiltration of glomus temporale tumors. *Am. J. Otol.* **1990**, *11*, 1–5.
31. Al Mefty, O.; Fox, J.L.; Rifai, A.; Smith, R.R. A combined infratemporal and posterior fossa approach for the removal of giant glomus tumors and chondrosarcomas. *Surg. Neurol.* **1987**, *28*, 423–431. [CrossRef] [PubMed]
32. Gottfried, O.N.; Liu, J.K.; Couldwell, W.T. Comparison of radiosurgery and conventional surgery for the treatment of glomus jugulare tumors. *Neurosurg. Focus* **2004**, *17*, 22–30. [CrossRef] [PubMed]
33. Whitfield, P.C.; Grey, P.; Hardy, D.G.; Moffat, D.A. The surgical management of patients with glomus tumours of the skull base. *Br. J. Neurosurg.* **1996**, *10*, 343–350. [CrossRef]
34. Mazzoni, A.; Sanna, M. A posterolateral approach to the skull base: The petro-occipital trans sigmoid approach. *Skull Base Surg.* **1995**, *5*, 157–167. [CrossRef] [PubMed]
35. Liu, J.K.; Sameshima, T.; Gottfried, O.N.; Couldwell, W.T.; Fukushima, T. The combined transmastoid retro-and infralabyrinthine transjugular transcondylar transtubercular high cervical approach for resection of glomus jugulare tumors. *Oper. Neurosurg.* **2006**, *59*, ONS115-25. [CrossRef] [PubMed]
36. Witiak, D.G.; Pensak, M.L. Limitations to mobilizing the intrapetrous carotid artery. *Ann. Otol. Rhinol. Laryngol.* **2002**, *111*, 343–348. [CrossRef] [PubMed]
37. Jackson, C.G.; McGrew, B.M.; Forest, J.A.; Netterville, J.L.; Hampf, C.F.; Glasscock, M.E. III. Lateral skull base surgery for glomus tumors: Long-term control. *Otol. Neurotol.* **2001**, *22*, 377–382. [CrossRef]
38. Zanoletti, E.; Mazzoni, A. Vagal paraganglioma. *Skull Base* **2006**, *16*, 161–167. [CrossRef]
39. Moe, K.S.; Li, D.; Linder, T.E.; Schmid, S.; Fisch, U. An update on the surgical treatment of temporal bone paraganglioma. *Skull Base Surg.* **1999**, *9*, 185–194. [CrossRef] [PubMed]
40. Pareschi, R.; Righini, S.; Destito, D.; Raucci, A.F.; Colombo, S. Surgery of glomus jugulare tumors. *Skull Base* **2003**, *13*, 149–157. [CrossRef]
41. Gejrot, T. Surgical treatment of glomus jugulare tumours with special reference to the diagnostic value of retrograde jugulography. *Acta Otolaryngol.* **1965**, *60*, 150–168. [CrossRef]

Disclaimer/Publisher's Note: The statements, opinions and data contained in all publications are solely those of the individual author(s) and contributor(s) and not of MDPI and/or the editor(s). MDPI and/or the editor(s) disclaim responsibility for any injury to people or property resulting from any ideas, methods, instructions or products referred to in the content.

MDPI AG
Grosspeteranlage 5
4052 Basel
Switzerland
Tel.: +41 61 683 77 34

Brain Sciences Editorial Office
E-mail: brainsci@mdpi.com
www.mdpi.com/journal/brainsci

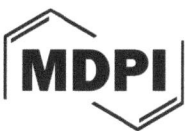

Disclaimer/Publisher's Note: The statements, opinions and data contained in all publications are solely those of the individual author(s) and contributor(s) and not of MDPI and/or the editor(s). MDPI and/or the editor(s) disclaim responsibility for any injury to people or property resulting from any ideas, methods, instructions or products referred to in the content.

www.ingramcontent.com/pod-product-compliance
Lightning Source LLC
LaVergne TN
LVHW072351090526
838202LV00019B/2519